MW00716917

SPRINGHOUSE

Professional Care Guide

Neoplastic Disorders

Springhouse Corporation
Springhouse, Pennsylvania

Staff

Senior Publisher
Matthew Cahill

Clinical Manager
Cindy Tryniszewski, RN, MSN

Art Director
John Hubbard

Senior Editor
June Norris

Clinical Editor
Beverly Ann Tscheschlog, RN

Editors
Edith McMahon (book editor), Crystal Norris, Elizabeth Weinstein

Designers
Stephanie Peters (senior associate art director), Lynn Foulk (book designer)

Copy Editors
Cynthia Breuninger (manager), Lynette High, Doris Weinstock, Lewis Adams

Typography
Diane Paluba (manager), Elizabeth Bergman, Joyce Rossi Biletz, Phyllis Marron, Robin Mayer, Valerie Rosenberger

Manufacturing
Deborah C. Meiris (director), T.A. Landis, Anna Brindisi

Production Coordinator
Patricia McCloskey

Editorial Assistants
Beverly Lane, Mary Madden, Dianne Tolbert

Indexer
Robin Hipple

The cover illustration depicts the dissemination of tumor cells into the blood circulation, which may lead to metastasis. Illustration by Kevin A. Somerville.

The clinical procedures described and recommended in this publication are based on research and consultation with medical and nursing authorities. To the best of our knowledge, these procedures reflect currently accepted clinical practice; nevertheless, they can't be considered absolute and universal recommendations. For individual application, all recommendations must be considered in light of the patient's clinical condition and, before administration of new or infrequently used drugs, in light of the latest package insert information. The authors and the publisher disclaim responsibility for any adverse effects resulting directly or indirectly from the suggested procedures, from any undetected errors, or from the reader's misunderstanding of the text.

©1995 by Springhouse Corporation. All rights reserved. No part of this publication may be used or reproduced in any manner whatsoever without written permission except for brief quotations embodied in critical articles and reviews. For information, write Springhouse Corporation, 1111 Bethlehem Pike, P.O. Box 908, Springhouse, PA 19477-0908. Authorization to photocopy items for internal or personal use, or the internal or personal use of specific clients, is granted by Springhouse Corporation for users registered with the Copyright Clearance Center (CCC) Transactional Reporting Service, provided that the fee of $.75 per page is paid directly to CCC, 27 Congress St., Salem, MA 01970. For those organizations that have been granted a license by CCC, a separate system of payment has been arranged. The fee code for users of the Transactional Reporting Service is 0874347785/95 $00.00 + $.75.

Printed in the United States of America

 A member of the Reed Elsevier plc group

PCG1-010395

Library of Congress Cataloging-in-Publication Data
Neoplastic disorders.
    p. cm. – (Professional care guides)
    Includes bibliographical references and index.
    1. Cancer – Nursing.   2. Nursing care plans.
      I. Springhouse Corporation.   II. Series.
    [DNLM: 1. Neoplasms – etiology – outlines.
    2. Neoplasms – diagnosis – outlines.
    3. Neoplasms – therapy – outlines.
QZ 18 N438 1995]
RC266.N46   1995
610.73′698 – dc20
DNLM/DLC   94-33985
ISBN: 0-87434-778-5   CIP

Contents

Contributors and consultants vii
Foreword viii

Chapter 1   **Introduction** 1
Self-test questions 15

Chapter 2   **Head, Neck, and Spinal Neoplasms** 17
Malignant brain tumors 17
Pituitary tumors 24
Laryngeal cancer 28
Thyroid cancer 32
Spinal neoplasms 36
Self-test questions 39

Chapter 3   **Thoracic Neoplasms** 43
Lung cancer 43
Breast cancer 50
Self-test questions 56

Chapter 4   **Abdominal and Pelvic Neoplasms** 59
Gastric cancer 59
Esophageal cancer 65
Pancreatic cancer 67
Colorectal cancer 73
Kidney cancer 78
Liver cancer 81
Bladder cancer 84
Gallbladder and bile duct cancers 89
Self-test questions 92

Chapter 5   **Genital Neoplasms** 95
Prostate cancer 95
Testicular cancer 99
Penile cancer 102
Cervical cancer 104
Uterine cancer 109
Vaginal cancer 115
Ovarian cancer 118
Cancer of the vulva 124
Fallopian tube cancer 127
Self-test questions 130

Chapter 6   **Bone Skin, and Soft-Tissue Neoplasms** 133
Primary malignant bone tumors 133
Multiple myeloma 138
Basal cell epithelioma 141
Squamous cell carcinoma 143
Malignant melanoma 147
Kaposi's sarcoma 153
Self-test questions 156

Chapter 7   **Blood and Lymph Neoplasms** 159
Hodgkin's disease 159
Malignant lymphomas 163
Mycosis fungoides 166
Acute leukemia 168
Chronic granulocytic leukemia 174
Chronic lymphocytic leukemia 177
Self-test questions 180

Selected References 184
Self-Test Answers and Rationales 186

Appendix A   **Chemotherapeutic Drugs** 200
Appendix B   **Chemotherapy Acronyms and Protocols** 239
Appendix C   ***ICD-9-CM* Classification of Neoplastic
Disorders** 263

Index 289

Contributors and Consultants

Marlene M. Ciranowicz, RN, MSN, CDE
Independent Nurse Consultant
Dresher, Pa.

Douglas D. DeCarolis, PharmD
Inpatient Clinical Coordinator
Minneapolis Veterans' Administration
Medical Center

Christine Ferrante, RN, MSN
Oncology Coordinator
Fitzgerald Mercy Hospital
Darby, Pa.

Richard Pazdur, MD, FACP
Assistant Vice President
for Academic Affairs
M.D. Anderson Cancer Center
University of Texas, Houston

Foreword

Today's changing health care climate has dramatically affected not only general medicine but also specialty care. Oncology—the specialty that encompasses the diagnosis, evaluation, and treatment of neoplastic disorders—has been particularly affected.

At a time when cancer therapies are growing in complexity, all health care professionals are increasingly pressed to provide these therapies at lower costs. To provide the best care at the least cost, health care professionals must have up-to-date information and skills to critically analyze treatment and its outcomes and to translate technology from inpatient to ambulatory settings.

Doctors, nurses, allied health care workers, and students are all well aware of the current scientific and socioeconomic influences shaping cancer care. For instance:
- Therapies are more aggressive and less life-threatening.
- Combination therapies, such as chemotherapy, surgery, and radiation, are in greater use.
- Technologic advances have extended from primary cancer care to supportive care.
- New equipment facilitates the delivery of chemotherapeutic drugs, blood products, and antibiotics safely and conveniently.
- Advances in drug therapy permit greater relief from the toxic effects of chemotherapeutic drugs and cancer-related pain.
- Patient teaching focuses on cancer prevention and early detection.

With this progress, though, comes a mandate to deliver better care in increasingly varied and complex settings. Fortunately, there's help at hand. *Neoplastic Disorders,* a part of the Professional Care Guide series, provides authoritative, easy-to-use, and up-to-date information for any health professional who cares for cancer patients. It begins by examining the causes, diagnosis, and treatment of cancer. Subsequent chapters address cancers of the head and neck, thorax, abdomen, pelvis, genitalia, and bone, skin, and soft tissue. A separate chapter covers leukemias and lymphomas. Lastly, the book's extensive appendices cover the full *ICD-9-CM* classification of neoplastic disorders, chemotherapeutic drugs (including dosage regimens, toxic reactions, and special considerations), and chemotherapy acronyms and protocols.

For convenience, each disorder entry in the book's seven chapters is organized consistently. Each one covers causes, signs and symptoms, diagnostic studies, treatments, and special considerations. For quick reference, staging charts appear for most cancers.

At the end of each chapter, you'll find a helpful self-test section. This section allows the reader to quickly evaluate understanding of the chapter's main concepts and clinical issues. Answers to these questions and the rationales appear at the back of the book.

In short, *Neoplastic Disorders* provides you with important information at a critical time. And it will help you deliver comprehensive, humane, and cost-effective care.

Richard Pazdur, MD, FACP
Assistant Vice President for
Academic Affairs
M.D. Anderson Cancer Center
University of Texas, Houston

CHAPTER 1

Introduction

Primarily a disease of older adults, cancer is second only to cardiovascular disease as the leading cause of death in the United States, accounting for more than 400,000 deaths annually. The disease results from a malignant transformation (carcinogenesis) of normal cells, causing them to enlarge and divide more rapidly than normal and serve no useful purpose.

The characteristic feature of cancer is the cell's ability to proliferate – rapidly, uncontrollably, and independently – from a prim ary site to other tissues where it establishes secondary foci (metastasis). Cancer cells metastasize through the blood or lymphatic system, by unintended transplantation from one site to another during surgery, and by local extension.

Classified by their histologic origin, tumors derived from epithelial tissues are called carcinomas; from epithelial and glandular tissues, adenocarcinomas; from connective, muscle, and bone tissues, sarcomas; from glial cells, gliomas; from pigmented cells, melanomas; and from plasma cells, myelomas. Cancer cells derived from erythrocytes are known as erythroleukemia; from lymphocytes, leukemia; and from lymphatic tissue, lymphoma.

What causes cancer?

Researchers think that cancer develops from the genes of a cell. They have identified about 100 cancer genes. Some are oncogenes, which activate cell division and influence embryonic development, and some are tumor suppressor genes, which halt cell division.

These genes are typically found in normal human cells, but certain kinds of mutations may transform the normal cells. Inherited defects may cause a genetic mutation, whereas exposure to a carcinogen may cause an acquired mutation. Current evidence indicates that carcinogenesis results from a complex interaction of carcinogens and accumulated mutations in several genes.

In animal studies of the ability of viruses to transform cells, some human viruses exhibit carcinogenic potential. For example, the Epstein-Barr virus, the cause of infectious mononucleosis, has been linked to lymphomas.

Of the known carcinogens, scientists consider radiation the most dangerous because it damages the genetic material known as deoxyribonucleic acid (DNA), possibly inducing genetically transferable abnormalities. Other factors, such as a person's tissue type and hormonal status, interact to potentiate radiation's carcinogenic effect.

Other substances that may damage DNA and induce specific forms of carcinogenesis include:
• asbestos – mesothelioma of the lung
• vinyl chloride – angiosarcoma of the liver
• aromatic hydrocarbons and benzopyrene (from polluted air) – lung cancer
• alkylating agents – leukemia
• tobacco – cancer of the lung, oral cavity and upper airways, esophagus, pancreas, kidneys, and bladder.

Diet, particularly a high-protein, high-fat diet, has also been implicated as a carcinogenic factor, especially in the development of GI cancer. Additives composed of nitrates and certain methods of food preparation – particularly charbroiling – are also recognized factors.

The role of hormones in carcinogenesis is still controversial, but it seems that excessive use of some hormones, especially estrogen, produces cancer in animals. Also, the synthetic estrogen diethylstilbestrol causes vaginal cancer in some daughters of women who were treated with it. It's unclear, however, whether changes in human hormonal balance retard or stimulate cancer development.

Some forms of cancer and precancerous lesions result from genetic predisposition either directly (as in Wilms' tumor and retinoblastoma) or indirectly (in association with inherited conditions such as Down's syndrome or immunodeficiency diseases). Expressed as autosomal recessive, X-linked, or autosomal dominant disorders, their common characteristics include:
• early onset of malignant disease
• increased incidence of bilateral cancer in paired organs (breasts, adrenal glands, kidneys) and the eighth cranial nerve (acoustic neuroma)

• increased incidence of multiple primary cancers in non-paired organs
• abnormal chromosome complement in tumor cells.

Immune tumor response

Other factors that interact to increase susceptibility to carcinogenesis are immunologic competence, age, nutritional status, hormonal balance, and response to stress. Theoretically, the body develops cancer cells continuously, but the immune system recognizes them as foreign cells and destroys them. This defense mechanism, known as immunosurveillance, has two major components: the cell-mediated immune response and the humoral immune response. These interacting responses promote antibody production, cellular immunity, and immunologic memory. Presumably, the intact human immune system is responsible for spontaneous regression of tumors.

Researchers believe that the cell-mediated immune response begins when T lymphocytes become sensitized by contact with a specific antigen. After repeated contacts, sensitized T cells release chemical factors called lymphokines, some of which begin to destroy the antigen. This reaction triggers the transformation of an additional population of T lymphocytes into killers of antigen-specific cells—in this case, cancer cells.

Similarly, the humoral immune response reacts to an antigen by triggering the release of antibodies from plasma cells and activating the serum complement system, which destroys the antigen-bearing cell. However, an opposing immune factor, a blocking antibody, can enhance tumor growth by protecting malignant cells from destruction by the immune system.

In therory, cancer arises when any one of several factors disrupts the immune system:
• Aging cells, when copying their genetic material, may begin to err, giving rise to mutations; the aging immune system may not recognize these mutations as foreign and thus may allow them to proliferate and form a malignant tumor.
• Cytotoxic drugs or steroids decrease antibody production and destroy circulating lymphocytes.
• Extreme stress or certain viral infections can depress the immune system.

• Increased susceptibility to infection often results from radiation, cytotoxic drug therapy, and lymphoproliferative and myeloproliferative diseases, such as lymphatic and myelocytic leukemia. These cause bone marrow depression, which can impair leukocyte function.

• Acquired immunodeficiency syndrome weakens cell-mediated immunity.

• Cancer itself is immunosuppressive; advanced cancer exhausts the immune response. (The absence of immune reactivity is known as anergy.)

Diagnostic methods

A thorough medical history and physical examination should precede sophisticated investigative procedures. Useful tests for the early detection and staging of tumors include X-ray, endoscopy, isotope scan, computed tomography scan, and magnetic resonance imaging.

However, the single most important diagnostic tool is a biopsy, which permits direct histologic study of tumor tissue. Biopsy samples can be taken by curettage, fluid aspiration (pleural effusion), needle aspiration biopsy (breast), dermal punch (skin or mouth), endoscopy (rectal polyps), and surgical excision (visceral tumors and nodes).

An important tumor marker, carcinoembryonic antigen (CEA), although not diagnostic by itself, can signal cancers of the large bowel, stomach, pancreas, lungs, and breasts, and sometimes sarcomas, leukemia, and lymphomas. CEA titers range from normal (less than 5 ng) to suspicious (5 to 10 ng) to highly suspicious (more than 10 ng). CEA provides a valuable baseline during chemotherapy to evaluate the extent of tumor spread, regulate drug dosage, aid determination of prognosis after surgery or radiation, and detect tumor recurrence.

While no more specific than CEA, alpha-fetoprotein, a fetal antigen uncommon in adults, can suggest testicular, ovarian, gastric, pancreatic, and primary lung cancers. Beta human chorionic gonadotropin may point to testicular cancer or choriocarcinoma. And although controversial, the prostate-specific antigen test may help evaluate prostate cancer.

Staging and grading

Choosing effective therapeutic options depends on correct staging of cancer, often with the internationally known TNM

Essential differences between benign and malignant tumors

	BENIGN	MALIGNANT
Growth	Expand slowly; push aside surrounding tissue but do not infiltrate	Usually infiltrate surrounding tissues rapidly, expanding in all directions
Limitation	Usually encapsulated	Seldom encapsulated; often poorly delineated
Recurrence	Rare after surgical removal	When removed surgically, commonly recur because of infiltration into surrounding tissues
Morphology	Cells closely resemble cells of tissue of origin	Cells may differ considerably from those of tissue of origin
Differentiation	Well-differentiated	Poor or no differentiation
Mitotic activity	Slight	Extensive
Tissue destruction	Usually slight	Extensive because of infiltration and metastatic lesion
Spread	No metastasis	Spread by blood or lymphatic systems to establish secondary tumors
Effect on body	Cachexia rare; usually not fatal but may obstruct vital organs, exert pressure, and produce excess hormones; can become malignant	Cachexia typical—anemia, loss of weight, weakness, general ill health; fatal if untreated

staging system (*t*umor size, *n*odal involvement, *m*etastatic progress). This classification system provides an accurate tumor description that can change as the disease progresses. TNM staging allows reliable comparison of treatments and survival rates among large population groups; it also identifies nodal involvement and metastasis of the disease.

Grading is another objective way to define a tumor. Grading takes into account resemblance of tumor tissue to normal cells (differentiation) and its estimated growth rate. Grading also identifies the lesion according to corresponding normal cells, such as lymphoid or mucinous lesions. (See *Essential differences between benign and malignant tumors.*)

Five major therapies	Cancer treatments include surgery, radiation, chemotherapy, biotherapy (also called immunotherapy), and hormonal therapy. Each therapy may be used alone or in combination, depending on the type, stage, localization, and responsiveness of the tumor and on limitations imposed by the patient's clinical status.
Surgery	Once the mainstay of cancer treatment, surgery is typically combined with other therapies. The surgical biopsy procedure is now used to obtain tissue for study; continuing surgery then removes the bulk of the tumor. Later, other therapies may be used to discourage proliferation of residual cells. Surgery can also relieve pain, correct obstruction, and alleviate pressure. Today's less radical surgical procedures (such as lumpectomy instead of radical mastectomy) are more acceptable to patients.
Radiation	This therapy aims to destroy the dividing cancer cells while damaging resting normal cells as little as possible. Both types of radiation, ionizing radiation and particle radiation, have cellular DNA as their target; however, particle radiation produces less skin damage.

Radiation treatment approaches include external beam radiation and intracavitary and interstitial implants. The latter therapy requires personal radiation protection for all staff members who come in contact with the patient. (See *Preparing the patient for external radiation therapy.*)

Normal and malignant cells respond to radiation differently, depending on blood supply, oxygen saturation, previous irradiation, and immune status. Generally, normal cells recover from radiation faster than malignant cells. The success of the treatment and amount of damage to normal tissue also vary with the intensity of the radiation. Although a large single dose of radiation has greater cellular effects than fractions of the same amount delivered sequentially, a protracted schedule allows time for normal tissue to recover in the intervals between individual sublethal doses.

Radiation may be used palliatively to relieve pain, obstruction, malignant effusions, cough, dyspnea, ulcerations, and hemorrhage; it can also promote the repair of pathologic fractures after surgical stabilization and delay tumor spread.

Preparing the patient for external radiation therapy

Follow the guidelines listed below to help relieve your patient's anxiety before he undergoes his first radiation treatment:

• Show the patient where radiation therapy takes place, and introduce him to the radiation therapist.

• Tell him to remove all metal objects (pens, buttons, or jewelry) that may interfere with therapy. Explain that the areas to be treated will be marked with ink and that *he must not scrub these areas* because it's important to radiate the same areas each time.

• Reinforce the explanation of the procedure and answer any questions the patient may have as honestly as you can. Realistically explain the benefits and adverse effects of radiation therapy that he may expect.

• Teach the patient to watch for and report any adverse reactions. Because radiation therapy may increase susceptibility to infection, warn him to avoid persons with colds or other infections during therapy.

• Reassure the patient that treatment is painless and won't make him radioactive. Stress that he'll be under constant surveillance during radiation administration and need only call out if he needs anything.

Combining radiation and surgery can minimize radical surgery, prolong survival, and preserve anatomic function. For example, preoperative doses of radiation shrink a tumor, making it operable while preventing further spread of the disease during surgery. After the wound heals, postoperative doses prevent residual cancer cells from multiplying or metastasizing.

Systemic effects, such as weakness, fatigue, anorexia, nausea, vomiting, and anemia, may subside with antiemetics, steroids, frequent small meals, fluid maintenance, and rest. They are seldom severe enough to require discontinuing radiation but may require a dosage adjustment. (For localized adverse effects, see *Adverse effects of radiation*, page 8.)

Radiation therapy involves frequent blood counts (particularly of white blood cells and platelets), especially if the target site involves areas of bone marrow production. Transdermal drug delivery (for example, using nitroglycerin, clonidine, or fentanyl) to irradiated skin should be avoided.

Radiation also requires special skin care, such as covering the irradiated area with loose cotton clothing and avoiding deodorants, colognes, and other topical agents during treatment. Advise the patient to shave with an elec-

Adverse effects of radiation

AREA RADIATED	EFFECT	MANAGEMENT
Abdomen, pelvis	Cramps, diarrhea	Administer opium tincture, (camphorated) and diphenoxylate with atropine; provide low-residue diet; maintain fluid and electrolyte balance.
Head	Alopecia	Encourage patient to wear wig or head covering.
	Mucositis	Give mouthwash with viscous lidocaine; give cool, carbonated drinks and ice pops; maintain soft, nonirritating diet.
	Moniliasis	Give nystatin mouthwash; avoid giving commercial mouthwash.
	Dental caries	Apply fluoride to teeth prophylactically; provide gingival care.
Chest	Lung tissue devitalization	Prohibit smoking; isolate patient from others with upper respiratory infections; provide humidifier if necessary.
	Pericarditis	Control arrhythmias with appropriate agents (procainamide, disopyramide phosphate); monitor for heart failure.
	Esophagitis	Give pain medication; provide total parenteral nutrition; maintain fluid balance.
Kidneys	Nephritis, lassitude, headache, edema, dyspnea on exertion, hypertensive nephropathy, azotemia, secondary anemia	Maintain fluid and electrolyte balance; watch for signs of renal failure.

tric razor only, to protect the skin from exposure to direct sunlight, to avoid temperature extremes, and to avoid swimming in chlorinated swimming pools.

Chemotherapy   A wide array of drugs may induce regression of a tumor and prevent its metastasis. Chemotherapy proves particularly useful in controlling residual disease. And as an adjunct to surgery or radiation therapy, it can induce long remissions and sometimes effect cures, especially in patients with childhood leukemia, Hodgkin's disease, choriocarcinoma, and testicular cancer. As palliative treatment, chemotherapy aims to improve the patient's quality of life by temporarily relieving pain or other symptoms.

Major chemotherapeutic drugs include the following:
• Alkylating agents and nitrosoureas inhibit cell growth and division by reacting with DNA.
• Antimetabolites prevent cell growth by competing with metabolites in the production of nucleic acid.
• Antitumor antibiotics block cell growth by binding with DNA and interfering with DNA-dependent ribonucleic acid synthesis.
• Plant alkaloids prevent cellular reproduction by disrupting cell mitosis.
• Steroid hormones inhibit the growth of hormone-susceptible tumors by changing their chemical environment.

Chemotherapeutic drugs can be given orally, S.C., I.M., I.V., intracavitarily, intrathecally, and by arterial infusion, depending on the drug and its pharmacologic action; usually, administration is intermittent to allow for bone marrow recovery between doses. Calculate dosage according to the patient's body surface area, with adjustments for general condition and degree of myelosuppression. When calculating dosage, make sure your information is current because dosages change periodically.

Although antineoplastic agents are toxic to cancer cells, they can also cause transient changes in normal tissues, especially among proliferating body cells. For example, antineoplastic agents typically suppress bone marrow, causing anemia, leukopenia, and thrombocytopenia; irritate GI epithelial cells, causing vomiting; and destroy the cells of the hair follicles and skin, causing alopecia and dermatitis.

Many I.V. drugs also cause venous sclerosis and pain on administration. If extravasated, they may cause deep cutaneous necrosis requiring debridement and skin grafting. (*Note:* Most drugs with the potential for direct tissue injury are now given through a central venous catheter.)

All patients undergoing chemotherapy need special care as follows:
• Watch for any signs of infection, especially if the patient is receiving simultaneous radiation treatment. Be alert for even a low-grade fever when the granulocyte count falls below 500/mm^3; take the patient's temperature often.
• Increase the patient's fluid intake before and throughout chemotherapy.

• Inform the patient of the possibility of temporary hair loss, and reassure him that his hair should grow back after therapy ends.

• Check the skin for petechiae, ecchymoses, chemical cellulitis, and secondary infection during treatment.

• Minimize tissue irritation and damage by checking needle placement before and during infusion if you administer the drug by a peripheral vein. Be sure to check for blood return before and during infusion of vesicants if the patient has a venous access device, a central venous line, or a peripherally inserted central catheter. Tell the patient to report any discomfort during infusion. If a vesicant extravasates, stop the infusion, aspirate the drug from the needle, and give the appropriate antidote. Administration of antidotes varies according to hospital policy.

• Encourage the patient to express his concerns, and provide simple and truthful information. Explain that not all patients who undergo chemotherapy experience nausea and vomiting and, for those who do, antiemetic drugs, relaxation therapy, and diet can minimize these problems.

Biotherapy

Formerly known as immunotherapy, biotherapy relies on agents known as biological response modifiers. Biological agents are usually combined with chemotherapeutic drugs or radiation therapy and are most effective in the early stages of cancer. Much of the work done in biotherapy is still experimental, so the availability of this treatment may be limited and its adverse effects are often unpredictable. However, several approaches are currently promising.

For example, some biological agents such as the interferons have a direct antitumor effect, whereas others can activate or influence the immune system. Biological agents have proved useful in treating hairy cell leukemia, renal cell carcinoma, and melanoma. The most widely used agents are the interferons and interleukin-2.

Advances have occurred in other areas of biotherapy also. Bone marrow transplantation restores hematologic and immunologic function in patients who have immunodeficiencies or acute leukemia who don't respond to conventional biotherapy.

When tagged with radioisotopes and injected into the body, biochemicals known as monoclonal antibodies help detect cancer by attaching to tumor cells. Soon these antibodies may be linked with toxins to destroy specific cancer cells without disturbing healthy cells.

Although not used to treat cancer directly, colony-stimulating factors may be used to support the patient with low blood counts related to chemotherapy.

Adverse effects of biotherapeutic agents include fever and flulike symptoms, fatigue, central nervous system effects (especially from the interferons), and capillary leak syndrome (most commonly associated with interleukin-2).

Hormonal therapy

Certain hormones affect the growth of certain cancer types. For example, the luteinizing-releasing hormone analogue leuprolide is now used to treat prostate cancer. Used long term, this hormone inhibits testosterone release and tumor growth. And tamoxifen, an antiestrogen hormonal agent, blocks estrogen receptors in breast tumor cells that require estrogen to thrive. Leuprolide produces such adverse effects as hot flashes, sweating, impotence, and decreased libido; tamoxifen's adverse effects include nausea, vomiting, and blood dyscrasias.

Maintaining nutrition and fluid balance

Tumors grow at the expense of normal tissue by competing for nutrients; consequently, the cancer patient commonly suffers from protein deficiency. Cancer treatments themselves produce fluid and electrolyte disturbances, such as vomiting and anorexia. Take the following steps to ensure adequate nutrition and fluid and electrolyte balance:

• Obtain a comprehensive dietary history to pinpoint nutritional problems and their origins, such as diabetes; help plan the patient's diet accordingly.

• Ask the dietitian to provide a liquid diet high in proteins, carbohydrates, and calories if the patient can't tolerate solid foods. If the patient has stomatitis, provide soft, bland, non-irritating foods.

• Encourage the patient's family to bring foods from home, if he requests.

• Make mealtime as relaxed and pleasant as possible. Encourage the patient to dine with visitors or other patients. Allow choices from a varied menu.

- If appropriate, you may suggest that the patient take a glass of wine before dinner to stimulate the appetite and aid relaxation.
- Urge the patient to drink juice or other caloric beverages instead of water.
- Suggest small, frequent meals if the patient can't tolerate normal ones.
- Avoid including strong-smelling foods in the patient's diet.

Providing tube feedings

The patient who has had recent head, neck, or GI surgery or who has pain when swallowing can receive nourishment through a nasogastric (NG) tube. If the patient still needs to use the tube after he's discharged, teach him how to insert it, how to test its position in his stomach by aspirating stomach contents, and how to use it to feed himself.

If an NG tube isn't appropriate, other alternatives are gastrostomy, jejunostomy, and, occasionally, esophagostomy. These procedures make it possible for you to feed the patient prescribed protein formulas and semiliquids, such as cream soups and eggnog; they also make it easier for the patient to feed himself.

Remember to forewarn the patient that if spilled gastric or intestinal juices come in contact with the abdominal skin, they will cause excoriation if they're not washed off immediately. Always flush the tube well with water following each feeding. Also, to provide adequate hydration, instill about 4 to 6 oz (118 to 177 ml) of water or another clear liquid between meals.

After jejunostomy, begin with very small feedings, slowly and carefully increasing the amounts. Provide additional fluids and calories during these days of limited food intake by supplementing jejunostomy feedings with I.V. fat emulsions.

Total parenteral nutrition

Commonly considered an important component of cancer care if the patient can't take enteral nutrition, total parenteral nutrition (TPN) can improve a severely debilitated patient's protein balance. In doing so, TPN characteristically strengthens and conditions the patient, allowing him to better tolerate surgery.

What's more, TPN can produce a slight weight gain in the patient receiving radiation therapy, provide optimum nutrition for wound healing, and help the patient combat infection after radical surgery.

Pain control

Typically, cancer patients have a great fear of overwhelming pain. Therefore, controlling pain is a major consideration at every stage of managing cancer—from localized cancer to advanced metastasis. In cancer patients, pain may result from inflammation of or pressure on pain-sensitive structures, tumor infiltration of nerves or blood vessels, or metastatic extension to bone. Such chronic and unrelenting pain can wear down the patient's tolerance to treatment, interfere with eating and sleeping, and color his life with anger, despair, and anxiety.

Narcotic analgesics, either alone or in combination with nonnarcotic analgesics or antianxiety agents, are the mainstay of pain relief in patients with advanced cancer. In terminal stages of cancer, effective narcotic dosages may be quite high, because drug tolerance invariably develops and the danger of addiction is unimportant. Provide such analgesics generously. Anticipate the need for pain relief, and provide it on a schedule that doesn't allow pain to break through. Don't wait until pain becomes severe to provide relief. Reassure the patient that you'll provide pain medication whenever he needs it. (See *Patient-controlled analgesia system,* page 14.)

Nonpharmacologic pain-relief techniques can be used alone or in combination with drug therapy. Popular nonpharmacologic techniques include cutaneous stimulation, relaxation, biofeedback, distraction, and guided imagery.

Other pain-relief measures include surgical excision of the tumor to relieve pressure on sensitive tissues and pain caused by inflamed necrotic tissue, treatment with antibiotics to combat inflammation, and radiation therapy to shrink metastatic tissue and control bone pain. When a tumor invades nerve tissue, effective pain control requires anesthetics, nerve blocks, electronic nerve stimulation with a dorsal column or transcutaneous electrical nerve stimulator, rhizotomy, or chordotomy.

Hospice approach

A holistic approach to patient care modeled after St. Christopher's Hospice in London, hospice care provides comprehensive physical, psychological, social, and spiritual care for

Patient-controlled analgesia system

An effective method of pain relief, the patient-controlled analgesia (PCA) system is used in some cancer care centers with encouraging results.

How PCA works

This system permits the patient to self-administer an analgesic by pressing a button at the bedside that activates a pump fitted with a prefilled syringe containing the analgesic. Small, intermittent doses of the analgesic administered I.V. maintain blood levels that ensure comfort and minimize sedation.

Dosages and time intervals (usually 8 to 10 minutes) that allow the patient to determine his comfort level are preset. The syringe is locked inside the pump as a safety feature. The system will only dispense the analgesic until the correct (pre-set) time interval has elapsed.

PCA advantages

Results of clinical studies indicate that patients who use PCA tend to titrate analgesic drugs effectively and maintain comfort without oversedation. They use less of the drug than the amount normally given by I.M. injection.

PCA provides several other advantages. Patients using this system:
• stay alert and active during daytime hours
• need not endure pain while waiting for an injection
• have reduced anxiety levels
• remain free from pain caused by injections
• need not call the nurse away from other clinical duties.

terminally ill patients. Although some hospices are located in inpatient settings, most hospice programs serve the terminally ill patient in his own home.

The goal of the hospice care team is to help the patient achieve as full a life as possible, with minimal pain, discomfort, and restriction. Of the many medications provided for pain control, morphine is considered the drug of choice.

Hospice care also emphasizes a coordinated team effort to help the patient and family members overcome the severe anxiety, fear, and depression that occur with terminal illness. Thus the hospice staff encourages family members to help with the patient's care, providing the patient with warmth and security and helping the family caregivers begin working out their grief before the patient dies.

Everyone involved must be committed to high-quality patient care, unafraid of emotional involvement, and comfortable with personal feelings about death and dying. Hospice care also requires open communication among team members for the evaluation of patient care and to help the staff members cope with their own feelings.

Psychological aspects

Few illnesses evoke as profound an emotional response as does cancer. A few patients face this difficult reality immediately. Many use denial as a coping mechanism and refuse to accept the diagnosis but find this stance difficult to maintain. As evidence of the tumor becomes inescapable, the patient may plunge into deep depression. Family members in denial may cope by encouraging unproven methods of cancer treatment. Some patients intellectualize their disease, enabling them to obscure its reality and regard it as unrelated to themselves. Generally, the patient who mentally objectifies his cancer will accept treatment.

Be aware of the possible behavioral responses so that you can identify them and then interact supportively with the patient and his family. For many cancers, you can offer realistic hope for long-term survival or remission; even in advanced disease, you can offer short-term achievable goals. Make sure you understand your own feelings about cancer. Then listen sensitively to the patient so you can offer understanding and support. When caring for a patient with terminal cancer, increase your effectiveness by seeking out someone to help you through your own grieving.

Self-test questions

You can quickly review your comprehension of this introductory chapter by answering the following questions. The answers to these questions and their rationales appear on pages 185 and 186.

1. Which of the following statements characterizes cancer in North America?
  a. It's second only to cardiovascular disease as the leading cause of death in adults.
  b. It's predominantly a disease of young and middle-aged adults.
  c. It's generally more common in women.
  d. It's the leading cause of death in children.

2. Cancer development involves the genes of a cell. Ap-

proximately how many cancer genes have researchers discovered?
- **a.** 100
- **b.** 150
- **c.** 200
- **d.** 400

3. Which of the following statements describes a difference between benign and malignant tumors?
- **a.** Benign tumors are usually poorly delineated, whereas malignant tumors are usually encapsulated.
- **b.** After surgical removal, benign tumors frequently recur whereas malignant tumors rarely recur.
- **c.** Benign tumors are not well differentiated; malignant tumors are.
- **d.** Benign tumors rarely cause cachexia, whereas cachexia is typical with malignant tumors.

4. Which of the following types of chemotherapeutic agents prevent cellular reproduction by disrupting cell mitosis?
- **a.** Alkylating agents
- **b.** Antimetabolites
- **c.** Antitumor antibiotics
- **d.** Plant alkaloids

5. When preparing a patient for external radiation therapy in areas of bone marrow production, you should inform him that:
- **a.** he will feel only mild bone pain during the treatment.
- **b.** he will be radioactive for 12 hours following each treatment.
- **c.** he will need frequent blood counts during the radiation period.
- **d.** he will not need chemotherapy.

CHAPTER 2

Head, Neck, and Spinal Neoplasms

Cancers of the head, neck, or spine are among the deadliest and most disfiguring. Involvement of speech and sense organs, as well as the central nervous system itself, can dramatically impair the patient's quality of life.

Malignant brain tumors

Malignant brain tumors (gliomas, meningiomas, and schwannomas) are slightly more common in men than in women. Their incidence is 4.5 per 100,000.

Malignant brain tumors may occur at any age. In adults, incidence is generally highest between ages 40 and 60. The most common tumor types in adults are gliomas and meningiomas; these tumors are usually supratentorial.

In children, incidence is generally highest before age 1 and then again between ages 2 and 12. The most common tumors in children are astrocytomas, medulloblastomas, ependymomas, and brain gliomas. In children, brain tumors represent one of the most common causes of death from cancer. (See *Comparing malignant brain tumors*, pages 18 to 20.)

Causes

What causes primary brain tumors isn't known. Some tumors may be congenitally acquired, such as epidermoid, dermoid, and teratoid tumors. Others may result from he-

alignant brain tumors

CLINICAL FEATURES

Glioblastoma multiforme *(spongioblastoma multiforme)*

• Peak incidence at 50 to 60 years; twice as common in men; most common glioma
• Unencapsulated, highly malignant; grows rapidly and infiltrates the brain extensively; may become enormous before diagnosed
• Occurs most often in cerebral hemispheres, especially frontal and temporal lobes (rarely in brain stem and cerebellum)
• Occupies more than one lobe of affected hemisphere; may spread to opposite hemisphere by corpus callosum; may metastasize into cerebrospinal fluid (CSF), producing tumors in distant parts of the nervous system

General
• Increased intracranial pressure (ICP) — nausea, vomiting, headache, papilledema
• Mental and behavioral changes
• Altered vital signs (increased systolic pressure; widened pulse pressure, respiratory changes)
• Speech and sensory disturbances
• In children, irritability, projectile vomiting

Localizing
• Midline: headache (frontal or occipital) — worse in morning; intensified by coughing, straining, or sudden head movements
• Temporal lobe: psychomotor seizures
• Central region: focal seizures
• Optic and oculomotor nerves: visual defects
• Frontal lobe: abnormal reflexes, motor responses

Astrocytoma

• Second most common malignant glioma (approximately 30% of all gliomas)
• Occurs at any age; incidence higher in men
• Occurs most often in white matter of cerebral hemispheres; may originate in any part of the central nervous system
• Cerebellar astrocytomas usually confined to one hemisphere

General
• Headache; mental activity changes
• Decreased motor strength and coordination
• Seizures; scanning speech
• Altered vital signs

Localizing
• Third ventricle: changes in mental activity and level of consciousness, nausea, pupillary dilation and sluggish light reflex; later — paresis or ataxia
• Brain stem and pons: early — ipsilateral trigeminal, abducens, and facial nerve palsies; later — cerebellar ataxia, tremors, other cranial nerve deficits
• Third or fourth ventricle or aqueduct of Sylvius: secondary hydrocephalus
• Thalamus or hypothalamus: variety of endocrine, metabolic, autonomic, and behavioral changes

Oligodendroglioma

• Third most common glioma
• Occurs in middle adult years; more common in women
• Slow-growing

General
• Mental and behavioral changes
• Decreased visual acuity and other visual disturbances
• Increased ICP

Localizing
• Temporal lobe: hallucinations, psychomotor seizures
• Central region: seizures (confined to one muscle group or unilateral)

Comparing malignant brain tumors *(continued)*

TUMOR	CLINICAL FEATURES
Oligodendroglioma *(continued)*	• Midbrain or third ventricle: pyramidal tract symptoms (dizziness, ataxia, paresthesia of the face) • Brain stem and cerebrum: nystagmus, hearing loss, dizziness, ataxia, paresthesia of the face, cranial nerve palsies, hemiparesis, suboccipital tenderness, loss of balance
Ependymoma	
• Rare glioma • Most common in children and young adults • Locates most often in fourth and lateral ventricles	*General* • Similar to oligodendroglioma • Increased ICP and obstructive hydrocephalus, depending on tumor size
Medulloblastoma	
• Rare glioma • Incidence highest in children ages 4 to 6 • Affects boys more than girls • Frequently metastasizes via CSF	*General* • Increased ICP *Localizing* • Brain stem and cerebrum: papilledema, nystagmus, hearing loss, flashing lights in vision, dizziness, ataxia, paresthesia of face, cranial nerve palsies (V, VI, VII, IX, and X, primarily sensory), hemiparesis, suboccipital tenderness; compression of supratentorial area produces other general and focal symptoms
Meningioma	
• Most common nongliomatous brain tumor (15% of primary brain tumors) • Peak incidence among 50-year-olds; rare in children; more common in women (ratio 3:2) • Arises from the meninges • Common locations include parasagittal area, sphenoidal ridge, anterior part of the base of the skull, cerebellopontile angle, spinal canal • Benign, well-circumscribed, highly vascular tumors that compress underlying brain tissue by invading overlying skull	*General* • Headache • Seizures (in two-thirds of patients) • Vomiting • Changes in mental activity • Similar to schwannomas *Localizing* • Skull changes (bony bulge) over tumor • Sphenoidal ridge, indenting optic nerve: unilateral visual changes and papilledema • Prefrontal parasagittal: personality and behavioral changes • Motor cortex: contralateral motor changes • Anterior fossa compressing both optic nerves and frontal lobes: headaches and bilateral vision loss • Pressure on cranial nerves causes varying symptoms

(continued)

ınant brain tumors *(continued)*

CLINICAL FEATURES

eurinoma, neurilemoma, cerebellopontile angle tumor)

• Accounts for approximately 10% of all intracranial tumors
• Higher incidence in women
• Onset of symptoms between ages 30 and 60
• Affects the craniospinal nerve sheath, usually cranial nerve VIII; also, V and VII, and to a lesser extent, VI and X on the same side as the tumor
• Benign, but often classified as malignant because of its growth patterns; slow-growing—may be present for years before symptoms occur

General
• Unilateral hearing loss with or without tinnitus
• Stiff neck and suboccipital discomfort
• Secondary hydrocephalus
• Ataxia and uncoordinated movements of one or both arms due to pressure on brain stem and cerebellum

Localizing
• Cranial nerve V: early—facial hypoesthesia or paresthesia on side of hearing loss; unilateral loss of corneal reflex
• Cranial nerve VI: diplopia or double vision
• Cranial nerve VII: paresis progressing to paralysis (Bell's palsy)
• Cranial nerve X: weakness of palate, tongue, and nerve muscles on same side as tumor

---

reditary factors, such as von Recklinghausen's disease or tuberous sclerosis.

Signs and symptoms

Brain tumors cause central nervous system (CNS) changes by invading and destroying tissues and by secondary effects—mainly compression of the brain, cranial nerves, and cerebral vessels; cerebral edema; and increased intracranial pressure (ICP). Generally, the symptoms of increased ICP vary with the type of tumor, its location, and the degree of invasion. Onset of symptoms is usually insidious, and brain tumors are commonly misdiagnosed.

Diagnosis

In many cases, a definitive diagnosis follows a tissue biopsy performed by stereotaxic surgery. In this procedure, a head ring is affixed to the skull, and an excisional device is guided to the lesion by a computed tomography (CT) scan or magnetic resonance imaging (MRI).

Other diagnostic tools include a patient history, a neurologic assessment, skull X-rays, a brain scan, a CT scan, MRI, and cerebral angiography. Lumbar puncture shows increased pressure and protein levels, decreased glucose levels and, occasionally, tumor cells in cerebrospinal fluid (CSF).

Treatment   Appropriate treatment includes removing a resectable tumor, reducing a nonresectable tumor, relieving cerebral edema or increased ICP and other symptoms, and preventing further neurologic damage.

The mode of therapy depends on the tumor's histologic type, radiosensitivity, and location and may include surgery, radiation, chemotherapy, or decompression of increased ICP with diuretics, corticosteroids, or possibly ventriculoatrial or ventriculoperitoneal shunting of CSF.

A glioma usually requires resection by craniotomy, followed by radiation therapy and chemotherapy. The combination of nitrosoureas (carmustine [BCNU] and lomustine [CCNU]) or procarbazine and postoperative radiation is more effective than radiation alone.

Surgical resection of low-grade cystic cerebellar astrocytomas brings long-term survival. Treatment of other astrocytomas includes repeated surgery, radiation therapy, and shunting of fluid from obstructed CSF pathways. Some astrocytomas are highly radiosensitive but others are radioresistant.

Treatment for oligodendrogliomas and ependymomas includes resection and radiation therapy; for medulloblastomas, resection and possibly intrathecal infusion of methotrexate or another antineoplastic drug. Meningiomas require resection, including dura mater and bone (operative mortality may reach 10% because of large tumor size).

For schwannomas, microsurgical technique allows complete dissection of the tumor and preservation of facial nerves. Although schwannomas are moderately radioresistant, postoperative radiation therapy is necessary.

Chemotherapy for malignant brain tumors includes the nitrosoureas that help break down the blood-brain barrier and allow other chemotherapeutic drugs to go through as well. Intrathecal and intra-arterial administration of drugs maximize drug actions.

Palliative measures for gliomas, astrocytomas, oligodendrogliomas, and ependymomas include dexamethasone for cerebral edema, and antacids and histamine receptor antagonists for stress ulcers. These tumors and schwannomas may also require anticonvulsants.

Special
considerations

- During your first contact with the patient, perform a comprehensive examination (including a complete neurologic evaluation) to provide baseline data. Obtain a thorough health history concerning onset of symptoms. Assist the patient and his family in coping with the treatment, potential disabilities, and changes in lifestyle resulting from his tumor.

Care during
hospitalization

Carefully document seizure activity (occurrence, nature, and duration).
- Maintain airway patency.
- Monitor patient safety.
- Administer anticonvulsant drugs as necessary.
- Check continuously for neurologic changes, and watch for increased ICP.
- Watch for sudden unilateral pupillary dilation with loss of light reflex; this ominous change indicates imminent transtentorial herniation.
- Monitor respiratory changes carefully (abnormal respiratory rate and depth may point to rising ICP or herniation of the cerebellar tonsils from an expanding infratentorial mass).
- Monitor the patient's temperature carefully. Fever commonly follows hypothalamic anoxia but might also indicate meningitis. Use hypothermia blankets preoperatively and postoperatively to keep the patient's temperature down and minimize cerebral metabolic demands.
- Administer steroids and osmotic diuretics such as mannitol to reduce cerebral edema. Fluids may be restricted to 1,500 ml/24 hours. Monitor fluid and electrolyte balance to avoid dehydration.
- Observe the patient for signs of stress ulcers: abdominal distention, pain, vomiting, and black, tarry stools. Administer antacids.

Care after
craniotomy

- Continue to monitor general neurologic status and watch for signs of increased ICP, such as an elevated bone flap and typical neurologic changes. To reduce the risk of increased ICP, restrict fluids to 1,500 ml/24 hours.
- To promote venous drainage and reduce cerebral edema after supratentorial craniotomy, elevate the head of the patient's bed about 30 degrees. Position him on his side to allow drainage of secretions and prevent aspiration.

• As appropriate, instruct the patient to avoid Valsalva's maneuver or isometric muscle contractions when moving or sitting up in bed; these can increase intrathoracic pressure and thereby increase ICP. Withhold oral fluids, which may provoke vomiting and consequently raise ICP.
• After infratentorial craniotomy, keep the patient flat for 48 hours, but logroll him every 2 hours to minimize complications of immobilization.
• Prevent other complications by paying careful attention to ventilatory status and to cardiovascular, GI, and musculoskeletal functions.

Other measures

• Radiation therapy is usually delayed until after the surgical wound heals, but it can induce wound breakdown even then. Therefore, you should observe the wound carefully for infection and sinus formation. Because radiation may cause brain inflammation, also watch for signs of rising ICP.
• Because carmustine (BCNU), lomustine (CCNU), and procarbazine—used as adjuncts to radiotherapy and surgery can possibly cause delayed bone marrow suppression, tell the patient to watch for and immediately report any signs of infection or bleeding that appear within 4 weeks after the start of chemotherapy.
• Before chemotherapy, give prochlorperazine or another antiemetic to minimize nausea and vomiting.
• Teach the patient and his family early signs of recurrence.
• Urge compliance with treatment.
• Because brain tumors may cause residual neurologic deficits that handicap the patient physically or mentally, begin rehabilitation early. Consult with occupational and physical therapists to encourage independence in daily activities.
• As necessary, provide aids for self-care and mobilization such as bathroom rails for wheelchair patients.
• If the patient is aphasic, arrange for consultation with a speech pathologist.

Pituitary tumors

Constituting 10% of intracranial neoplasms, pituitary tumors originate most often in the anterior pituitary (adenohypophysis). They occur in adults of both sexes, usually during the third and fourth decades of life. The three tissue types of pituitary tumors include chromophobe adenoma (90%), basophil adenoma, and eosinophil adrenoma.

Pituitary tumors aren't malignant in the strict sense, but because their growth is invasive, they're considered a neoplastic disease. The prognosis is fair to good, depending on the extent to which the tumor spreads beyond the sella turcica.

Causes

Although the exact cause is unknown, a predisposition to pituitary tumors may be inherited through an autosomal dominant trait.

Chromophobe adenoma may be associated with production of corticotropin, melanocyte-stimulating hormone, growth hormone, and prolactin; basophil adenoma, with evidence of excess corticotropin production and, consequently, with signs of Cushing's syndrome; eosinophil adenoma, with excessive growth hormone.

Signs and symptoms

As pituitary adenomas grow, they replace normal glandular tissue and enlarge the sella turcica, which houses the pituitary gland. The resulting pressure on adjacent intracranial structures produces these typical neurologic manifestations:
• frontal headache
• visual symptoms, beginning with blurring and progressing to field cuts (hemianopias) and then unilateral blindness
• cranial nerve involvement (III, IV, VI) from lateral extension of the tumor, resulting in strabismus; double vision, with compensating head tilting and dizziness; conjugate deviation of gaze; nystagmus; lid ptosis; and limited eye movements
• increased intracranial pressure (ICP)—secondary hydrocephalus
• personality changes or dementia, if the tumor breaks through to the frontal lobes

• seizures
• rhinorrhea, if the tumor erodes the base of the skull
• pituitary apoplexy secondary to hemorrhagic infarction of the adenoma. Such hemorrhage may lead to both cardiovascular and adrenocortical collapse.
  Endocrine manifestations may include:
• hypopituitarism, to some degree, in all patients with adenoma, becoming more obvious as the tumor replaces normal gland tissue. Symptoms include amenorrhea, decreased libido and impotence in men, skin changes (waxy appearance, decreased wrinkles, and pigmentation), loss of axillary and pubic hair, lethargy, weakness, increased fatigability, intolerance to cold, and constipation (because of decreased corticotropin and thyroid-stimulating hormone production)
• addisonian crisis, precipitated by stress and resulting in nausea, vomiting, hypoglycemia, hypotension, and circulatory collapse
• diabetes insipidus, resulting from extension to the hypothalamus
• prolactin-secreting adenomas (in 70% to 75%), with amenorrhea and galactorrhea; also growth hormone-secreting adenomas, with acromegaly; and corticotropin-secreting adenomas, with Cushing's syndrome.

Diagnosis

• *Skull X-rays with tomography* show enlargement of the sella turcica or erosion of its floor; if growth hormone secretion predominates, X-rays show enlarged paranasal sinuses and mandible, thickened cranial bones, and separated teeth.
• *Carotid angiography* shows displacement of the anterior cerebral and internal carotid arteries if the tumor mass is enlarging; it also rules out intracerebral aneurysm.
• *Computed tomography scan* may confirm the existence of the adenoma and accurately depict its size.
• *Cerebrospinal fluid (CSF) analysis* may show increased protein levels.
• *Endocrine function tests* may contribute helpful information, but results are often ambiguous and inconclusive.
• *Magnetic resonance imaging* differentiates among healthy, benign, and malignant tissues as well as arteries and veins.

Treatment

Surgical options include transfrontal removal of large tumors impinging on the optic apparatus and transsphenoidal

Transsphenoidal pituitary surgery

This shows placement of bivalve speculum and rongeur for pituitary gland removal.

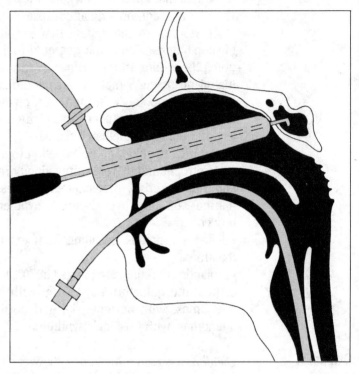

resection for smaller tumors confined to the pituitary fossa. The transsphenoidal approach permits selective removal of the tumor while preserving normal pituitary tissue. (See *Transsphenoidal pituitary surgery.*) Radiation is the primary treatment for small, nonsecretory tumors that don't extend beyond the sella turcica or for patients who may be poor postoperative risks; otherwise, it's an adjunct to surgery.

Postoperative treatment includes hormone replacement with cortisone and thyroid and sex hormones, correction of electrolyte imbalance, and insulin therapy as needed.

Drug therapy may include bromocriptine, an ergot derivative that shrinks prolactin-secreting and growth hormone-secreting tumors. Cyproheptadine, an antiserotonin

Postcraniotomy care

• Monitor vital signs (especially level of consciousness), and perform a baseline neurologic assessment from which to plan further care and evaluate progress.
• Maintain the patient's airway; suction as necessary.
• Monitor intake and output carefully.

• Give the patient nothing by mouth for 24 to 48 hours to prevent aspiration and vomiting, which increases intracranial pressure.
• Observe for cerebral edema, bleeding, and cerebrospinal fluid leakage.
• Provide a restful, quiet environment.

---

drug, can reduce increased corticosteroid levels in the patient with Cushing's syndrome.

Adjuvant radiotherapy is used when only partial removal of the tumor is possible. Cryohypophysectomy (freezing the area with a probe inserted by the transsphenoidal route) is a promising alternative to surgical dissection of the tumor.

Special considerations

• Conduct a comprehensive health history and physical assessment to establish the onset of neurologic and endocrine dysfunction and provide baseline data for later comparison. (See *Postcraniotomy care.*)
• Establish a supportive, trusting relationship with the patient and family to assist them in coping with the diagnosis, treatment, and potential long-term changes. Make sure they understand that the patient needs lifelong evaluations and, possibly, hormone replacement.
• Reassure the patient that some of the distressing symptoms caused by pituitary dysfunction (for example, altered sexual drive, impotence, infertility, loss of hair, and emotional lability) will disappear with treatment.
• Maintain a safe, clutter-free environment for the visually impaired or acromegalic patient. Reassure him that he'll probably recover his sight.
• Position patients who have undergone supratentorial or transsphenoidal hypophysectomy with the head of the bed elevated about 30 degrees, to promote venous drainage from the head and reduce cerebral edema.
• Place the patient on his side to allow drainage of secretions and prevent aspiration.

• Withhold oral fluids, which can cause vomiting and subsequent increased ICP. Don't allow a patient who has had transsphenoidal surgery to blow his nose. Watch for CSF drainage from the nose and for signs of infection from the contaminated upper respiratory tract.
• Inform the patient that he'll lose his sense of smell.
• Regularly compare the patient's postoperative neurologic status with your baseline assessment.
• Monitor intake and output to detect fluid and electrolyte imbalance.
• Before discharge, encourage the patient to wear a medical identification bracelet or necklace that identifies his hormone deficiencies and their proper treatment.

Laryngeal cancer

The most common form of laryngeal cancer is squamous cell carcinoma (95%); rare forms include adenocarcinoma, sarcoma, and others. Such cancer may be intrinsic or extrinsic. An intrinsic tumor is on the true vocal cord and does not have a tendency to spread because underlying connective tissues lack lymph nodes. An extrinsic tumor is on some other part of the larynx and tends to spread early. Laryngeal cancer is five times more common in males than in females; most victims are between ages 50 and 65.

Causes

In laryngeal cancer, major predisposing factors include smoking and alcoholism; minor factors include chronic inhalation of noxious fumes and familial tendency.
    Laryngeal cancer is classified according to its location:
• supraglottis (false vocal cords)
• glottis (true vocal cords)
• subglottis (downward extension from vocal cords [rare]).

Signs and symptoms

In intrinsic laryngeal cancer, the dominant and earliest symptom is hoarseness that persists longer than 3 weeks; in extrinsic cancer, it's a lump in the throat or pain or burning in the throat when drinking citrus juice or hot liquid. Later clinical effects of metastasis include dysphagia, dysp, cough, enlarged cervical lymph nodes, and pain radiating to the ear.

Diagnosis

Any hoarseness that lasts longer than 2 weeks requires visualization of the larynx by laryngoscopy.

Firm diagnosis also requires xeroradiography, biopsy, laryngeal tomography, computed tomography scan, or laryngography to define the borders of the lesion, and a chest X-ray to detect metastasis. (See *Staging laryngeal cancer,* page 30.)

Treatment

Early lesions are treated with laser surgery or radiation and advanced lesions with laser surgery, radiation, and chemotherapy. In early stages, laser surgery can excise precancerous lesions; in advanced stages, it can help relieve obstruction caused by tumor growth.

Surgical procedures vary with tumor size and can include cordectomy, partial or total laryngectomy, supraglottic laryngectomy, or total laryngectomy with laryngoplasty.

The treatment goal is to eliminate the cancer and preserve speech. If speech preservation isn't possible, speech rehabilitation may include esophageal speech or prosthetic devices; surgical techniques to construct a new voice box are still experimental.

Radiation and surgery may cause residual airway obstruction, loss of taste, or xerostomia.

Special considerations

• Provide psychological support and good preoperative and postoperative care to minimize complications and speed recovery.

Care before laryngectomy

• Instruct the patient to maintain good oral hygiene. If appropriate, instruct a male patient to shave off his beard.
• Encourage the patient to express his concerns before surgery. Help him choose a temporary nonspeaking communication method (such as writing).
• If appropriate, arrange for a laryngectomee to visit the patient. Explain postoperative procedures (suctioning, nasogastric [NG] tube feeding, and care of his laryngectomy tube) and their results (breathing through the neck, speech alteration).

geal cancer

The T stages cover supraglottic, glottic, and subglottic tumors.

Primary tumor
TX — primary tumor not assessable
T0 — no evidence of primary tumor
Tis — carcinoma in situ

Supraglottic tumor stages
T1 — tumor confined to one subsite in supraglottis; vocal cords retain motion
T2 — tumor extends to other sites in supraglottis or to glottis; vocal cords retain motion
T3 — tumor confined to larynx, but vocal cords lose motion; or tumor extends to the postcricoid area, the pyriform sinus, or the preepiglottic space, and vocal cords lose motion; or both
T4 — tumor extends through thyroid cartilage or extends to tissues beyond the larynx (such as the oropharynx or soft tissues of the neck), or both

Glottic tumor stages
T1 — tumor confined to vocal cords, which retain normal motion; may involve anterior or posterior commissural
T2 — tumor extends to supraglottis or subglottis or both; vocal cords may lose motion
T3 — tumor confined to larynx, but vocal cords lose motion
T4 — tumor extends through thyroid cartilage or extends to tissues beyond the larynx (such as the oropharynx or soft tissues of the neck), or both

Subglottic tumor stages
T1 — tumor confined to subglottis
T2 — tumor extends to vocal cords; vocal cords may lose motion
T3 — tumor confined to larynx with vocal cord fixation
T4 — tumor extends through cricoid or thyroid cartilage or extends to tissues beyond the larynx, or both

Regional lymph nodes
NX — regional lymph nodes can't be assessed
N0 — no evidence of regional lymph node metastasis
N1 — metastasis in a single ipsilateral lymph node, 3 cm or less in greatest dimension
N2 — metastasis in one or more ipsilateral lymph nodes, or in bilateral or contralateral nodes, larger than 3 cm but less than 6 cm in greatest dimension
N3 — metastasis in a node larger than 6 cm in greatest dimension

Distant metastasis
MX — distant metastasis not assessable
M0 — no evidence of distant metastasis
M1 — distant metastasis

Staging categories
Laryngeal cancer progresses from mild to severe as follows:
Stage 0 — Tis, N0, M0
Stage I — T1, N0, M0
Stage II — T2, N0, M0
Stage III — T3, N0, M0; T1, N1, M0; T2, N1, M0; T3, N1, M0
Stage IV — T4, N0 or N1, M0; any T, N2 or N3, M0; any T, any N, M1

• Also prepare the patient for other functional losses: He won't be able to smell, blow his nose, whistle, gargle, sip, or suck on a straw.

Care after partial laryngectomy

• Give I.V. fluids and, usually, tube feedings for the first 2 days postoperatively; then resume oral fluids.
• Keep the tracheostomy tube (inserted during surgery) in place until edema subsides.
• Keep the patient from using his voice until he has medical permission (usually 2 to 3 days postoperatively). Then caution him to whisper until healing is complete.

Care after total laryngectomy

• As soon as the patient returns to his bed, place him on his side and elevate his head 30 to 45 degrees. When you move him, remember to support his neck.
• The patient will probably have a laryngectomy tube in place until his stoma heals (about 7 to 10 days). This tube is shorter and thicker than a tracheostomy tube but requires the same care. Watch for crusting and secretions around the stoma, which can cause skin breakdown. To prevent crust formation, provide adequate room humidification. Remove crusting with petrolatum, antimicrobial ointment, and moist gauze.
• Teach stoma care.
• Watch for and report complications: fistula formation (redness, swelling, or secretions on the suture line), carotid artery rupture (bleeding), and tracheostomy stenosis (constant shortness of breath). A fistula may form between the reconstructed hypopharynx and the skin. This eventually heals spontaneously but may take weeks or months.
• Carotid artery rupture may occur in patients who have had preoperative radiation, particularly those with a fistula that constantly bathes the carotid artery with oral secretions. If carotid rupture occurs, apply pressure to the site; call for help immediately and take patient to the operating room for carotid ligation.
• Tracheostomy stenosis occurs weeks to months after laryngectomy; treatment includes fitting the patient with successively larger tracheostomy tubes until he can tolerate insertion of a large one. If the patient has a fistula, feed him through an NG tube; otherwise, food will leak through the fistula and delay healing.

• Monitor vital signs (be especially alert for fever, which indicates infection). Record fluid intake and output and watch for dehydration.

• Give frequent mouth care.

• Suction gently; do not attempt deep suctioning, which could penetrate the suture line. Suction through both the tube and the patient's nose because the patient can no longer blow air through his nose. Remember to suction his mouth gently.

• After insertion of a drainage catheter (usually connected to a blood drainage system or a GI drainage system), don't stop suctioning until drainage is minimal. After catheter removal, check dressings for drainage.

• Give analgesics as needed.

• If the patient has an NG feeding tube, check tube placement and elevate the patient's head to prevent aspiration.

• Reassure the patient that speech rehabilitation may help him speak again. Encourage contact with the International Association of Laryngectomees and other sources of support.

• Support the patient through some inevitable grieving. If the depression seems severe, consider making a psychiatric referral.

Thyroid cancer

Thyroid carcinoma occurs in all age-groups, especially in people who have had radiation treatment to the neck area. Papillary and follicular carcinomas are most common and are usually associated with prolonged survival. Papillary carcinoma accounts for half of all thyroid cancers in adults; it is most common in young adult females and metastasizes slowly. It is the least virulent form of thyroid cancer. Follicular carcinoma is less common than papillary carcinoma but more likely to recur and metastasize to the regional nodes and through blood vessels into the bones, liver, and lungs.

Medullary carcinoma originates in the parafollicular cells derived from the last branchial pouch and contains amyloid and calcium deposits. It can produce calcitonin, histaminase, corticotropin (producing Cushing's syndrome), and prostaglandins E_2 and F_3 (producing diarrhea). This rare form of thyroid cancer is familial, associated with pheochromocytoma, and completely curable when detected before it causes symptoms. Untreated, it progresses rapidly. Seldom curable by resection, giant cell and spindle cell cancer (anaplastic tumor) resists radiation and metastasizes rapidly.

Causes

Predisposing factors include radiation exposure, prolonged thyroid-stimulating hormone (TSH) stimulation (through radiation or heredity), familial predisposition, and chronic goiter.

Signs and symptoms

The primary signs of thyroid cancer are a painless nodule, a hard nodule in an enlarged thyroid gland, or palpable lymph nodes with thyroid enlargement. Eventually, the pressure of such a nodule or enlargement causes hoarseness, dysphagia, dyspnea, and pain on palpation.

If the tumor is large enough to destroy the gland, hypothyroidism follows, with its typical symptoms of low metabolism (mental apathy and sensitivity to cold). However, if the tumor stimulates excess thyroid hormone production, it induces symptoms of hyperthyroidism (sensitivity to heat, restlessness, and hyperactivity). Other clinical features include diarrhea, anorexia, irritability, vocal cord paralysis, and symptoms of distant metastasis.

Diagnosis

The first clue to thyroid cancer is usually an enlarged, palpable node in the thyroid gland, neck, lymph nodes of the neck, or vocal cords. A patient history of radiation therapy or a family history of thyroid cancer supports the diagnosis. However, tests must rule out nonmalignant thyroid enlargements, which are much more common.

Thyroid scan differentiates between functional nodes (rarely malignant) and hypofunctional nodes (commonly malignant) by measuring how readily nodules trap isotopes compared with the rest of the thyroid gland. In thyroid cancer, the scintiscan shows a "cold," nonfunctioning nodule.

Other tests include needle biopsy, computed tomography scan, ultrasonic scan, chest X-ray, and serum alkaline phosphatase and serum calcitonin assays to diagnose medullary cancer. Calcitonin assay is a reliable clue to silent

Staging thyroid cancer

The classification and staging systems adopted by the American Joint Committee on Cancer describe thyroid cancer according to the tumor's (T) size and extent at its origin, its invasion of regional (cervical and upper mediastinal) lymph nodes (N), and the disease's metastasis (M) to other structures.

Primary tumor
TX—primary tumor can't be assessed
T0—no evidence of primary tumor
T1—tumor 1 cm or less in greatest dimension and limited to the thyroid
T2—tumor more than 1 cm but less than 4 cm in greatest dimension and limited to the thyroid
T3—tumor more than 4 cm and limited to the thyroid
T4—tumor of any size that extends beyond the thyroid

Regional lymph nodes
NX—regional lymph nodes can't be assessed
N0—no evidence of regional lymph node metastasis
N1—regional lymph node metastasis
N1a—metastasis in ipsilateral cervical nodes
N1b—metastasis in bilateral, midline, or contralateral cervical or mediastinal lymph nodes

Distant metastasis
MX—distant metastasis can't be assessed
M0—no evidence of distant metastasis
M1—distant metastasis

Staging categories for papillary or follicular cancer
Papillary or follicular cancer progresses from mild to severe as follows:
Stage I—any T, any N, M0 (patient under age 45); T1, N0, M0 (patient age 45 or over)
Stage II—any T, any N, M1 (patient under age 45); T2, N0, M0; T3, N0, M0 (patient age 45 or over)
Stage III—T4, N0, M0; any T, N1, M0 (patient age 45 or over)
Stage IV—any T, any N, M1 (patient age 45 or over)

Staging categories for medullary cancer
Medullary cancer progresses from mild to severe as follows:
Stage I—T1, N0, M0
Stage II—T2, N0, M0; T3, N0, M0; T4, N0, M0
Stage III—any T, N1, M0
Stage IV—any T, any N, M1

Staging categories for undifferentiated cancer
All cases are Stage IV.
Stage IV—any T, any N, any M

---

medullary carcinoma. (For more information, see *Staging thyroid cancer.*)

Treatment

• Total or subtotal thyroidectomy, with modified node dissection (bilateral or unilateral) on the side of the primary cancer (papillary or follicular cancer)

• Total thyroidectomy and radical neck excision (for medullary or giant cell and spindle cell cancer)
• Radiation (^{131}I), with external radiation (for inoperable cancer and sometimes postoperatively in lieu of radical neck excision) or alone (for metastasis)
• Adjunctive thyroid suppression, with exogenous thyroid hormones suppressing TSH production, and simultaneous administration of an adrenergic blocking agent, such as propranolol, increasing tolerance to surgery and radiation
• Chemotherapy for symptomatic, widespread metastasis is limited but doxorubicin is sometimes beneficial.

Special considerations

• Before surgery, tell the patient to expect temporary voice loss or hoarseness lasting several days after surgery.
• After surgery when the patient regains consciousness, keep him in semi-Fowler's position, with his head neither hyperextended nor flexed, to avoid pressure on the suture line. Support his head and neck with sandbags and pillows; when you move him, continue this support with your hands.
• After monitoring vital signs, check the patient's dressing, neck, and back for bleeding. If he complains that the dressing feels tight, loosen it and call the doctor immediately.
• Check serum calcium levels daily; hypocalcemia may develop if parathyroid glands are removed.
• Watch for and report other complications: hemorrhage and shock (elevated pulse rate and hypotension), tetany (carpopedal spasm, twitching, and seizures), thyroid storm (high fever, severe tachycardia, delirium, dehydration, and extreme irritability), and respiratory obstruction (dyspnea, crowing respirations, retraction of neck tissues).
• Keep a tracheotomy set and oxygen equipment handy in case of respiratory obstruction. Use continuous steam inhalation in the patient's room until his chest is clear.
• The patient may need I.V. fluids or a soft diet, but many patients can tolerate a regular diet within 24 hours of surgery.
• After extensive tumor and lymph node surgery, provide care in the same way that you would after other radical neck surgery.

Spinal neoplasms

Spinal neoplasms may be any one of many tumor types similar to intracranial tumors; they involve the cord or its roots and, if untreated, can eventually cause paralysis. As primary tumors, they originate in the meningeal coverings, the parenchyma of the cord or its roots, the intraspinal vasculature, or the vertebrae. They can also occur as metastatic foci from primary tumors.

Causes

Primary tumors of the spinal cord may be extramedullary (occurring outside the spinal cord) or intramedullary (occurring within the cord itself). Extramedullary tumors may be intramural (meningiomas and schwannomas), which account for 60% of all primary spinal cord neoplasms; or extramural (metastatic tumors from breasts, lungs, prostate, leukemia, or lymphomas), which account for 25% of these neoplasms.

Intramedullary tumors, or gliomas (astrocytomas or ependymomas), are comparatively rare, accounting for only about 10%; in children, they're low-grade astrocytomas.

Spinal cord tumors are rare compared with intracranial tumors (a ratio of 1:4). They occur with equal frequency in both men and women, with the exception of meningiomas, which occur most often in women. Spinal cord tumors can occur anywhere along the length of the cord or its roots.

Signs and symptoms

Extramedullary tumors produce symptoms by pressing on nerve roots, the spinal cord, and spinal vessels; intramedullary tumors, by destroying the parenchyma and compressing adjacent areas. Because intramedullary tumors may extend over several spinal cord segments, their symptoms are more variable than those of extramedullary tumors.

The following clinical effects are likely with all spinal cord neoplasms:

• Pain—Most severe directly over the tumor, radiates around the trunk or down the limb on the affected side, and is unrelieved by bed rest

• Motor symptoms—Asymmetrical spastic muscle weakness, decreased muscle tone, exaggerated reflexes, and a positive

Babinski's sign. If the tumor is at the level of the cauda equina, muscle flaccidity, muscle wasting, weakness, and progressive diminution in tendon reflexes are characteristic.

• Sensory deficits – Contralateral loss of pain, temperature, and touch sensation (Brown-Séquard syndrome). These losses are less obvious to the patient than functional motor changes. Caudal lesions invariably produce paresthesia in the nerve distribution pathway of the involved roots.

• Bladder symptoms – Urine retention is an inevitable late sign with cord compression. Early signs include incomplete emptying or difficulty with the urinary stream, which is usually unnoticed or ignored. Cauda equina tumors cause bladder and bowel incontinence due to flaccid paralysis.

• Constipation.

Diagnosis

• *Lumbar puncture* shows clear yellow cerebrospinal fluid (CSF) as a result of increased protein levels if the flow is completely blocked. If the flow is partially blocked, protein levels rise, but the fluid is only slightly yellow in proportion to the CSF protein level. A Papanicolaou test of the CSF may show malignant cells of metastatic carcinoma.

• *X-rays* show distortions of the intervertebral foramina, changes in the vertebrae or collapsed areas in the vertebral body, and localized enlargement of the spinal canal, indicating an adjacent block.

• *Myelography* identifies the level of the lesion by outlining it if the tumor is causing partial obstruction; it shows anatomic relationship to the cord and the dura. If obstruction is complete, the injected dye can't flow past the tumor. (This study is dangerous if cord compression is nearly complete, because withdrawal or escape of CSF will actually allow the tumor to exert greater pressure against the cord.)

• *Radioisotope bone scan* demonstrates metastatic invasion of the vertebrae by showing a characteristic increase in osteoblastic activity.

• *Computed tomography scan* and *magnetic resonance imaging* show cord compression and tumor location.

• *Frozen section biopsy* at surgery identifies the tissue type.

Treatment

Generally, treatment of spinal cord tumors includes decompression or radiation. Laminectomy is indicated for primary tumors that produce spinal cord or cauda equina compression; it's *not* usually indicated for metastatic tumors.

If the tumor is slowly progressive, or if it's treated before the cord degenerates from compression, symptoms are likely to disappear, and complete restoration of function is possible. In a patient with metastatic carcinoma or lymphoma who suddenly experiences complete transverse myelitis with spinal shock, functional improvement is unlikely, even with treatment, and his outlook is ominous.

If the patient has incomplete paraplegia of rapid onset, emergency surgical decompression may save cord function. Steroid therapy minimizes cord edema until surgery can be performed.

Partial removal of intramedullary gliomas, followed by radiation, may temporarily ease symptoms. Metastatic extramural tumors can be controlled with radiation, analgesics, and, in the case of hormone-mediated tumors (breast and prostate), appropriate hormonal therapy.

Transcutaneous electrical nerve stimulation (TENS) may control radicular pain from spinal cord tumors and is an alternative to opiate analgesics. In TENS, an electrical charge applied to the skin stimulates large-diameter nerve fibers and inhibits transmission of pain impulses through small-diameter nerve fibers.

Special considerations

• When caring for patients with spinal cord tumors, emphasize emotional support and skilled intervention during acute and chronic phases, early recognition of recurrence, prevention and treatment of complications, and maintenance of quality of life.

• On your first contact with the patient, you should perform a complete neurologic evaluation to obtain baseline data for planning future care and evaluating changes in his clinical status.

• Care for the patient with a spinal cord tumor is basically the same as that for the patient with spinal cord injury and requires psychological support, rehabilitation (including bowel and bladder retraining), and prevention of infection and skin breakdown.

• After laminectomy, care includes checking neurologic status frequently, changing position by logrolling, administering

analgesics, monitoring frequently for infection, and aiding in early walking.
• Help the patient and his family to understand and cope with the diagnosis, treatment, potential disabilities, and necessary changes in lifestyle.
• Take safety precautions for the patient with impaired sensation and motor deficits. Use side rails if the patient is bedridden; if he's not, encourage him to wear flat shoes, and remove scatter rugs and clutter to prevent falls.
• Encourage the patient to be independent in performing daily activities. Avoid aggravating pain by moving the patient slowly and by making sure his body is well aligned when giving personal care. Advise him to use TENS to block radicular pain.
• Administer steroids and antacids for cord edema after radiation therapy. Monitor for sensory or motor dysfunction, which indicates the need for more steroids.
• Enforce bed rest for the patient with vertebral body involvement until he can safely walk, because body weight alone can cause cord collapse and cord laceration from bone fragments.
• Logroll and position the patient on his side every 2 hours to prevent pressure ulcers and other complications of immobility.
• If the patient is to wear a back brace, make sure he does wear it whenever he gets out of bed.

Self-test questions

You can quickly review your comprehension of this chapter on head, neck, and spinal neoplasms by answering the following questions. The answers to these questions and their rationales appear on pages 186 to 188.

Case history questions

Linda Frank, a 23-year-old patient with no known neurologic condition, experiences a seizure at work and is rushed to the hospital. During the examination, the patient states that she has experienced severe headaches at the base of her skull with increasing frequency but attributed the headaches to stress. She also mentions that her ability to see clearly has decreased over the past several weeks. She den-

ies any other abnormal neurologic signs and symptoms. Papilledema is noted during the ophthalmic portion of the physical examination. Suspecting a brain tumor, the doctor orders an extensive diagnostic workup. Test results confirm the presence of a brain tumor.

1. Generally, signs of a brain tumor result from which of the following pathological changes?
   a. Progressive loss of protein in cerebral spinal fluid
   b. Increased intracranial pressure
   c. Compression of a vertebral artery
   d. Destruction of a pyramidal tract

2. Biopsy reveals the tumor to be an oligodendroglioma. Which of the following statements is true regarding oligodendrogliomas?
   a. It's a slow-growing tumor.
   b. It's the second most common malignant glioma.
   c. It occurs more commonly in men.
   d. It primarily occurs in young adults.

Jim Jackson has a 30-year history of smoking and seeks medical attention for persistent hoarseness. Mr. Jackson informs the doctor that the hoarseness has been present more than 6 weeks. No other abnormalities are noted during the examination. The doctor orders a laryngoscopy, which reveals a laryngeal lesion. A biopsy reveals the lesion to be malignant.

3. Laryngeal cancer is classified by:
   a. cell type.
   b. severity of symptoms.
   c. location of the tumor.
   d. size of the tumor.

4. The patient is scheduled for a partial laryngectomy. How long after surgery must he wait before he can speak?
   a. 6 to 8 hours
   b. 12 to 18 hours
   c. 24 to 36 hours
   d. 48 to 72 hours

Sue McGuire, a 32-year-old mother, seeks medical attention after discovering a painless but hard nodule on the left side of her neck. She denies experiencing hoarseness, dysphagia, dyspnea, or pain on palpation. However, she does report increasing bouts of fatigue and cold sensitivity as well as an overall sluggish feeling. A comprehensive history and physical examination accompanied by a complete diagnostic workup reveal thyroid cancer.

5. Which of the following forms of thyroid cancer is the least virulent?
   a. Papillary carcinoma
   b. Follicular carcinoma
   c. Medullary carcinoma
   d. Spindle cell carcinoma

6. When obtaining a medical history from a patient with a neck nodule, what predisposing factor associated with thyroid cancer should you note?
   a. Presence of subacute granulomatous thyroiditis
   b. Age over 65
   c. Past history of radiation exposure
   d. Excessive intake of iodized salt

Additional questions

7. Which neurologic symptom does a patient with a pituitary tumor typically report?
   a. Frontal headache
   b. Hearing loss
   c. Balance instability
   d. Taste impairment

8. Which of the following functions will the patient undergoing transsphenoidal surgery lose permanently?
   a. Bladder control
   b. Bowel control
   c. Sense of smell
   d. Night vision

9. Most spinal cord neoplasms occur with equal frequency in both men and women. Which of the following spinal cord neoplasms occurs most often in women?
  a. Schwannomas
  b. Meningiomas
  c. Astrocytomas
  d. Ependymomas

10. If a spinal cord tumor completely blocks cerebrospinal fluid (CSF) flow, which abnormality will become apparent when a spinal tap is performed?
  a. CSF can't be aspirated.
  b. CSF will appear clear yellow.
  c. CSF will appear cloudy.
  d. CSF pressure will not be measurable.

CHAPTER 3

Thoracic Neoplasms

The lungs and breasts are the most common sites for thoracic cancer. Soft-tissue sarcomas, although rare, may also develop in the chest region.

Lung cancer

Typically, lung cancer develops within the wall or epithelia of the bronchial tree. Its most common types are epidermoid (squamous cell) carcinoma, small-cell (oat cell) carcinoma, adenocarcinoma, and large-cell (anaplastic) carcinoma. Although the prognosis is usually poor, it varies with the extent of spread at the time of diagnosis and the cell-type growth rate. Only 13% of patients with lung cancer survive 5 years after diagnosis. Lung cancer is the most common cause of cancer death in men and is fast becoming the most common cause in women, even though it's largely preventable. (See *Distribution of the six most common cancer sites,* page 44.)

Causes

Most experts agree that lung cancer results from inhalation of carcinogenic pollutants by a susceptible host. Who, though, is most susceptible? Any smoker over age 40, especially if he began to smoke before age 15, has smoked a whole pack or more per day for 20 years, or works with or near asbestos.

Pollutants in tobacco smoke cause progressive lung cell degeneration. Lung cancer is 10 times more common in smokers than in nonsmokers; indeed, 80% of lung cancer patients are smokers. Cancer risk is determined by the num-

Distribution of the six most common cancer sites

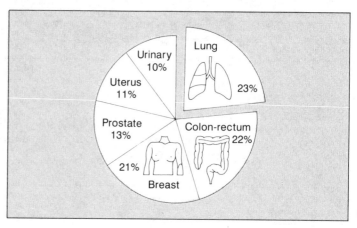

ber of cigarettes smoked daily, the depth of inhalation, how early in life smoking began, and the nicotine content of cigarettes. Two other factors also increase susceptibility: exposure to carcinogenic industrial and air pollutants (asbestos, uranium, arsenic, nickel, iron oxides, chromium, radioactive dust, and coal dust), and familial susceptibility.

Signs and symptoms

Because early-stage lung cancer usually produces no symptoms, this disease is often advanced at diagnosis. The following late-stage symptoms often lead to diagnosis:
• With epidermoid and small-cell carcinomas – smoker's cough, hoarseness, wheezing, dyspnea, hemoptysis, and chest pain
• With adenocarcinoma and large-cell carcinoma – fever, weakness, weight loss, anorexia, and shoulder pain.
   Besides their obvious interference with respiratory function, lung tumors may also alter the production of hormones that regulate body function or homeostasis. Clinical conditions that result from such changes are known as hormonal paraneoplastic syndromes:
• With large-cell carcinoma – gynecomastia.
• With large-cell carcinoma and adenocarcinoma – hypertrophic pulmonary osteoarthropathy (bone and joint pain

from cartilage erosion due to abnormal production of growth hormone).
• With small-cell carcinoma – Cushing's and carcinoid syndromes.
• With epidermoid tumors – hypercalcemia.

Metastatic symptoms vary greatly, depending on the effect of tumors on intrathoracic and distant structures:
• bronchial obstruction (hemoptysis, atelectasis, pneumonitis, dyspnea)
• recurrent nerve invasion (hoarseness, vocal cord paralysis)
• chest wall invasion (piercing chest pain, increasing dyspnea, severe shoulder pain radiating down arm)
• local lymphatic spread (cough, hemoptysis, stridor, pleural effusion)
• phrenic nerve involvement (dyspnea, shoulder pain, and unilateral paralyzed diaphragm with paradoxical motion)
• esophageal compression (dysphagia)
• vena caval obstruction (venous distention and edema of face, neck, chest, and back)
• pericardial involvement (pericardial effusion, tamponade, arrhythmia)
• cervical thoracic sympathetic nerve involvement (miosis, ptosis, exophthalmos, reduced sweating).

Distant metastasis may involve any part of the body, most commonly the central nervous system, liver, and bone.

Diagnosis

Typical clinical findings may strongly suggest lung cancer, but firm identification requires further evidence from the following:
• *Chest X-ray* usually shows an advanced lesion, but it can detect a lesion up to 2 years before symptoms appear. It also indicates tumor size and location. (See *Staging lung cancer,* page 46.)
• *Sputum cytology,* which is 75% reliable, requires a specimen coughed up from the lungs and tracheobronchial tree, not from postnasal secretions or saliva.
• *Computed tomography (CT) scan* of the chest may help to delineate the tumor's size and its relationship to surrounding structures.
• *Bronchoscopy* can locate the tumor site. Bronchoscopic washings provide material for cytologic and histologic ex-

Staging lung cancer

Using the TNM (*tumor, node, metastasis*) classification system, the American Joint Committee on Cancer stages lung cancer as follows:

Primary tumor
TX—primary tumor can't be assessed, or malignant tumor cells detected in sputum or bronchial washings but undetected by X-ray or bronchoscopy
T0—no evidence of primary tumor
Tis—carcinoma in situ
T1—tumor 3 cm or less in greatest dimension, surrounded by normal lung or visceral pleura; no bronchoscopic evidence of cancer closer to the center of the body than the lobar bronchus
T2—tumor larger than 3 cm; or one that involves the main bronchus and is 2 cm or more from the carina; or one that invades the visceral pleura; or one that's accompanied by atelectasis or obstructive pneumonitis that extends to the hilar region but doesn't involve the entire lung
T3—tumor of any size that extends into neighboring structures, such as the chest wall, diaphragm, or mediastinal pleura; or tumor in the main bronchus that doesn't involve but is less than 2 cm from the carina; or tumor that's accompanied by atelectasis or obstructive pneumonitis of the entire lung
T4—tumor of any size that invades the mediastinum, heart, great vessels, trachea, esophagus, vertebral body, or carina; or tumor with malignant pleural effusion

Regional lymph nodes
NX—regional lymph nodes can't be assessed
N0—no detectable metastasis to lymph nodes
N1—metastasis to the ipsilateral peribronchial or hilar lymph nodes or both
N2—metastasis to the ipsilateral mediastinal and the subcarinal lymph nodes or both
N3—metastasis to the contralateral mediastinal or hilar lymph nodes, the ipsilateral or contralateral scalene nodes, or the supraclavicular lymph nodes

Distant metastasis
MX—distant metastasis can't be assessed
M0—no evidence of distant metastasis
M1—distant metastasis

Staging categories
Lung cancer progresses from mild to severe as follows:
Occult carcinoma—TX, N0, M0
Stage 0—Tis, N0, M0
Stage I—T1, N0, M0; T2, N0, M0
Stage II—T1, N1, M0; T2, N1, M0
Stage IIIA—T1, N2, M0; T2, N2, M0; T3, N0, M0; T3, N1, M0; T3, N2, M0
Stage IIIB—any T, N3, M0; T4, any N, M0
Stage IV—any T, any N, M1

amination. The flexible fiber-optic bronchoscope increases test effectiveness.
• *Needle biopsy* of the lungs uses biplanar fluoroscopic visual control to detect peripherally located tumors. This allows firm diagnosis in 80% of patients.

• *Tissue biopsy* of accessible metastatic sites includes supraclavicular and mediastinal node and pleural biopsy.

• *Thoracentesis* allows chemical and cytologic examination of pleural fluid.

Additional studies include preoperative mediastinoscopy or mediastinotomy to rule out involvement of mediastinal lymph nodes (which would preclude curative pulmonary resection).

Other tests to detect metastasis include bone scan, bone marrow biopsy (recommended in small-cell carcinoma), and CT scan of the brain or abdomen.

After histologic confirmation, staging determines the extent of the disease and helps in planning treatment and predicting prognosis.

Treatment

Recent treatment—which consists of combinations of surgery, radiation, and chemotherapy—may improve prognosis and prolong survival. Nevertheless, because treatment usually begins at an advanced stage, it is largely palliative.

Surgery is the primary treatment for stage I, stage II, or selected stage III squamous cell carcinoma, adenocarcinoma, and large-cell carcinoma, unless the tumor is nonresectable or other conditions (such as cardiac disease) rule out surgery. Surgery may include partial removal of a lung (wedge resection, segmental resection, lobectomy, or radical lobectomy) or total removal (pneumonectomy, or radical pneumonectomy).

Preoperative radiation therapy may reduce tumor bulk to allow for surgical resection. Preradiation chemotherapy helps improve response rates. Radiation therapy is ordinarily recommended for stage I and stage II lesions, if surgery is contraindicated, and for stage III lesions when the disease is confined to the involved hemithorax and the ipsilateral supraclavicular lymph nodes.

Generally, radiation therapy is delayed until 1 month after surgery, to allow the wound to heal, and is then directed to the part of the chest most likely to develop metastasis. High-dose radiation therapy or radiation implants may also be used.

Chemotherapy combinations of fluorouracil, vincristine, mitomycin, cisplatin, and vindesine produce a response rate of about 40% but have a minimal effect on overall survival.

Promising combinations for treating small-cell carcinomas include cyclophosphamide with doxorubicin and vincristine; cyclophosphamide with doxorubicin, vincristine, and etoposide; and etoposide with cisplatin, cyclophosphamide, and doxorubicin. Clinical trials are currently in progress using taxol.

In laser therapy, still largely experimental, laser energy is directed through a bronchoscope to destroy local tumors.

Special considerations

• Provide comprehensive supportive care and patient teaching to minimize complications and speed recovery from surgery, radiation, and chemotherapy.

Care before thoracic surgery

• Supplement and reinforce the information given to the patient by the health care team about the disease and the surgical procedure.
• Explain expected postoperative procedures, such as insertion of an indwelling catheter, use of an endotracheal tube or chest tube (or both), dressing changes, and I.V. therapy.
• To avoid as many complications after surgery as possible, teach the patient how to perform coughing, deep diaphragmatic breathing, and range-of-motion (ROM) exercises.
• Reassure the patient that analgesics will be provided and proper positioning will be implemented to control postoperative pain.
• Inform the patient that he may take nothing by mouth after midnight the night before surgery, that he will shower with a soaplike antibacterial agent the night or morning before surgery, and that he'll be given preoperative medications, such as a sedative and an anticholinergic to dry secretions.

Care after thoracic surgery

• Maintain a patent airway, and monitor chest tubes to reestablish normal intrathoracic pressure and prevent postoperative and pulmonary complications.
• Check vital signs every 15 minutes during the first hour after surgery, every 30 minutes during the next 4 hours, and then every 2 hours. Watch for abnormal respiration and other changes.
• Suction the patient often, and encourage him to begin deep breathing and coughing as soon as possible.

• Check secretions often. Initially, sputum will be thick and dark with blood, but it should become thinner and grayish-yellow within a day.

• Monitor and record closed chest drainage. Keep chest tubes patent and draining effectively. Fluctuation in the water seal chamber on inspiration and expiration indicates that the chest tube is patent. Watch for air leaks. Either the chest tube or the drainage system may need replacement.

• Position the patient on the surgical side to promote drainage and lung reexpansion.

• Watch for foul-smelling discharge and excessive drainage on dressing. Usually, the dressing is removed after 24 hours, unless the wound appears infected.

• Monitor intake and output. Maintain adequate hydration.

• Watch for and treat infection, shock, hemorrhage, atelectasis, dyspnea, mediastinal shift, and pulmonary embolus.

• To prevent pulmonary embolus, apply antiembolism stockings and encourage ROM exercises.

Care during chemotherapy and radiation

• Explain possible adverse effects of radiation and chemotherapy. Watch for, treat, and, when possible, try to prevent them.

• Ask the dietary department to provide soft, nonirritating foods that are high in protein, and encourage the patient to eat high-calorie between-meal snacks.

• Give antiemetics and antidiarrheals as needed.

• Schedule patient care activities in a way that helps the patient conserve his energy.

• During radiation therapy, administer skin care to minimize skin breakdown. If the patient receives radiation therapy in an outpatient setting, warn him to avoid tight clothing, exposure to the sun, and harsh ointments on his chest.

• Teach the patient exercises to help prevent shoulder stiffness.

• Educate high-risk patients in ways to reduce their chances of developing lung cancer.

• Refer smokers who want to quit to local branches of the American Cancer Society and Smokenders, or suggest group therapy, individual counseling, or hypnosis.

• Encourage patients with recurring or chronic respiratory infections and those with chronic lung disease who detect any change in the character of a cough to see their doctor promptly for evaluation.

Breast cancer

The most common type of cancer affecting women, breast cancer is the number two killer (after lung cancer) of women ages 35 to 54. It occurs in men, but rarely. The 5-year survival rate has improved from 53% in the 1940s to 70% in the 1980s because of earlier diagnosis and the variety of treatment modes now available. The death rate, however, has not changed in the past 50 years.

Lymph node involvement is the most valuable prognostic predictor. With adjuvant therapy, 70% to 75% of women with negative nodes will survive 10 years or more, as compared with 20% to 25% of women with positive nodes.

Although breast cancer may develop any time after puberty, it's most common after age 50.

Causes

The cause of breast cancer isn't known, but its high incidence in women implicates estrogen. Certain predisposing factors are clear; women at *high risk* include those who:
• have a family history of breast cancer.
• have long menstrual cycles or began menses early or menopause late.
• have never been pregnant.
• were first pregnant after age 31.
• have had unilateral breast cancer.
• have endometrial or ovarian cancer.
• were exposed to low-level ionizing radiation.

Many other possible predisposing factors have been investigated, including estrogen therapy, antihypertensives, high-fat diet, obesity, and fibrocystic disease of the breasts.

Women at *lower risk* include those who:
• were pregnant before age 20.
• had multiple pregnancies.
• are Indian or Asian.

Pathophysiology

Breast cancer occurs more often in the left breast than the right, and more often in the upper outer quadrant. Growth rates vary. Theoretically, slow-growing breast cancer may take up to 8 years to become palpable at ⅜″ (1 cm) in size. It spreads by way of the lymphatic system and the bloodstream, through the right heart to the lungs, and eventually to the other breast, the chest wall, liver, bone, and brain.

Many refer to the estimated growth rate of breast cancer as "doubling time," or the time it takes the malignant cells to double in number. Estimated survival time for breast cancer is based on tumor size and spread; the number of involved nodes is the single most important factor in predicting survival time.

Classified by histologic appearance and location of the lesion, breast cancer may be:
• adenocarcinoma – arising from the epithelia
• intraductal – developing within the ducts (includes Paget's disease)
• infiltrating – occurring in parenchymal tissue of the breast
• inflammatory (rare) – reflecting rapid tumor growth, in which the overlying skin becomes edematous, inflamed, and indurated
• lobular carcinoma in situ – reflecting tumor growth involving lobes of glandular tissue
• medullary or circumscribed – large tumor with rapid growth rate.

These histologic classifications should be coupled with a staging or nodal status classification system for a clearer understanding of the extent of the cancer. The most commonly used system for staging cancer, both before and after surgery, is the TNM (*tumor-node-metastasis*) system. (See *Staging breast cancer*, page 52.)

Signs and symptoms

Warning signals of possible breast cancer include:
• a lump or mass in the breast (about 25% are malignant)
• change in symmetry or size of the breast
• change in skin, thickening, scaly skin around the nipple, dimpling, edema (peau d'orange), or ulceration
• change in skin temperature (a warm, hot, or pink area; suspect cancer in a nonlactating woman past childbearing age until proven otherwise)
• unusual drainage or discharge
• change in the nipple, such as itching, burning, or erosion
• pain (not usually a symptom of breast cancer unless the tumor is advanced, but it should be investigated)
• bone metastasis, pathologic bone fractures, and hypercalcemia
• edema of the arm.

Staging breast cancer

Cancer staging helps form a prognosis and a treatment plan. For breast cancer, most clinicians use the TNM (*tumor, node, metastasis*) system developed by the American Joint Committee on Cancer.

Primary tumor
TX—primary tumor can't be assessed
T0—no evidence of primary tumor
Tis—carcinoma in situ: intraductal carcinoma, lobular carcinoma in situ, or Paget's disease of the nipple with no tumor
T1—tumor 2 cm or less in greatest dimension
T1a—tumor 0.5 cm or less in greatest dimension
T1b—tumor more than 0.5 cm but not more than 1 cm in greatest dimension
T1c—tumor more than 1 cm but not more than 2 cm in greatest dimension
T2—tumor more than 2 cm but not more than 5 cm in greatest dimension
T3—tumor more than 5 cm in greatest dimension
T4—tumor of any size that extends to the chest wall or skin
T4a—tumor extends to the chest wall
T4b—tumor accompanied by edema (including peau d'orange), ulcerated breast skin, or satellite skin nodules on the same breast
T4c—both T4a and T4b
T4d—inflammatory carcinoma

Regional lymph nodes
NX—regional lymph nodes can't be assessed
N0—no evidence of nodal involvement
N1—movable ipsilateral axillary nodal involvement
N2—ipsilateral axillary nodal involvement with nodes fixed to one another or to other structures
N3—ipsilateral internal mammary nodal involvement

Distant metastasis
MX—distant metastasis can't be assessed
M0—no evidence of distant metastasis
M1—distant metastasis (including metastasis to ipsilateral supraclavicular nodes)

Staging categories
Breast cancer progresses from mild to severe as follows:
Stage 0—Tis, N0, M0
Stage I—T1, N0, M0
Stage IIA—T0, N1, M0; T1, N1, M0; T2, N0, M0
Stage IIB—T2, N1, M0; T3, N0, M0
Stage IIIA—T0, N2, M0; T1, N2, M0; T2, N2, M0; T3, N1 or N2, M0
Stage IIIB—T4, any N, M0; any T, N3, M0
Stage IV—any T, any N, M1

Diagnosis

The most reliable method of detecting breast cancer is the regular breast self-examination, followed by immediate evaluation of any abnormality. Other diagnostic measures include mammography, needle biopsy, and surgical biopsy.

Mammography is indicated for any woman whose physical examination might suggest breast cancer. It should be done as a baseline on women between ages 35 and 39; every 1 to 2 years for women ages 40 to 49; and annually on women who are over age 50, who have a family history of breast cancer, or who have had unilateral breast cancer, to check for new disease. However, the value of mammography is questionable for women under age 35 (because of the density of the breasts), except those who are strongly suspected of having breast cancer.

False-negative results can occur in as many as 30% of all tests for breast cancer. Consequently, with a suspicious mass, a negative mammogram is disregarded, and a fine-needle aspiration or surgical biopsy is done. Ultrasonography, which can distinguish a fluid-filled cyst from a tumor, can also be used instead of an invasive surgical biopsy.

A bone scan, a computed tomography scan, measurement of alkaline phosphatase levels, liver function studies, and a liver biopsy can detect distant metastasis. A hormonal receptor assay done on the tumor can determine if the tumor is estrogen- or progesterone-dependent. (This test guides decisions to use therapy that blocks the action of the estrogen hormone that supports tumor growth.)

Treatment

Therapy should take into consideration the stage of the disease, the woman's age and menopausal status, and the disfiguring effects of the surgery. Treatment may include one or any combination of lumpectomy, radical mastectomy, chemotherapy, radiation, and hormonal therapy.

• Lumpectomy also aids in determining tumor cell type. It is often done on an outpatient basis and is the only surgery some patients require, especially those with a small tumor and no evidence of maxillary node involvement. Radiation therapy is typically combined with this surgery.

A two-stage procedure, in which the surgeon removes the lump, confirms that it's malignant, and discusses treatment options, allows the patient to participate in her treatment plan. If the tumor is diagnosed as malignant, such planning may be done before surgery. In lumpectomy and dissection of the maxillary lymph nodes, the tumor and the maxillary lymph nodes are removed, leaving the breast intact.

• A simple mastectomy removes the breast but not the lymph nodes or pectoral muscles. Modified radical mastectomy removes the breast and the maxillary lymph nodes. Radical mastectomy (performed less often) removes the breast, pectoralis major and minor, and the maxillary lymph nodes. Reconstructive surgery can create a breast mound if the patient doesn't have evidence of advanced disease.

• Chemotherapy is used either as adjuvant or primary therapy, depending on several factors, including TNM staging and estrogen receptor status. The most commonly used antineoplastic drugs are cyclophosphamide, fluorouracil, methotrexate, doxorubicin, vincristine, taxol, and prednisone. A common drug combination is cyclophosphamide, methotrexate, and fluorouracil, which is used in both premenopausal and postmenopausal women.

Tamoxifen, an estrogen antagonist, is the adjuvant treatment of choice for postmenopausal patients with positive estrogen receptor status.

• Peripheral stem cell therapy may be used for advanced breast cancer.

• Primary radiation therapy *before or after* tumor removal is effective for small tumors in early stages with no evidence of distant metastasis; it's also used to prevent or treat local recurrence. Presurgical radiation to the breast helps "sterilize" the field, making a tumor in inflammatory breast cancer more surgically manageable.

• Breast cancer patients may also receive estrogen, progesterone, androgen, or antiandrogen aminoglutethimide therapy. The success of these drug therapies, along with growing evidence that breast cancer is a systemic, not local, disease, has led to a decline in ablative surgery.

Special considerations

• To provide good care for a breast cancer patient, begin with a history, assess the patient's feelings about her illness, and determine what she knows about it and what she expects.

Preoperative care

• If a mastectomy is scheduled, in addition to the routine preoperative preparation (for example, skin preparations and not allowing the patient anything by mouth), teach the patient how to deep-breathe and cough to prevent pulmonary complications and how to rotate her ankles to help prevent thromboembolism.

Postoperative arm and hand care

Hand exercises for the patient who is prone to lymphedema can begin on the day of surgery. Plan arm exercises to anticipate potential problems with the suture line. The following are some precautions to help avoid lymphedema:
• Have the patient open her hand and close it tightly six to eight times every 3 hours while she's awake.
• Elevate the arm on the affected side on a pillow above the heart level.
• Encourage the patient to wash her face and comb her hair; these are effective exercises.

• Measure and record the circumference of the patient's arm 2″ (5 cm) above her elbow. Indicate the exact place you measured. By remeasuring a month after surgery, and at intervals during and following radiation therapy, you will be able to determine whether lymphedema is present. The patient may complain that her arm is heavy—an early sign of lymphedema.
• Instruct the patient that when she gets home, she can elevate her arm and hand by supporting them on the back of a chair or a couch.

• Tell the patient she can ease her pain by lying on the affected side, or by placing a hand or pillow on the incision. Preoperatively, show her where the incision will be made.
• Inform the patient that she'll receive medication to relieve pain. Adequate pain relief encourages coughing and turning and promotes general well-being. Positioning a small pillow anteriorly under the patient's arm provides comfort.
• Encourage the patient to get out of bed as soon as the anesthesia wears off or the first evening after surgery.
• Explain that after mastectomy, an incisional drain or suction device (Hemovac) will be used to remove accumulated serosanguineous fluid and to decrease tension on the suture line, thereby promoting healing.
• Teach the patient how to prevent lymphedema of the arm, an early complication of any breast cancer treatment that involves lymph node dissection. (See *Postoperative arm and hand care.*)

Postoperative care

• Inspect the dressing anteriorly and posteriorly; check for bleeding. Measure and record the amount and note the color of drainage. Expect drainage to be bloody during the first 4 hours and afterward to become serous.
• Check circulatory status (blood pressure, pulse, respirations, and bleeding).

• Monitor intake and output for at least 48 hours after general anesthesia.

• Inspect the incision. Encourage the patient to look at her incision, perhaps when the first dressing is removed.

• Help the patient prevent lymphedema. Tell her to exercise her hand and arm on the affected side regularly and to avoid activities that might cause infection in this hand or arm. Infection increases the chance of developing lymphedema. Prevention is important because lymphedema can't be treated effectively.

• Advise the patient to ask her doctor about reconstructive surgery or to call the local or state medical society for the names of plastic reconstructive surgeons who regularly perform surgery to create breast mounds.

• Inform the patient that the American Cancer Society's Reach to Recovery group can provide instruction, emotional support, and a list of area stores that sell prostheses.

• Give psychological support. Many patients fear cancer and disfigurement and worry about loss of sexual function.

• Explain that breast surgery doesn't interfere with sexual function and that the patient may resume sexual activity as soon as she desires after surgery. She may experience "phantom breast syndrome" (a tingling or a pins-and-needles sensation in the area of the amputated breast tissue) or depression following mastectomy.

Self-test questions

You can quickly review your comprehension of the chapter on thoracic neoplasms by answering the following questions. The answers to these questions and their rationales appear on pages 188 and 189.

Case history questions

One morning while getting dressed, Ted Baxter, who has a long history of smoking, coughs up a small amount of blood-tinged sputum. Frightened, he makes an appointment to see his family doctor right away. After performing a history review and physical examination, the doctor sends Mr. Baxter to radiology for a chest X-ray. The X-ray shows a lesion in the

*lower lobe of his left lung. Suspecting lung cancer, the doc-
tor orders sputum for cytology, a bronchoscopy, and a needle biopsy of the lesion. Test results reveal the lung lesion to
be epidermoid carcinoma.*

1. Smoking, a major risk factor for lung cancer, is usually
noted in the patient's history in about what percentage of
patients with lung cancer?
  a. 35%
  b. 50%
  c. 65%
  d. 80%

2. You should monitor a patient with epidermoid carcinoma of the lung for which of the following metabolic abnormalities?
  a. Gynecomastia
  b. Cushing's syndrome
  c. Hypercalcemia
  d. Hyponatremia

3. Which of the following chemotherapy combinations may
the patient with lung cancer receive?
  a. Fluorouracil and cisplatin
  b. Carboplatin, cyclophosphamide
  c. Doxorubicin, cisplatin, etoposide
  d. Doxorubicin, bleomycin, vinblastine, dacarbazine

4. After thoracic surgery to remove a cancerous lung lesion
and adjacent lung tissue, the correct patient position is?
  a. prone.
  b. supine.
  c. on the surgical side.
  d. on the nonsurgical side.

*During a routine breast self-examination, Joan Carr, who is
postmenopausal, finds a lump in her right breast. She seeks
medical attention immediately, knowing her risk for breast
cancer is higher than average because her mother and sis-
ter have had the disease. Her doctor orders a mammogram
and needle biopsy of the lump. Test results confirm the diagnosis of breast cancer.*

5. Which of the following statements characterizes breast cancer?
   a. Breast cancer occurs most often in the upper outer quadrant of the breast.
   b. Breast cancer occurs most often in the right breast.
   c. Women who experienced menopause early are at higher risk for breast cancer.
   d. Hispanic women have the lowest risk for breast cancer.

6. What is the single most important factor in predicting survival time for a patient with breast cancer?
   a. Tumor size
   b. Type of breast cancer present
   c. History of breast cancer in other breast
   d. Number of lymph nodes involved

7. Following a modified radical mastectomy, the patient has an incisional drain in place. What color should the drainage be 24 hours after surgery?
   a. Bloody
   b. Serous
   c. Milky white to gray
   d. Yellowish

8. The postmastectomy patient may prevent lymphedema of the affected arm by:
   a. wearing tightly fitted rubber gloves when washing dishes.
   b. avoiding use of lanolin hand cream.
   c. performing arm and hand exercises daily.
   d. dangling the affected arm every 3 to 4 hours daily.

CHAPTER 4

Abdominal and Pelvic Neoplasms

Cancers in the abdomen and pelvis can obstruct the affected organ, disrupt its secretory or absorptive functions, and obstruct the flow of GI contents.

Gastric cancer

Although gastric cancer is common throughout the world and affects people of all races, it kills more Japanese, Icelanders, Chileans, and Austrians than people of other nationalities. And it strikes men over age 40 more commonly than it does women and other age-groups.

Over the past 25 years in the United States, the incidence of gastric cancer has fallen 50%, with the resulting death rate now one-third of what it was 30 years ago. The prognosis depends on the cancer's stage at the time of diagnosis; however, the overall 5-year survival rate is approximately 15%.

Causes

What causes gastric cancer isn't known. The disease is commonly associated with gastritis accompanied by gastric atrophy, which is now thought to result from, rather than precede, gastric cancer. Predisposing factors include environmental influences, such as smoking and excessive alcohol intake. Genetic factors have also been implicated because gastric cancer occurs more frequently in people with type A blood than in those with type O; similarly, it oc-

Sites of gastric cancer

The illustration below shows how frequently gastric cancer occurs in different parts of the stomach.

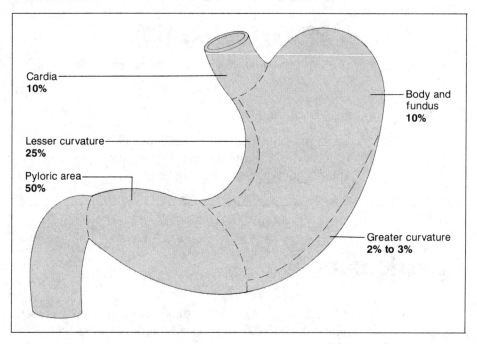

Cardia
10%

Body and
fundus
10%

Lesser curvature
25%

Pyloric area
50%

Greater curvature
2% to 3%

curs more frequently in people with a family history of gastric cancer. Dietary factors, including types of food preparation, physical properties of some foods, and certain methods of food preservation (especially smoking, pickling, or salting), also seem related.

Based on gross appearance, gastric cancer can be classified as polypoid, ulcerating, ulcerating and infiltrating, or diffuse. The parts of the stomach affected by gastric cancer, listed in order of decreasing frequency, are the pylorus and antrum, the lesser curvature, the cardia, the body of the stomach, and the greater curvature. (See *Sites of gastric cancer*.)

Gastric cancer infiltrates rapidly to the regional lymph nodes, omentum, liver, and lungs by the following routes: the walls of the stomach, duodenum, and esophagus; the lymphatic system; adjacent organs; the bloodstream; and the peritoneal cavity.

The decreased incidence of gastric cancer in the United States has been attributed, without proof, to Americans' relatively balanced diet and to widespread refrigeration, which reduces nitrate-producing bacteria in food.

Signs and symptoms

Early clues to gastric cancer are chronic dyspepsia and epigastric discomfort, followed in later stages by weight loss, anorexia, a feeling of fullness after eating, anemia, and fatigue. If the carcinoma is in the cardia, the first symptom may be dysphagia and, later, vomiting (often coffee-ground vomitus). Affected patients may also have blood in their stools.

The course of gastric cancer may be insidious or fulminating. Unfortunately, the patient typically treats himself with antacids until the symptoms of advanced cancer appear.

Diagnosis

In gastric cancer, diagnosis depends primarily on reinvestigations of any persistent or recurring GI changes and complaints. To rule out other conditions producing similar symptoms, diagnostic evaluation must include the testing of blood, stool, and stomach fluid samples.

Diagnosis typically requires various studies, including the following:

• *Barium X-rays* of the GI tract with fluoroscopy show changes in the GI tract (such as a tumor or a filling defect in the outline of the stomach, loss of flexibility and distensibility, and abnormal gastric mucosa with or without ulceration).

• *Gastroscopy* with fiber-optic endoscopy helps rule out other diffuse gastric mucosal abnormalities by allowing direct visualization and gastroscopic biopsy to evaluate gastric mucosal lesions.

• *Photography* with fiber-optic endoscopy provides a permanent record of gastric lesions that can later be used to determine disease progression and effect of treatment.

Certain other studies may rule out specific organ metastasis: computed tomography scans, chest X-rays, liver and bone scans, and liver biopsy. (See *Staging gastric cancer,* page 62.)

Staging gastric cancer

Both the prognosis and treatment of gastric cancer depend on its type and stage. Using the TNM (*tumor*, *node*, *metastasis*) system, the American Joint Committee on Cancer describes the following stages of gastric cancer.

Primary tumor
TX—primary tumor can't be assessed
T0—no evidence of primary tumor
Tis—carcinoma in situ; intraepithelial tumor; doesn't penetrate the lamina propria
T1—tumor penetrates the lamina propria or submucosa
T2—tumor penetrates the muscularis propria or subserosa
T3—tumor penetrates the serosa (visceral peritoneum) without invading adjacent structures
T4—tumor invades adjacent structures

Regional lymph nodes
NX—regional lymph nodes can't be assessed
N0—no evidence of regional lymph node metastasis
N1—involvement of perigastric lymph nodes within 3 cm of the edge of the primary tumor

N2—involvement of the perigastric lymph nodes more than 3 cm from the edge of the primary tumor, or in lymph nodes along the left gastric, common hepatic, splenic, or celiac arteries

Distant metastasis
MX—distant metastasis can't be assessed
M0—no evidence of distant metastasis
M1—distant metastasis

Staging categories
Gastric cancer stages progress from mild to severe as follows:
Stage 0—Tis, N0, M0
Stage IA—T1, N0, M0
Stage IB—T1, N1, M0; T2, N0, M0
Stage II—T1, N2, M0; T3, N0, M0
Stage IIIA—T2, N2, M0; T3, N1, M0; T4, N0, M0
Stage IIIB—T3, N2, M0; T4, N1, M0
Stage IV—T4, N2, M0; any T, any N, M1

Treatment

Surgery is usually the treatment of choice. Excision of the lesion with appropriate margins is possible in more than one-third of patients. Even in patients whose disease isn't considered surgically curable, resection offers palliation and improves potential benefits from chemotherapy and radiation.

The nature and extent of the lesion determine which kind of surgery is most appropriate. Common surgical procedures include subtotal gastric resection (subtotal gastrectomy) and total gastric resection (total gastrectomy). When the cancer involves the pylorus and antrum, gastric resection removes the lower stomach and duodenum (gastrojejunostomy or Billroth II). If metastasis has occurred, the omentum and spleen may also be removed.

If gastric cancer has spread to the liver, peritoneum, or lymph glands, palliative surgery may include gastrostomy, jejunostomy, or a gastric or partial gastric resection. Such surgery may temporarily relieve vomiting, nausea, pain, and dysphagia, while allowing enteral nutrition to continue.

Chemotherapy for GI cancer may help to control symptoms and prolong survival. Adenocarcinoma of the stomach has responded to several agents, including fluorouracil, carmustine, doxorubicin, cisplatin, methotrexate, and mitomycin. Antiemetics can control nausea, which increases as the cancer advances. In the more advanced stages, sedatives and tranquilizers may be necessary to control overwhelming anxiety. Narcotics are often necessary to relieve severe and unremitting pain.

Radiation has been particularly useful when combined with chemotherapy in patients who have unresectable or partially resectable disease. It should be administered on an empty stomach and shouldn't be used preoperatively because it may damage viscera and impede healing.

Treatment with antispasmodics and antacids may help relieve GI distress.

Special considerations

• Before surgery, prepare the patient for its effects and for postsurgical procedures, such as insertion of a nasogastric (NG) tube for drainage and I.V. lines.

• Reassure the patient who is having a partial gastric resection that he may eventually be able to eat normally, and prepare the patient who is having a total gastrectomy for slow recovery and only partial return to a normal diet.

• Include the family in all phases of the patient's care.

• Emphasize the importance to the patient of changing position every 2 hours and of performing deep breathing.

• After surgery, give meticulous supportive care to promote recovery and prevent complications.

• After any type of gastrectomy, pulmonary complications may result and oxygen may be needed. Regularly assist the patient with turning, coughing, and deep breathing. Turning the patient hourly and administering analgesic narcotics may prevent pulmonary problems. Incentive spirometry may also be needed for complete lung expansion. Proper positioning is important as well: semi-Fowler's position facilitates breathing and drainage.

• After gastrectomy, little (if any) drainage comes from the NG tube because no secretions form after stomach removal. Without a stomach for storage, many patients experience dumping syndrome.

• Intrinsic factor is absent from gastric secretions, leading to malabsorption of vitamin B_{12}. To prevent vitamin B_{12} deficiency, the patient must take a replacement vitamin for the rest of his life as well as an iron supplement.

• During radiation treatment, encourage the patient to eat high-calorie, well-balanced meals.

• Offer fluids, such as ginger ale, to minimize such radiation adverse effects as nausea and vomiting.

• Patients who experience poor digestion and absorption after gastrectomy need a special diet: frequent feedings of small amounts of clear liquids, increasing to small, frequent feedings of bland food.

• After total gastrectomy, patients must eat small meals for the rest of their lives. (Some patients need pancreatin and sodium bicarbonate after meals to prevent or control steatorrhea and dyspepsia.)

• Wound dehiscence and delayed healing, stemming from decreased protein levels, anemia, and avitaminosis, may occur. Preoperative vitamin and protein replacement can prevent such complications. Observe the wound regularly for redness, swelling, failure to heal, or warmth. Parenteral administration of vitamin C may improve wound healing.

• Vitamin deficiency may result from obstruction, diarrhea, or an inadequate diet. Ascorbic acid, thiamine, riboflavin, nicotinic acid, and vitamin K supplements may be beneficial.

• Good nutrition promotes weight gain, strength, independence, a positive outlook, and tolerance for surgery, radiation therapy, or chemotherapy. Aside from meeting caloric needs, nutrition must provide adequate protein, fluid, and potassium intake to facilitate glycogen and protein synthesis. Anabolic agents, such as methandrostenolone, may induce nitrogen retention. Steroids, antidepressants, wine, or brandy may boost the appetite.

• When all treatments have failed, concentrate on keeping the patient comfortable and free of pain, and provide as much psychological support as possible.

• If the patient is going home, discuss continuing care needs with the caregiver, or refer the patient to an appropriate home health care agency. Encourage the patient and the caregivers to express their feelings and concerns. Answer their questions honestly with tact and sensitivity.

Esophageal cancer

Most common in men over age 60, esophageal cancer is nearly always fatal. This disease occurs worldwide, but incidence varies geographically. It's most common in Japan, China, the Middle East, and parts of South Africa.

Causes

Although the cause of esophageal cancer is unknown, predisposing factors include chronic irritation caused by heavy smoking and excessive use of alcohol, stasis-induced inflammation as in achalasia or stricture, and nutritional deficiency. Esophageal tumors are usually fungating and infiltrating. Most arise in the squamous cell epithelium; a few are adenocarcinomas; fewer still are melanomas and sarcomas.

Regardless of type, esophageal cancer is usually fatal, with a 5-year survival rate below 10% and regional metastasis occurring early via submucosal lymphatics. Metastasis produces such serious complications as tracheoesophageal fistulas, mediastinitis, and aortic perforation. Common sites of distant metastasis include the liver and lungs.

Signs and symptoms

Dysphagia and weight loss are the most common presenting symptoms. Dysphagia is mild and intermittent at first, but it soon becomes constant. Pain, hoarseness, coughing, and esophageal obstruction follow. Cachexia usually develops.

Diagnosis

X-rays of the esophagus, with barium swallow and motility studies, reveal structural and filling defects and reduced peristalsis.

Endoscopic examination of the esophagus, punch and brush biopsies, and exfoliative cytologic tests confirm esophageal tumors. (See *Staging esophageal cancer,* page 66.)

Staging esophageal cancer

Using the TNM (*tumor, node, metastasis*) system, the American Joint Committee on Cancer has established the following stages for esophageal cancer.

Primary tumor
TX—primary tumor can't be assessed
T0—no evidence of primary tumor
Tis—carcinoma in situ
T1—tumor invades lamina propria or submucosa
T2—tumor invades muscularis propria
T3—tumor invades adventitia
T4—tumor invades adjacent structures

Regional lymph nodes
NX—regional lymph nodes can't be assessed
N0—no regional lymph node metastasis
N1—regional lymph node metastasis

Distant metastasis
MX—distant metastasis can't be assessed
M0—no known distant metastasis
M1—distant metastasis

Staging categories
Esophageal cancer progresses from mild to severe as follows:
Stage 0—Tis, N0, M0
Stage I—T1, N0, M0
Stage IIA—T2, N0, M0; T3, N0, M0
Stage IIB—T1, N1, M0; T2, N1, M0
Stage III—T3, N1, M0; T4, any N, M0
Stage IV—any T, any N, M1

Treatment

Whenever possible, treatment includes resection to maintain a passageway for food. This may require such radical surgery as esophagogastrectomy with jejunal or colonic bypass grafts. Palliative surgery may include a feeding gastrostomy. Other therapies may consist of radiation; chemotherapy with various combinations of cisplatin, methotrexate, carboplatin, doxorubicin, and fluorouracil; or installation of prosthetic tubes to bridge the tumor and alleviate dysphagia.

Treatment complications may be severe. Surgery may precipitate an anastomotic leak, a fistula, pneumonia, and empyema. Rarely, radiation may cause esophageal perforation, pneumonitis and pulmonary fibrosis, or myelitis of the spinal cord. Prosthetic tubes may dislodge and perforate the mediastinum or erode the tumor.

Special considerations

• Before surgery, answer the patient's questions and let him know what to expect after surgery, such as gastrostomy tubes, closed chest drainage, and nasogastric suctioning.
• After surgery, monitor vital signs. Be alert for unexpected changes. If surgery included an esophageal anastomosis,

keep the patient flat on his back to avoid tension on the suture line.

• Promote adequate nutrition and evaluate the patient's nutritional and hydration status for possible supplementary parenteral feedings.

• Prevent aspiration of food by placing the patient in Fowler's position for meals and allowing plenty of time to eat. Provide high-calorie, high-protein, pureed food as needed. Because the patient will probably regurgitate some food, clean his mouth carefully after each meal. Keep mouthwash handy.

• If the patient has a gastrostomy tube, give food slowly—using gravity—in prescribed amounts (usually 200 to 500 ml). Offer something to chew before each feeding, to promote gastric secretions and a semblance of normal eating.

• Instruct the family in gastrostomy tube care (checking tube patency before each feeding, providing skin care around the tube, and keeping the patient upright during and after feedings).

• Provide emotional support for the patient and family; refer them to appropriate organizations, such as the American Cancer Society.

Pancreatic cancer

A deadly GI cancer, pancreatic cancer progresses rapidly. Pancreatic tumors are almost always duct cell adenocarcinomas and most arise in the head of the pancreas. Rarer tumors are those of the body and tail of the pancreas and islet cell tumor. (See *Types of pancreatic cancer,* page 68, and *Islet cell tumors,* page 69.) The two main tissue types are cylinder cell and large, fatty, granular cell.

Causes

Pancreatic cancer occurs most commonly in men between ages 35 and 70. Geographically, the incidence is highest in Israel, the United States, Sweden, and Canada.

Types of pancreatic cancer

TYPE AND PATHOLOGY	CLINICAL FEATURES
Head of pancreas • Tumor often obstructs ampulla of Vater and common bile duct • Tumor directly metastasizes to duodenum • Adhesions anchor tumor to spine, stomach, and intestines.	• Jaundice (dominant sign) — slowly progressive, unremitting; may cause skin (especially of the face and genitals) to turn olive green or black • Pruritus — often severe • Weight loss — rapid and severe (as great as 30 lbs [13.6 kg]); may lead to emaciation, weakness, and muscle atrophy • Slowed digestion, gastric distention, nausea, diarrhea, and steatorrhea with clay-colored stools • Liver and gallbladder enlargement from lymph node metastasis to biliary tract and duct wall results in compression and obstruction; gallbladder may be palpable (Courvoisier's sign). • Dull, nondescript, continuous abdominal pain radiating to right upper quadrant; relieved by bending forward • GI hemorrhage and biliary infection common
Body and tail of pancreas • Large nodular masses become fixed to retropancreatic tissues and spine. • Direct invasion of spleen, left kidney, suprarenal gland, diaphragm • Involvement of celiac plexus results in thrombosis of splenic vein and spleen infarction.	**Body** • Pain (dominant symptom) — usually epigastric, develops slowly and radiates to back; relieved by bending forward or sitting up; intensified by lying supine; most intense 3 to 4 hours after eating; when celiac plexus is involved, pain is more intense and lasts longer • Venous thrombosis and thrombophlebitis — frequent; may precede other symptoms by months • Splenomegaly (from infarction), hepatomegaly (occasionally), and jaundice (rarely) **Tail** Symptoms resulting from metastasis: • Abdominal tumor (most common finding) that produces a palpable abdominal mass; abdominal pain radiating to left hypochondrium and left chest • Anorexia leading to weight loss, emaciation, and weakness • Splenomegaly and upper GI bleeding

Evidence suggests that pancreatic cancer is linked to inhalation or absorption of the following carcinogens, which are then excreted by the pancreas:
• cigarettes
• foods high in fat and protein
• food additives
• industrial chemicals, such as benzidine, and urea.

Possible predisposing factors are chronic pancreatitis, diabetes mellitus, and chronic alcohol abuse.

Signs and symptoms

The most common features of pancreatic cancer are weight loss, abdominal or low back pain, jaundice, and diarrhea.

Islet cell tumors

Relatively uncommon, islet cell tumors (insulinomas) may be benign or malignant and produce symptoms in three stages:
• *slight hypoglycemia* —fatigue, restlessness, malaise, and excessive weight gain.
• *compensatory secretion of epinephrine* —pallor, clamminess, perspiration, palpitations, finger tremors, hunger, decreased temperature, increased pulse and blood pressure.

• *severe hypoglycemia* —ataxia, clouded sensorium, diplopia, episodes of violence and hysteria.

Usually, insulinomas metastasize to the liver alone but may metastasize to bone, the brain, and the lungs. Death results from a combination of hypoglycemic reactions and widespread metastasis. Treatment consists of enucleation of the tumor (if benign) and chemotherapy with streptozocin or resection to include pancreatic tissue (if malignant).

Other generalized effects include fever, skin lesions (usually on the legs), and emotional disturbances, such as depression, anxiety, and premonition of fatal illness.

Diagnosis

Definitive diagnosis requires a laparotomy with a biopsy. (See *Staging pancreatic cancer,* page 70.) Other tests used to detect pancreatic cancer include the following:
• *Ultrasound* can identify a mass but not its histologic features.
• *Computed tomography scan* is similar to ultrasound but shows greater detail.
• *Angiography* shows the vascular supply of the tumor.
• *Endoscopic retrograde cholangiopancreatography* allows visualization, instillation of contrast medium, and specimen biopsy.
• *Magnetic resonance imaging* shows tumor size and location in great detail.

Laboratory tests supporting this diagnosis include serum bilirubin (increased); serum amylase and serum lipase (occasionally elevated); prothrombin time (prolonged); alanine aminotransferase and aspartate aminotransferase (elevated levels indicate necrosis of liver cells); alkaline phosphatase (marked elevation occurs with biliary obstruction); plasma insulin radioimmunoassay (shows measurable serum insulin in the presence of islet cell tumors); hemoglobin and hematocrit (may show mild anemia); fasting blood glucose (may indicate hypoglycemia or hyperglycemia); and stools

Staging pancreatic cancer

Using the TNM (*tumor, node, metastasis*) system, the American Joint Committee on Cancer has established the following stages for pancreatic cancer.

Primary tumor
TX—primary tumor can't be assessed
T0—no evidence of primary tumor
T1—tumor limited to the pancreas
T1a—tumor 2 cm or less in greatest dimension
T1b—tumor more than 2 cm in greatest dimension
T2—tumor penetrates the duodenum, bile duct, or peripancreatic tissues
T3—tumor penetrates the stomach, spleen, colon, or adjacent large vessels

Regional lymph nodes
NX—regional lymph nodes can't be assessed

N0—no evidence of regional lymph node metastasis
N1—regional lymph node metastasis

Distant metastasis
MX—distant metastasis can't be assessed
M0—no known distant metastasis
M1—distant metastasis

Staging categories
Pancreatic cancer progresses from mild to severe as follows:
Stage I—T1, N0, M0; T2, N0, M0
Stage II—T3, N0, M0
Stage III—any T, N1, M0
Stage IV—any T, any N, M1

(occult blood may point to ulceration in GI tract or ampulla of Vater).

Treatment

Because this disease has usually metastasized widely at diagnosis, treatment of pancreatic cancer is rarely successful. Therapy consists of surgery and, possibly, radiation and chemotherapy.

Small advances have been made in the survival rate with surgery:
• Total pancreatectomy may increase survival time by removing a localized tumor or by controlling postoperative gastric ulceration.
• Cholecystojejunostomy, choledochoduodenostomy, and choledochojejunostomy have partially replaced radical resection to bypass obstructing common bile duct extensions, thereby decreasing the incidence of jaundice and pruritus.
• Whipple's operation, or pancreatoduodenectomy, has a high mortality but can produce wide lymphatic clearance, except with tumors located near the portal vein, superior mesenteric vein and artery, and celiac axis. This rarely used

procedure removes the head of the pancreas, the duodenum, and portions of the body and tail of the pancreas, stomach, jejunum, pancreatic duct, and distal portion of the bile duct.
• Gastrojejunostomy is performed if radical resection isn't indicated and duodenal obstruction is expected to develop later.

Although pancreatic cancer generally responds poorly to chemotherapy, recent studies using combinations of fluorouracil, streptozocin, ifosfamide, and doxorubicin show a trend toward longer survival time. Other medications used in pancreatic cancer include:
• antibiotics (oral, I.V., or I.M.) – to prevent infection and relieve symptoms
• anticholinergics – particularly propantheline, to decrease GI tract spasm and motility and reduce pain and secretions
• antacids (oral or by nasogastric [NG] tube) – to decrease secretion of pancreatic enzymes and to suppress peptic activity, thereby reducing stress-induced damage to gastric mucosa
• diuretics – to mobilize extracellular fluid from ascites
• insulin – to provide adequate exogenous insulin supply after pancreatic resection
• narcotics – to relieve pain, but only after analgesics fail because morphine, meperidine, and codeine can lead to biliary tract spasm and increase common bile duct pressure
• pancreatic enzymes – (average dose is 0.5 to 1 mg with meals) to assist in digestion of proteins, carbohydrates, and fats when pancreatic juices are insufficient because of surgery or obstruction.

Radiation therapy is usually ineffective except as an adjunct to chemotherapy or as a palliative measure.

Special considerations

• Provide comprehensive supportive care to prevent surgical complications, increase patient comfort, and help the patient and his family cope with inevitable death.
• Before surgery, ensure that the patient is medically stable, particularly regarding nutrition (this may take 4 to 5 days). If the patient can't tolerate oral feedings, provide total parenteral nutrition and I.V. fat emulsions to correct deficiencies and maintain positive nitrogen balance.

• Give blood transfusions (to combat anemia), vitamin K (to overcome prothrombin deficiency), antibiotics (to prevent postoperative complications), and gastric lavage (to maintain gastric decompression).

• Tell the patient about expected postoperative procedures and expected adverse effects of radiation and chemotherapy.

• After surgery, watch for and report complications, such as fistulas, pancreatitis, fluid and electrolyte imbalance, infection, hemorrhage, skin breakdown, nutritional deficiency, hepatic failure, renal insufficiency, and diabetes.

• If the patient is receiving chemotherapy, treat adverse effects symptomatically.

• Monitor fluid balance, abdominal girth, metabolic state, and weight daily. In weight loss, replace nutrients I.V., P.O., or with an NG tube; in weight gain (due to ascites), impose dietary restrictions, such as a low-sodium or fluid-retention diet as ordered. Maintain a 2,500-calorie diet.

• Serve small, frequent nutritious meals by enlisting the dietitian's services. Administer an oral pancreatic enzyme at mealtimes if needed. Give an antacid to prevent stress ulcers.

• To prevent constipation, administer laxatives, stool softeners, and cathartics; modify diet; and increase fluid intake. To increase GI motility, position the patient properly at mealtime and help him walk when he can.

• Ensure adequate rest and sleep. Assist with range-of-motion (ROM) and isometric exercises as appropriate.

• Administer pain medication, antibiotics, and antipyretics. Note time, site (if injected), and response.

• Watch for signs of hypoglycemia or hyperglycemia; administer glucose or an antidiabetic agent as ordered. Monitor blood glucose and urine sugar and acetone levels and the patient's response to treatment.

• Document progression of jaundice.

• Provide meticulous skin care to avoid pruritus and necrosis. Prevent excoriation in a pruritic patient by clipping his nails and having him wear cotton gloves.

• Watch for signs of upper GI bleeding; test stools and vomitus for occult blood, and keep a flow sheet of hemoglobin and hematocrit values. To control active bleeding, promote gastric vasoconstriction with medication. Replace any fluid loss. Ease discomfort from pyloric obstruction with an NG tube.

• To prevent thrombosis, apply antiembolism stockings and assist in ROM exercises. If thrombosis occurs, elevate the patient's legs and give an anticoagulant or aspirin.

• Encourage the patient to verbalize his fears. Promote family involvement and offer the assistance of a counselor. Help the patient and his family deal with the reality of death.

Colorectal cancer

The second most common visceral neoplasm in the United States and Europe, colorectal cancer is equally distributed between men and women.

Colorectal malignant tumors are almost always adenocarcinomas. About half of these are sessile lesions of the rectosigmoid area; the rest are polypoid lesions.

Colorectal cancer tends to progress slowly and remains localized for a long time. Consequently, it's potentially curable in 75% of patients if early diagnosis allows resection before nodal involvement. With improved diagnosis, the overall 5-year survival rate is nearing 50%.

Causes

The exact cause of colorectal cancer is unknown, but studies showing concentration in areas of higher economic development suggest a relationship to diet (excess animal fat, particularly beef, and low fiber). Other factors that magnify the risk of developing colorectal cancer include the following:

• other diseases of the digestive tract
• age (over 40)
• history of ulcerative colitis (average interval before onset of cancer is 11 to 17 years)
• familial polyposis (cancer almost always develops by age 50).

Signs and symptoms

Colorectal cancer's signs and symptoms result from local obstruction and, in later stages, from direct extension to adjacent areas (the bladder, prostate, ureters, vagina, and sacrum) and distant metastasis (usually to the liver). In the early stages, signs and symptoms are typically vague and depend on the anatomic location and function of the bowel segment containing the tumor. Later, they generally include pallor, cachexia, ascites, hepatomegaly, or lymphangiectasis.

On the right side of the colon (which absorbs water and electrolytes), early tumor growth causes no signs of obstruction, because the tumor tends to grow along the bowel rather than surround the lumen and the fecal content in this area is normally liquid. It may, however, cause black, tarry stools; anemia; and abdominal aching, pressure, or dull cramps. As the disease progresses, the patient develops weakness, fatigue, exertional dyspnea, vertigo and, eventually, diarrhea, obstipation, anorexia, weight loss, vomiting, and other signs of intestinal obstruction. In addition, a tumor on the right side may be palpable.

On the left side, a tumor causes signs of an obstruction even in early stages because in this area stools are of a formed consistency. It commonly causes rectal bleeding (often ascribed to hemorrhoids), intermittent abdominal fullness or cramping, and rectal pressure. As the disease progresses, the patient develops obstipation, diarrhea, or "ribbon" or pencil-shaped stools. Typically, he notices that passage of a stool or flatus relieves the pain. At this stage, bleeding from the colon becomes obvious, with dark or bright red blood in the feces and mucus in or on the stools.

With a rectal tumor, the first symptom is a change in bowel habits, often beginning with an urgent need to defecate on arising ("morning diarrhea") or obstipation alternating with diarrhea. Other signs are blood or mucus in stools and a sense of incomplete evacuation. Late in the disease, pain begins as a feeling of rectal fullness that later becomes a dull, and sometimes constant, ache confined to the rectum or sacral region.

Diagnosis

Only tumor biopsy can verify colorectal cancer, but other tests help detect it:
• *Digital examination* can detect almost 15% of colorectal cancers.
• *Hemoccult (guaiac) test* can detect blood in stools.

Staging colorectal cancer

Named for pathologist Cuthbert Dukes, the Dukes colorectal cancer classification system assigns tumors to four stages. These stages (with substages) reflect the extent of bowel mucosa and bowel wall infiltration, lymph node involvement, and metastasis.

Stage A
Malignant cells are confined to the bowel mucosa, and the lymph nodes contain no cancer cells. Treated promptly, about 80% of these patients remain disease-free 5 years later.

Stage B
Malignant cells extend through the bowel mucosa but remain within the bowel wall. The lymph nodes are normal. In substage B_2, all bowel wall layers and immediately adjacent structures contain malignant cells, but the lymph nodes remain normal. About 50% of patients with substage B_2 survive for 5 or more years.

Stage C
Malignant cells extend into the bowel wall and the lymph nodes. In substage C_2, malignant cells extend through the entire thickness of the bowel wall and into the lymph nodes. The 5-year survival rate for patients with stage C disease is about 25%.

Stage D
Malignant cells have metastasized to distant organs by way of the lymph nodes and mesenteric vessels; they typically lodge in the lungs and liver. Only 5% of patients with stage D cancer survive 5 or more years.

• *Proctoscopy* or *sigmoidoscopy* can detect up to 66% of colorectal cancers.

• *Colonoscopy* permits visual inspection (and photographs) of the colon up to the ileocecal valve and provides access for polypectomies and biopsies of suspected lesions.

• *Computed tomography scan* helps to detect areas affected by metastasis.

• *Barium X-ray*, utilizing a dual contrast agent and air, can locate lesions that are undetectable manually or visually. Barium examination should *follow* endoscopy or excretory urography because the barium sulfate interferes with these tests.

• *Carcinoembryonic antigen*, though not specific or sensitive enough for early diagnosis, is helpful in monitoring patients before and after treatment to detect metastasis or recurrence. (See *Staging colorectal cancer*.)

Treatment

The most effective treatment for colorectal cancer is surgery to remove the malignant tumor, adjacent tissues, and any lymph nodes that may contain cancer cells. The type of surgery depends on the location of the tumor:
• Cecum and ascending colon—right hemicolectomy (for advanced disease) may include resection of the terminal segment of the ileum, cecum, ascending colon, and right half of the transverse colon with corresponding mesentery
• Proximal and middle transverse colon—right colectomy to include transverse colon and mesentery corresponding to midcolic vessels or segmental resection of transverse colon and associated midcolic vessels
• Sigmoid colon—surgery is usually limited to sigmoid colon and mesentery
• Upper rectum—anterior or low anterior resection (newer method, using a stapler, allows for resections much lower than were previously possible)
• Lower rectum—abdominoperineal resection and permanent sigmoid colostomy.

Chemotherapy is indicated for patients with metastasis, residual disease, or a recurrent inoperable tumor. Drugs used in such treatment commonly include fluorouracil with levamisole, leucovorin, methotrexate, or streptozocin. Patients whose tumor has extended to regional lymph nodes may receive fluorouracil and levamisole for 1 year postoperatively.

Radiation therapy induces tumor regression and may be used before or after surgery or combined with chemotherapy, especially fluorouracil.

Special
considerations

• Before surgery, monitor the patient's diet modifications, laxatives, enemas, and antibiotics—all used to clean the bowel and to decrease abdominal and perineal cavity contamination during surgery.
• If the patient is having a colostomy, teach him and his family about the procedure. Emphasize that the stoma will be red, moist, and swollen and that postoperative swelling will eventually subside.
• Show them a diagram of the intestine before and after surgery, stressing how much of the bowel will remain intact. Supplement your teaching with instructional aids. Arrange a postsurgical visit from a recovered ostomate.

• Prepare the patient for a postoperative I.V. line, a nasogastric tube, and an indwelling urinary catheter.

• Discuss the importance of cooperating during coughing and deep-breathing exercises.

• After surgery, explain to the patient's family the importance of their positive reactions to the patient's adjustment. Consult with an enterostomal therapist, if available, to help set up a regimen for the patient.

• Encourage the patient to look at the stoma and participate in its care as soon as possible. Teach good hygiene and skin care. Allow him to shower or bathe as soon as the incision heals.

• If appropriate, instruct the patient with a sigmoid colostomy to do his own irrigation as soon as he can after surgery. Advise him to schedule irrigation for the time of day when he normally evacuated before surgery. Many patients find that irrigating every 1 to 3 days is necessary for regulation.

• If flatus, diarrhea, or constipation occurs, eliminate suspected causative foods from the patient's diet; they may be reintroduced later.

• After several months, many ostomates establish control with irrigation and no longer need to wear a pouch. A stoma cap or gauze sponge placed over the stoma protects it and absorbs mucoid secretions.

• Before he achieves such control, advise the patient that he can resume physical activities, including sports, provided no threat of injury to the stoma or surrounding abdominal muscles exists. However, he should avoid heavy lifting because herniation or prolapse may occur through weakened muscles in the abdominal wall.

• A structured, gradually progressive exercise program to strengthen abdominal muscles may be instituted under medical supervision.

• If appropriate, refer the patient to a home health agency for follow-up care and counseling. Suggest sexual counseling for male patients; most are impotent after an abdominoperineal resection.

• Instruct anyone who's had colorectal cancer that he is at increased risk for another primary cancer and should have yearly screening and testing as well as follow a high-fiber diet.

Staging kidney cancer

Using the TNM (*tumor, node, metastasis*) system, the American Joint Committee on Cancer has established the following stages for kidney cancer.

Primary tumor
TX—primary tumor can't be assessed
T0—no evidence of primary tumor
T1—tumor 2.5 cm or less in greatest dimension and limited to the kidney
T2—tumor greater than 2.5 cm in greatest dimension and limited to the kidney
T3—tumor extends into major veins or invades adrenal gland or perinephric tissues, but not beyond Gerota's fascia
T3a—tumor extends into adrenal gland or perinephric tissues, but not beyond Gerota's fascia
T3b—tumor grossly extends into renal veins or vena cava
T4—tumor extends beyond Gerota's fascia

Regional lymph nodes
NX—regional lymph nodes can't be assessed
N0—no evidence of regional lymph node metastasis
N1—metastasis in a single lymph node, 2 cm or less in greatest dimension

N2—metastasis in a single lymph node, between 2 and 5 cm in greatest dimension, or metastasis to several lymph nodes, none more than 5 cm in greatest dimension
N3—metastasis in a lymph node, more than 5 cm in greatest dimension

Distant metastasis
MX—distant metastasis can't be assessed
M0—no known distant metastasis
M1—distant metastasis

Staging categories
Kidney cancer progresses from mild to severe as follows:
Stage I—T1, N0, M0
Stage II—T2, N0, M0
Stage III—T1, N1, M0; T2, N1, M0; T3a, N0, M0; T3a, N1, M0; T3b, N0, M0; T3b, N1, M0
Stage IV—T4, any N, M0; any T, N2, M0; any T, N3, M0; any T, any N, M1

Kidney cancer

Also known as nephrocarcinoma, renal cell carcinoma, hypernephroma, or Grawitz's tumor, kidney cancer usually occurs in older adults, with about 85% of tumors originating in the kidneys and others resulting from metastasis from other primary sites. Renal pelvic tumors and Wilms' tumor occur primarily in children. Kidney tumors, which usually are large, firm, nodular, encapsulated, unilateral, and solitary, can be separated histologically into clear cell, granular, and spindle cell types. (See *Staging kidney cancer.*)

Overall, the prognosis for kidney cancer has improved considerably, with the 5-year survival rate now at approximately 50% of patients.

Causes

The causes of kidney cancer aren't known. However, this type of cancer is increasing, possibly as a result of exposure to environmental carcinogens as well as increased longevity. Even so, this cancer accounts for only about 2% of all adult cancers. Kidney cancer is twice as common in men as in women and usually strikes after age 40.

Signs and symptoms

Kidney cancer produces a classic clinical triad—hematuria, pain, and a palpable mass—but any one may be the first sign of cancer. Microscopic or gross hematuria (which may be intermittent) suggests that the cancer has spread to the renal pelvis. Constant abdominal or flank pain may be dull or, if the cancer causes bleeding or blood clots, acute and colicky. The mass is generally smooth, firm, and nontender. All three signs coexist in only about 10% of patients.

Other symptoms include fever (perhaps from hemorrhage or necrosis), hypertension (from compression of the renal artery with renal parenchymal ischemia), rapidly progressing hypercalcemia (possibly from ectopic parathyroid hormone production by the tumor), and urine retention. Weight loss, edema in the legs, nausea, and vomiting signal advanced disease.

Diagnosis

Studies to identify kidney cancer usually include computed tomography scans, excretory urography, ultrasound, cystoscopy (to rule out associated bladder cancer), and nephrotomography or renal angiography to distinguish a kidney cyst from a tumor.

Related tests include liver function studies showing increased levels of alkaline phosphatase, bilirubin, alanine aminotransferase, and aspartate aminotransferase and prolonged prothrombin time. Such results may point to liver metastasis, but if metastasis hasn't occurred, these abnormalities reverse after tumor resection.

Routine laboratory findings of hematuria, anemia (unrelated to blood loss), polycythemia, hypercalcemia, and increased erythrocyte sedimentation rate call for more testing to rule out kidney cancer.

Treatment

Radical nephrectomy, with or without regional lymph node dissection, offers the only chance of cure. Because the disease is radiation-resistant, radiation is used only if the cancer spreads to the perinephric region or the lymph nodes or if the primary tumor or metastatic sites can't be fully excised. In these cases, high radiation doses are used.

Chemotherapy has been only erratically effective against kidney cancer. Chlorambucil, fluorouracil, cyclophosphamide, vinblastine, lomustine, vincristine, cisplatin, tamoxifen, teniposide, interferons, and hormones, such as medroxyprogesterone and testosterone, have been used, usually with poor results. Biotherapy (lymphokine-activated killer cells with recombinant interleukin-2) shows promise but causes adverse reactions. Interferon is somewhat effective in advanced disease.

Special considerations

• Provide meticulous postoperative care, supportive treatment during other therapy, and psychological support to hasten recovery and minimize complications.
• Before surgery, assure the patient that his body will adapt to the loss of a kidney.
• Teach the patient about such expected postoperative procedures as diaphragmatic breathing, coughing properly, splinting his incision, and others.
• After surgery, encourage diaphragmatic breathing and coughing.
• Assist the patient with leg exercises, and turn him every 2 hours.
• Check dressings often for excessive bleeding. Watch for signs of internal bleeding, such as restlessness, sweating, and increased pulse rate.
• Place the patient on the operative side to allow the pressure of adjacent organs to fill the dead space at the surgical site, improving dependent drainage. If possible, help the patient walk within 24 hours after surgery.
• Maintain adequate fluid intake, and monitor intake and output. Monitor laboratory results for anemia, polycythemia, or abnormal blood values that may point to bone or liver involvement or may result from radiation or chemotherapy.
• Symptomatically treat adverse effects of medication.
• Stress compliance with the prescribed outpatient treatment regimen.

Liver cancer

Also called primary and metastatic hepatic carcinoma, liver cancer is a rare form of cancer with a high mortality. It accounts for roughly 2% of all cancers in the United States and for 10% to 50% in Africa and parts of Asia. Liver cancer is most prevalent in men (particularly over age 60); incidence increases with age. It is rapidly fatal, usually within 6 months, from GI hemorrhage, progressive cachexia, hepatic failure, or metastasis.

Most primary liver tumors (90%) originate in the parenchymal cells and are hepatomas (hepatocellular carcinoma, primary lower-cell carcinoma). Some primary tumors originate in the intrahepatic bile ducts and are known as cholangiomas (cholangiocarcinoma, cholangiocellular carcinoma). Rarer tumors include a mixed-cell type, Kupffer's cell sarcoma, and hepatoblastomas (which occur almost exclusively in children and are usually resectable and curable).

The liver is one of the most common sites of metastasis from other primary cancers, particularly of the colon, rectum, stomach, pancreas, esophagus, lung, breast, or skin. In the United States, metastatic liver carcinoma occurs over 20 times more often than primary liver carcinoma and, after cirrhosis, is the leading cause of liver-related death. At times, liver metastasis may appear as a solitary lesion, the first sign of recurrence after a remission.

Causes

The immediate cause of liver cancer is unknown, but it may be a congenital disease in children. Adult liver cancer may result from environmental exposure to carcinogens, such as the chemical compound aflatoxin (a mold that grows on rice and peanuts), thorium dioxide (a contrast medium formerly used in liver radiography), Senecio alkaloids, and possibly androgens and oral estrogens.

Roughly 30% to 70% of patients with hepatomas also have cirrhosis. (Hepatomas are 40 times more likely to develop in a cirrhotic liver than in a normal one.) Whether cirrhosis is a premalignant state, or alcohol and malnutrition predispose the liver to develop hepatomas, is still unclear. Another risk factor is exposure to the hepatitis B virus, although this is likely to change with the availability of the hepatitis B vaccine.

Signs and symptoms

Clinical effects of liver cancer include:
• a mass in the right upper quadrant
• tender, nodular liver on palpation
• severe pain in the epigastrium or the right upper quadrant
• bruit, hum, or rubbing sound if tumor involves a large part of the liver
• weight loss, weakness, anorexia, fever
• occasional jaundice or ascites
• occasional evidence of metastasis through venous system to lungs, from lymphatics to regional lymph nodes, or by direct invasion of portal veins
• dependent edema.

Diagnosis

The confirming test for liver cancer is liver biopsy by needle or open biopsy. Liver cancer is difficult to diagnose in the presence of cirrhosis, but several tests can help identify it:
• *Serum alanine aminotransferase, aspartate aminotransfase, alkaline phosphatase, lactate dehydrogenase, and bilirubin* all show abnormal liver function.
• *Alpha-fetoprotein* rises to a level above 500 mcg/ml.
• *Chest X-ray* may rule out metastasis.
• *Liver scan* may show filling defects.
• *Arteriography* may define large tumors.
• *Electrolyte studies* may indicate increased sodium retention (resulting in functional renal failure), hypoglycemia, leukocytosis, hypercalcemia, or hypocholesterolemia.

Treatment

Because liver cancer is often in an advanced stage at diagnosis, few hepatic tumors are resectable. A resectable tumor must be a single tumor in one lobe, without cirrhosis, jaundice, or ascites. Resection is done by lobectomy or partial hepatectomy.

Radiation therapy for unresectable tumors is usually palliative. But because of the liver's low tolerance for radiation, this therapy has not increased survival.

Another method of treatment is chemotherapy with I.V. fluorouracil, methotrexate, streptozocin, lomustine, or doxorubicin or with regional infusion of fluorouracil or floxuridine (catheters are placed directly into the hepatic artery or left brachial artery for continuous infusion for 7 to 21 days, or permanent implantable pumps are used on an outpatient basis for long-term infusion).

Appropriate treatment for liver metastasis may include resection by lobectomy or chemotherapy with mitomycin or fludarabine (results similar to those in hepatoma). Liver transplantation is now an alternative for some patients.

Special considerations

• Emphasize comprehensive supportive care and emotional support for the patient with liver cancer.
• Control edema and ascites. Monitor the patient's diet throughout treatment. Most patients need a special diet that restricts sodium, fluids (no alcohol allowed), and protein.
• Weigh the patient daily, and note intake and output accurately.
• Watch for signs of ascites — peripheral edema, orthopnea, or dyspnea on exertion. If ascites is present, measure and record abdominal girth daily. To increase venous return and prevent edema, elevate the patient's legs whenever possible.
• Monitor respiratory function. Note any increase in respiratory rate or shortness of breath. Bilateral pleural effusion (noted on chest X-ray) is common, as is metastasis to the lungs. Watch carefully for signs of hypoxemia from intrapulmonary arteriovenous shunting.
• Relieve fever. Administer sponge baths and aspirin suppositories if there are no signs of GI bleeding. Avoid acetaminophen because the diseased liver can't metabolize it. High fever indicates infection and requires antibiotics.
• Give meticulous skin care. Turn the patient frequently and keep his skin clean to prevent pressure ulcers. Apply lotion to prevent chafing, and administer an antipruritic, such as diphenhydramine for severe itching.
• Watch for encephalopathy. Many patients develop end-stage symptoms of ammonia intoxication, including confusion, restlessness, irritability, agitation, delirium, asterixis, lethargy, and, finally, coma.
• Monitor the patient's serum ammonia level, vital signs, and neurologic status. Be prepared to control ammonia accumulation with sorbitol (to induce osmotic diarrhea), neomycin (to reduce bacterial flora in the GI tract), lactulose (to control bacterial elaboration of ammonia), and sodium polystyrene sulfonate (to lower potassium level).

• If a transhepatic catheter is used to relieve obstructive jaundice, irrigate it frequently with prescribed solution (normal saline or, sometimes, 5,000 units of heparin in 500 ml of dextrose 5% in water).
• Monitor vital signs frequently for any indication of bleeding or infection.
• After surgery, give standard postoperative care. Watch for intraperitoneal bleeding and sepsis, which may precipitate coma.
• Monitor for renal failure by checking urine output and blood urea nitrogen and creatinine levels hourly.
• Remember that throughout the course of this intractable illness, your primary concern is to keep the patient as comfortable as possible.

Bladder cancer

Benign or malignant bladder tumors (papillomas) can develop on the surface of the bladder wall or grow within the bladder wall (generally more virulent) and quickly invade underlying muscles. Most bladder tumors (90%) are transitional cell carcinomas, arising from the transitional epithelium of mucous membranes. Less common are adenocarcinomas, epidermoid carcinomas, squamous cell carcinomas, sarcomas, tumors in bladder diverticula, and carcinoma in situ. Bladder tumors are most prevalent in people over age 50 (men more than women) and are more common in densely populated industrial areas.

Causes

Certain environmental carcinogens, such as beta-naphthylamine, benzidine, tobacco, and nitrates, predispose people to transitional cell tumors. Thus, workers in certain industries, such as rubber workers, weavers and leather finishers, aniline dye workers, hairdressers, petroleum workers, and spray painters, are at high risk for such tumors. The period between exposure to the carcinogen and development of symptoms is about 18 years.

Squamous cell carcinoma of the bladder is most common in geographic areas where schistosomiasis is endemic. It's also associated with chronic bladder irritation and infection (for example, from kidney stones, indwelling urinary catheters, and cystitis caused by cyclophosphamide).

Signs and symptoms

In early stages, approximately 25% of patients with bladder tumors have no symptoms. Commonly, the first sign is gross, painless, intermittent hematuria (often with clots in the urine). Patients with invasive lesions often have suprapubic pain after voiding. Other symptoms include bladder irritability, urinary frequency, nocturia, and dribbling.

Diagnosis

Only cystoscopy and biopsy confirm bladder cancer. Cystoscopy should be performed when hematuria first appears. When it is performed under anesthesia, a bimanual examination is usually done to determine if the bladder is fixed to the pelvic wall. A thorough history and physical examination may help determine whether the tumor has invaded the prostate or the lymph nodes. (See *Comparing staging systems for bladder cancer,* page 86.)

The following tests can provide essential information about the tumor:

• *Urinalysis* can detect blood in the urine and malignant cytology.

• *Excretory urography* can identify a large, early-stage tumor or an infiltrating tumor, delineate functional problems in the upper urinary tract, assess hydronephrosis, and detect rigid deformity of the bladder wall.

• *Retrograde cystography* evaluates bladder structure and integrity. Test results help to confirm the diagnosis.

• *Pelvic arteriography* can reveal tumor invasion into the bladder wall.

• *Computed tomography scan* reveals the thickness of the involved bladder wall and detects enlarged retroperitoneal lymph nodes.

• *Ultrasonography* can detect metastasis beyond the bladder and can distinguish a bladder cyst from a tumor.

Treatment

Superficial bladder tumors are removed by transurethral (cystoscopic) resection and fulguration (electrical destruc-

Comparing staging systems for bladder cancer

Staging helps determine the most appropriate treatment for bladder cancer. One of two staging systems may be used: the TNM (*tumor, node, metastasis*) system or the JSM (*Jewett-Strong-Marshall*) system. The JSM system grades cancers 0 and A through D. Both systems distinguish superficial bladder cancers from invasive bladder cancers, which penetrate bladder muscle and may spread to other sites.

TNM	STAGE	JSM
Superficial tumor		
TX	Primary tumor can't be assessed	–
T0	No tumor	0
Tis	Carcinoma in situ	0
Ta	Noninvasive papillary tumor	0
Invasive tumor		
T1	Tumor invades subepithelial connective tissue and lamina propria	A
T2	Tumor invades superficial muscle (inner half)	B_1
T3a	Tumor invades deep muscle	B_2
T3b	Tumor invades perivesical fat	C
T4	Tumor invades prostate, uterus, vagina, pelvic wall, or abdominal wall	D_1
NX	Regional lymph nodes can't be assessed	–
N0	No evidence of lymph node involvement	–
N1	Metastasis in a single lymph node, 2 cm or less in greatest dimension	D_1
N2	Metastasis in a single lymph node, between 2 and 5 cm in greatest dimension, or metastases to several lymph nodes, none greater than 5 cm in greatest dimension	–
N3	Metastasis in a lymph node more than 5 cm in greatest dimension	–
MX	Distant metastasis can't be assessed	–
M0	No evidence of distant metastasis	–
M	Distant metastasis	D_2

tion). This procedure is adequate when the tumor has not invaded the muscle.

Intravesicular chemotherapy is also used for superficial tumors (especially those which occur in many sites) and for preventing tumor recurrence. This treatment involves washing the bladder directly with antineoplastic drugs. Commonly used agents include thiotepa, doxorubicin, mitomycin, and bacille Calmette-Guérin.

If additional tumors develop, fulguration may have to be repeated every 3 months for years. However, if the tumors penetrate the muscle layer or recur frequently, cystoscopy with fulguration is no longer appropriate.

Tumors too large to be treated through a cystoscope require segmental bladder resection to remove a full-thickness section of the bladder. This procedure is feasible only if the tumor isn't near the bladder neck or ureteral orifices. Bladder instillations of thiotepa after transurethral resection may also help control such tumors.

For infiltrating bladder tumors, radical cystectomy is the treatment of choice. The week before cystectomy, treatment may include external beam radiation to the bladder. Surgery involves removal of the bladder and perivesical fat, lymph nodes, urethra, prostate and seminal vesicles (in males), and uterus and adnexa (in females). The surgeon forms a urinary diversion, usually an ileal conduit. The patient must then wear an external pouch continuously. Other diversions include ureterostomy, nephrostomy, vesicostomy, ileal bladder, ileal loop, and sigmoid conduit.

Men are impotent following radical cystectomy and urethrectomy, because these procedures damage the sympathetic and parasympathetic nerves that control erection and ejaculation. At a later date, the patient may desire a penile implant to make sexual intercourse (without ejaculation) possible.

Treatment for patients with advanced bladder cancer includes cystectomy to remove the tumor, radiation therapy, and systemic chemotherapy with such drugs as cyclophosphamide, fluorouracil, doxorubicin, and cisplatin. This combination sometimes is successful in arresting bladder cancer. Cisplatin is the most effective single agent.

Investigational treatments and photodynamic therapy include intravesicular administration of interferon alfa-2a and alfa-2b and tumor necrosis factor. Photodynamic therapy involves I.V. injection of a photosensitizing agent such as hematoporphyrin ether, which malignant cells readily absorb. Then a cystoscopic laser device introduces laser energy into the bladder, exposing the malignant cells to laser light, which kills them. Because this treatment also produces photosensitivity in normal cells, the patient must totally avoid sunlight for about 30 days.

Special
considerations

• Before surgery, select a stoma site that the patient can see (this is usually in the rectus muscle to minimize the risk of herniation). Do so by assessing the abdomen in various positions.

• After surgery, encourage the patient to look at the stoma. If he has difficulty doing this, leave the room briefly while the stoma is exposed. Provide a mirror to make viewing easier.

• To obtain a specimen for culture and sensitivity testing, catheterize the patient, using sterile technique. Insert the lubricated tip of the catheter into the stoma about 2″ (5 cm). In many hospitals, a double telescoping catheter is available for ileal conduit catheterization.

• Advise the patient with a urinary stoma that he may participate in most activities except for heavy lifting and contact sports.

• When a patient with a urinary diversion is discharged, arrange for follow-up home health care or refer him to an enterostomal therapist, who will help coordinate the patient's care.

• Teach the patient about his urinary stoma. Encourage his spouse, a friend, or a relative to attend the teaching session. Advise this person beforehand that a negative reaction to the stoma can impede the patient's adjustment.

• First, show the patient how to prepare and apply the pouch, which may be reusable or disposable. If he chooses the reusable type, he'll need at least two.

• To select the right pouch size, measure the stoma and order a pouch with an opening that clears the stoma with a ⅛″ (0.3-cm) margin.

• Instruct the patient to remeasure the stoma after he goes home, in case the size changes. The pouch should have a drainage valve at the bottom. Tell the patient to empty the pouch when it's one-third full or every 2 to 3 hours.

• To ensure a good skin seal, select a skin barrier that contains synthetics and little or no karaya gum (which urine tends to destroy). Check the pouch frequently to make sure that the skin seal remains intact. A good skin seal with a skin barrier may last for 3 to 6 days, so change the pouch only that often. Tell the patient he can wear a loose-fitting elastic belt to help secure the pouch.

• The ileal conduit stoma reaches its permanent size 2 to 4 months after surgery. Because the intestine normally produces mucus, mucus will appear in the draining urine.

• Tell the patient to keep the skin around the stoma clean and free of irritation. After removing the pouch, he should wash the skin with water and mild soap. Then he should rinse well with clear water to remove soap residue, and then gently pat the skin dry without rubbing. Instruct him to place a gauze sponge soaked with a mixture of one part vinegar and three parts water over the stoma for a few minutes to prevent uric acid crystal buildup.

• Advise the patient that while preparing the skin to place a rolled-up dry sponge over the stoma to collect draining urine. Tell him to coat the skin with a silicone skin protector and cover it with the collection pouch. If skin irritation or breakdown occurs, apply a layer of antacid precipitate to the clean, dry skin before coating with the skin protector.

• Teach the patient that he can level uneven surfaces on his abdomen, such as gullies, scars, or wedges, with a variety of specially prepared products or skin barriers.

• Everyone at high risk for bladder cancer—for example, chemical workers and people with a history of benign bladder tumors or persistent cystitis—should have periodic cytologic examinations and learn about the danger of disease-causing agents.

• Refer ostomates to such resources as the American Cancer Society and the United Ostomy Association.

Gallbladder and bile duct cancers

Gallbladder cancer is rare, accounting for less than 1% of all cancers. It's normally found coincidentally in patients with cholecystitis; 1 in 400 cholecystectomies reveals malignancy. This disease is most prevalent in females over age 60. It's rapidly progressive and usually fatal; patients seldom live a year after diagnosis. The poor prognosis is due to late diagnosis; gallbladder cancer is usually not diagnosed until after cholecystectomy, when it is often in an advanced, metastatic stage.

Extrahepatic bile duct cancer is the cause of approximately 3% of all cancer deaths in the United States. It occurs in both men and women (incidence is slightly higher in men) between ages 60 and 70. The usual site is at the bifurcation in the common duct. Cancer at the distal end of the common duct is often confused with cancer of the pancreas. Characteristically, metastatis occurs in local lymph nodes, the liver, lungs, and peritoneum.

Causes

Many consider gallbladder cancer a complication of gallstones. However, this inference rests on circumstantial evidence from postmortem examinations showing that 60% to 90% of gallbladder cancer patients also have gallstones; but postmortem data from patients with gallstones show gallbladder cancer in only 0.5%.

Adenocarcinoma is the predominant tissue type in gallbladder cancer, accounting for 85% to 95% of cancers; squamous cell cancer accounts for 5% to 15%. Mixed-tissue types are rare.

Lymph node metastasis is present in 25% to 70% of patients at diagnosis. Direct extension to the liver is common (in 46% to 89%); direct extension to both the cystic and the common bile ducts, stomach, colon, duodenum, and jejunum also occurs and produces obstructions. Metastasis also takes place by portal or hepatic veins to the peritoneum, ovaries, and lower lung lobes.

The cause of extrahepatic bile duct cancer isn't known; however, statistics report an unexplained increased incidence of this cancer in patients with ulcerative colitis. This association may be due to a common cause—perhaps an immune mechanism or chronic use of certain drugs by the colitis patient.

Signs and symptoms

Clinically, gallbladder cancer is almost indistinguishable from cholecystitis: pain in the epigastrium or right upper quadrant, weight loss, anorexia, nausea, vomiting, and jaundice. However, chronic, progressively severe pain in an afebrile patient suggests malignancy. In patients with simple gallstones, pain is sporadic. Another telling clue to cancer is a palpable gallbladder (right upper quadrant) with obstructive jaundice. Some patients may also have hepatosplenomegaly.

Progressive profound jaundice is commonly the first sign of obstruction due to extrahepatic bile duct cancer. The jaundice is usually accompanied by chronic pain in the epigastrium or the right upper quadrant, radiating to the back. Other common symptoms, if associated with active cholecystitis, include pruritus, skin excoriations, anorexia, weight loss, chills, and fever.

Diagnosis

The following tests support this diagnosis when they suggest hepatic dysfunction and extrahepatic biliary obstruction:
• *baseline studies* (complete blood count, routine urinalysis, electrolyte studies, enzymes)
• *liver function tests* (serum bilirubin, urine bile and bilirubin, and urobilinogen levels are elevated in more than 50% of patients; serum alkaline phosphatase levels are also elevated)
• *occult blood in stools* (linked to the associated anemia)
• *cholecystography* (may show stones or calcification)
• *cholangiography* (may locate common duct obstruction)
• *magnetic resonance imaging* (detects tumors).

The following tests help compile data that confirm extrahepatic bile duct cancer:
• *liver function studies* (indicate biliary obstruction: elevated levels of bilirubin [5 to 30 mg/dl], alkaline phosphatase, and blood cholesterol; prolonged prothrombin time)
• *endoscopic retrograde cannulization of the pancreas* (identifies the tumor site and allows access for obtaining a biopsy specimen).

Treatment

Surgical treatment of gallbladder cancer is palliative and includes such procedures as cholecystectomy, common bile duct exploration, T-tube drainage, and wedge excision of hepatic tissue. If the cancer invades gallbladder musculature, the survival rate is less than 5%, even with resection. Cases of long-term survival (4 to 5 years) have been reported, but few survive longer than 6 months after surgery.

Surgery may relieve the obstruction and jaundice that result from extrahepatic bile duct cancer. The procedure depends on the cancer site and may include cholecystoduodenostomy or T-tube drainage of the common duct.

Other palliative measures for both kinds of cancers include radiation, radiation implants (for local and incisional recurrences), and chemotherapy (with combinations of fluorouracil, doxorubicin, and lomustine). All have limited effects.

Special considerations

• After biliary resection, monitor vital signs, and use strict aseptic technique when caring for the incision and the surrounding area.
• Place the patient in low Fowler's position.
• Encourage deep breathing and coughing (the high incision makes the patient want to take shallow breaths). Using analgesics and splinting his abdomen with a pillow or an abdominal binder may aid in greater respiratory efforts.
• Monitor bowel sounds and bowel movements. Observe the patient's tolerance of his diet.
• Provide analgesics as needed.
• Check intake and output carefully. Watch for electrolyte imbalance; monitor I.V. solutions to avoid overloading the cardiovascular system.
• Monitor the nasogastric tube (in place for 24 to 72 hours postoperatively to relieve distention) and the T tube. Record amount and color of drainage each shift. Secure the T tube to minimize tension on it and prevent its being pulled out.
• Help the patient and his family cope with their reactions to the diagnosis by offering information and support.
• Teach the patient how to manage the biliary catheter.
• Advise the patient of the adverse effects of chemotherapy and radiation therapy, and monitor him for these effects.

Self-test questions

You can quickly review your comprehension of this chapter on abdominal and pelvic neoplasms by answering the following questions. The correct answers to these questions and their rationales appear on pages 189 to 191.

Case history questions

In response to pleading from his wife, Arlen Harris, who has chronic dyspepsia, makes an appointment with the family doctor. *He tells the doctor that he has had increasing bouts of dyspepsia for the past several months and until recently found antacids effective.*

When weighed, Mr. Harris expresses surprise that he has lost 7 lb (3.2 kg) since his last checkup because he hadn't been dieting. He denies ever seeing blood in his stools. No abnormal findings are revealed during the physical examination. Concerned over the patient's history, however, the doctor orders a GI workup. Diagnostic studies reveal a malignant gastric tumor.

1. Which part of the stomach does gastric cancer most commonly affect?
  a. Pylorus
  b. Cardia
  c. Body of the stomach
  d. Greater curvature

2. Mr. Harris is scheduled for the Billroth II procedure to remove the tumor and adjacent tissue, which involves:
  a. partial removal of the stomach.
  b. total removal of the stomach.
  c. removal of the upper stomach and gallbladder.
  d. removal of the lower stomach and duodenum.

3. If Mr. Harris had an unresectable gastric tumor, radiation therapy might have been prescribed. When receiving radiation therapy, a patient should prepare by:
  a. eating immediately before treatment.
  b. maintaining an empty stomach until after treatment.
  c. drinking a glass of milk 1 hour before treatment.
  d. taking an antacid 30 minutes after treatment.

Additional questions

4. Which of the following is a risk factor for esophageal cancer?
  a. Hypoglycemia
  b. Achalasia
  c. Ulcerative colitis
  d. Anorexia nervosa

5. Which type of cancer most commonly affects the pancreas?

    a. Duct cell adenocarcinoma
    b. Insulinoma
    c. Acinar cell carcinoma
    d. Cystadenocarcinoma

6. A patient with colorectal cancer undergoes a colon resection with a sigmoid colostomy. How often will he have to irrigate his colostomy?
    a. Twice daily
    b. At least once a day
    c. Every 1 to 3 days as needed
    d. Only when constipation occurs

7. Which of the following statements about kidney cancer is true?
    a. Kidney cancer accounts for about 8% of adult cancers.
    b. Kidney cancer is twice as common in men as in women.
    c. Kidney cancer usually strikes after age 60.
    d. The 5-year survival rate for kidney cancer is approximately 20%.

8. A patient with liver cancer will need to restrict dietary intake of:
    a. protein.
    b. potassium.
    c. polyunsaturated fats.
    d. fat-soluble vitamins.

9. The first sign of bladder cancer usually is:
    a. suprapubic pain with full bladder.
    b. urinary tract infection.
    c. incontinence.
    d. hematuria.

10. Which of the following organs may be affected by metastasis of gallbladder cancer?
    a. Brain
    b. Kidneys
    c. Testes
    d. Lungs

CHAPTER 5

Genital Neoplasms

Besides their impact on physiologic function, cancers of the reproductive system have profound implications for the patient's body image and self-esteem.

Prostate cancer

The most common neoplasm in men over age 50, prostate cancer ranks as the second leading cause of male cancer death. Adenocarcinoma is its most common form; only rarely does it occur as a sarcoma. About 85% of prostate cancers originate in the posterior part of the prostate gland; the rest occur near the urethra. Malignant prostate tumors seldom result from the benign enlargement that commonly develops around the prostatic urethra in elderly men. Prostate cancer seldom produces symptoms until it's advanced.

Causes

Although androgens regulate prostate growth and function and may also speed tumor growth, a definite link between increased androgen levels and prostate cancer hasn't been found. When primary prostate lesions metastasize, they typically invade the prostatic capsule and then spread along the ejaculatory ducts in the space between the seminal vesicles or perivesicular fascia.

Prostate cancer accounts for about 18% of all cancers. Unaffected by socioeconomic status or fertility, incidence is highest in blacks and lowest in Asians. Incidence also increases with age more rapidly than any other cancer.

Signs and
symptoms

Prostate cancer's signs and symptoms appear only in the advanced stages and include difficulty initiating a urinary stream, dribbling, urine retention, unexplained cystitis and, rarely, hematuria.

Diagnosis

• *Digital rectal examination* may reveal a small, hard nodule that may help diagnose prostate cancer before symptoms develop. The American Cancer Society advises a yearly digital examination for men over age 40, a yearly blood test to detect prostate-specific antigen (PSA) in men over age 50, and an ultrasound follow-up of any abnormal results.
• *Biopsy* confirms the diagnosis.
• *PSA* levels will be elevated in all cases of prostate cancer.
• *Serum acid phosphatase* levels will be elevated in two-thirds of men with metastatic prostate cancer. Therapy aims to return the serum acid phosphatase level to normal; a subsequent rise points to recurrence.
• *Alkaline phosphatase* levels are elevated in bone metastasis.
• *Bone scan* is positive in bone metastasis.
• *Magnetic resonance imaging, computed tomography scan,* and *excretory urography* may also aid diagnosis.

Treatment

Management of prostate cancer depends on clinical assessment, tolerance of therapy, expected life span, and the stage of the disease. (See *Staging prostate cancer.*) Appropriate treatment must be chosen carefully because prostate cancer usually affects older men, who commonly have coexisting disorders, such as hypertension, diabetes, or cardiac disease.

Therapy varies with each stage of the disease and generally includes radiation, prostatectomy, orchiectomy to reduce androgen production, and hormone therapy with synthetic estrogen (diethylstilbestrol [DES]) and antiandrogens, such as cyproterone, megestrol, and flutamide. Radical prostatectomy is usually effective for localized lesions.

Radiation therapy is used to cure some locally invasive lesions and to relieve pain from metastatic bone involvement. A single injection of the radionuclide strontium 89 is also used to treat pain caused by bone metastasis.

If hormone therapy, surgery, and radiation therapy aren't feasible or successful, chemotherapy (using combinations of

Staging prostate cancer

Developed by the American Joint Committee on Cancer, descriptive categories, known as the TNM (*tumor*, *node*, *metastasis*) cancer staging system, interpret prostate cancer's progress.

Primary tumor
TX—primary tumor can't be assessed
T0—no evidence of primary tumor
T1—tumor an incidental histologic finding
T1a—three or fewer microscopic foci of cancer
T1b—more than three microscopic foci of cancer
T2—tumor limited to the prostate gland
T2a—tumor less than 1.5 cm in greatest dimension, with normal tissue on at least three sides
T2b—tumor larger than 1.5 cm in greatest dimension or present in more than one lobe
T3—unfixed tumor extends into the prostatic apex or into or beyond the prostatic capsule, bladder neck, or seminal vesicle
T4—tumor fixed or invades adjacent structures not listed in T3

Regional lymph nodes
NX—regional lymph nodes can't be assessed
N0—no evidence of regional lymph node metastasis

N1—metastasis in a single lymph node, 2 cm or less in greatest dimension
N2—metastasis in a single lymph node, between 2 and 5 cm in greatest dimension, or metastasis to several lymph nodes, none more than 5 cm in greatest dimension
N3—metastasis in a lymph node more than 5 cm in greatest dimension

Distant metastasis
MX—distant metastasis can't be assessed
M0—no known distant metastasis
M1—distant metastasis

Staging categories
Prostate cancer progresses from mild to severe as follows:
Stage 0 or Stage I—T1a, N0, M0; T2a, N0, M0
Stage II—T1b, N0, M0; T2b, N0, M0
Stage III—T3, N0, M0
Stage IV—T4, N0, M0; any T, N1, M0; any T, N2, M0; any T, N3, M0; any T, any N, M1

---

cyclophosphamide, doxorubicin, fluorouracil, cisplatin, etoposide, and vindesine) may be tried. However, current drug therapy offers limited benefits. Combining several treatment methods may be most effective.

Special considerations

• Plan your care of the patient with prostate cancer to emphasize psychological support, postoperative care, and treatment of radiation's adverse effects.

• Before prostatectomy, explain the expected aftereffects of surgery (such as impotence and incontinence) and radiation. Discuss tube placement and dressing changes.

• Teach the patient to do perineal exercises 1 to 10 times an hour. Have him squeeze his buttocks together, hold this position for a few seconds, and then relax.

• After prostatectomy or suprapubic prostatectomy, regularly check the dressing, incision, and drainage systems for excessive bleeding; also watch the patient for signs of bleeding (pallor, falling blood pressure, or rising pulse rate) and infection.

• Maintain adequate fluid intake.

• Give antispasmodics to control postoperative bladder spasms. Give analgesics as needed.

• Urinary incontinence is common after surgery; keep the patient's skin clean, dry, and free of drainage and urine.

• Encourage perineal exercises within 24 to 48 hours after surgery.

• Provide meticulous catheter care – especially if a three-way catheter with a continuous irrigation system is in place. Check the tubing for kinks and blockages, especially if the patient reports pain. Warn him not to pull on the catheter.

• After transurethral resection, watch for signs of urethral stricture (dysuria, decreased force and caliber of urinary stream, and straining to urinate) and for abdominal distention (from urethral stricture or catheter blockage). Irrigate the catheter as ordered.

• After perineal prostatectomy, avoid taking a rectal temperature or inserting any kind of rectal tube. Provide pads to absorb urine leakage, a rubber ring for the patient to sit on, and sitz baths for pain and inflammation.

• After perineal and retropubic prostatectomy, explain that urine leakage after catheter removal is normal and will subside.

• When a patient receives hormonal therapy, watch for adverse effects. Gynecomastia, fluid retention, nausea, and vomiting are common with DES. Thrombophlebitis may also occur, especially with DES.

• After radiation therapy, watch for common adverse effects: proctitis, diarrhea, bladder spasms, and urinary frequency. Internal radiation usually results in cystitis in the first 2 to 3 weeks. Urge the patient to drink at least 2,000 ml of fluid daily. Provide analgesics and antispasmodics as needed.

Testicular cancer

Malignant testicular tumors primarily affect young to middle-aged men and are the most common solid tumor in this group. (In children, testicular tumors are rare.) Most testicular tumors originate in gonadal cells. About 40% are seminomas – uniform, undifferentiated cells resembling primitive gonadal cells. The remainder are nonseminomas – tumor cells showing various degrees of differentiation.

The prognosis varies with the cell type and disease stage. When treated with surgery and radiation, almost all patients with localized disease survive beyond 5 years.

Causes

The cause of testicular cancer isn't known, but incidence is higher in men with cryptorchidism (even when surgically corrected) and in men whose mothers used diethylstilbestrol during pregnancy. Testicular cancer is rare in nonwhite males and accounts for less than 1% of all male cancer deaths. It spreads through the lymphatic system to the iliac, preaortic, and mediastinal lymph nodes, with metastasis to the lungs, liver, viscera, and bone.

Signs and symptoms

The first sign is usually a firm, painless, smooth testicular mass, varying in size and sometimes producing a sense of testicular heaviness. When such a tumor causes chorionic gonadotropin or estrogen production, gynecomastia and nipple tenderness may result. In advanced stages, signs and symptoms include ureteral obstruction, abdominal mass, cough, hemoptysis, shortness of breath, weight loss, fatigue, pallor, and lethargy.

Diagnosis

Two effective means of detecting a testicular tumor are regular self-examinations and testicular palpation during routine physical examination. Transillumination can distinguish between a tumor (which doesn't transilluminate) and a hydrocele or spermatocele (which does). Follow-up measures should include an examination for gynecomastia and abdominal masses.

Diagnostic tests include excretory urography to detect ureteral deviation resulting from preaortic node involvement, urinary or serum luteinizing hormone levels, blood tests, lymphangiography, ultrasound, and abdominal computed tomography scan. Serum alpha-fetoprotein and beta-human chorionic gonadotropin levels — indicators of testicular tumor activity — provide a baseline for measuring response to therapy and determining the prognosis.

Surgical excision and biopsy of the tumor and testis permits histologic verification of the tumor cell type — essential for effective treatment. Inguinal exploration determines the extent of nodal involvement.

Treatment

The extent of surgery, radiation, and chemotherapy varies with tumor cell type and stage. (See *Staging testicular cancer.*) Surgery includes orchiectomy and retroperitoneal node dissection. Most surgeons remove the testis, not the scrotum (to allow for a prosthetic implant). Hormone replacement therapy is sometimes necessary after bilateral orchiectomy.

Radiation of the retroperitoneal and homolateral iliac nodes follows removal of a seminoma. All positive nodes receive radiation after removal of a nonseminoma. A patient with retroperitoneal extension receives prophylactic radiation to the mediastinal and supraclavicular nodes.

Essential for tumors beyond Stage 0, chemotherapy consists of combinations of bleomycin, etoposide, and cisplatin; cisplatin, vindesine, and bleomycin; cisplatin, vinblastine, and bleomycin; or cisplatin, vincristine, methotrexate, bleomycin, and leucovorin. Chemotherapy and radiation followed by autologous bone marrow transplantation may help unresponsive patients.

Special considerations

• Plan your care so that it addresses both the patient's psychological and physical needs.
• Before orchiectomy, reassure the patient that sterility and impotence need not follow unilateral orchiectomy, that synthetic hormones can restore hormonal balance, and that most surgeons don't remove the scrotum. In many cases, a testicular prosthesis can correct anatomic disfigurement.

Staging testicular cancer

Using the TNM (*tumor*, *node*, *metastasis*) system, the American Joint Committee on Cancer has established the following stages for testicular cancer.

Primary tumor
TX—primary tumor can't be assessed (this stage is used in the absence of radical orchiectomy)
T0—histologic scar or no evidence of primary tumor
Tis—intratubular tumor: preinvasive cancer
T1—tumor limited to testicles, including the rete testis
T2—tumor extends beyond tunica albuginea or into epididymis
T3—tumor extends into spermatic cord
T4—tumor invades scrotum

Regional lymph nodes
NX—regional lymph nodes can't be assessed
N0—no evidence of regional lymph node metastasis
N1—metastasis in a single lymph node, 2 cm or less in greatest dimension

N2—metastasis in a single lymph node, between 2 and 5 cm in greatest dimension, or metastasis to several lymph nodes, none more than 5 cm in greatest dimension
N3—metastasis in a lymph node more than 5 cm in greatest dimension

Distant metastasis
MX—distant metastasis can't be assessed
M0—no known distant metastasis
M1—distant metastasis

Staging categories
Testicular cancer progresses from mild to severe as follows:
Stage 0—Tis, N0, M0
Stage I—T1, N0, M0; T2, N0, M0
Stage II—T3, N0, M0; T4, N0, M0
Stage III—any T, N1, M0
Stage IV—any T, N2, M0; any T, N3, M0; any T, any N, M1

• After orchiectomy, for the first day after surgery, apply an ice pack to the scrotum and provide analgesics as needed.
• Check for excessive bleeding, swelling, and signs of infection.
• Provide a scrotal athletic supporter to minimize pain during ambulation.
• During chemotherapy, give antiemetics as needed for nausea and vomiting. Encourage small, frequent meals to maintain oral intake despite anorexia. Establish a mouth care regimen and check for stomatitis. Watch for signs of myelosuppression. If the patient receives vinblastine, assess for neurotoxicity (peripheral paresthesia, jaw pain, and muscle cramps). If he receives cisplatin, check for ototoxicity. To prevent renal damage, encourage increased fluid intake and

provide I.V. fluids, a potassium supplement, and diuretics as needed.

Penile cancer

Circumcised men in modern cultures are rarely affected by penile cancer; when it does occur, it's usually in men who are over age 50. The most common form, epidermoid squamous cell carcinoma, is usually found in the glans but may also occur on the corona glandis, and, rarely, in the preputial cavity. This cancer produces ulcerative or papillary (wartlike, nodular) lesions, which may become quite large before spreading beyond the penis; such lesions may destroy the glans prepuce and invade the corpora.

Prognosis varies according to staging at time of diagnosis. If begun early enough, radiation therapy increases the 5-year survival rate to over 60%; surgery only, to over 55%. Unfortunately, many men delay treatment of penile cancer, because they fear disfigurement and loss of sexual function.

Causes

The exact cause of penile cancer is unknown; however, it's generally associated with poor personal hygiene and phimosis in uncircumcised men. This may account for the low incidence among Jews and people of other cultures that practice circumcision at birth or shortly thereafter. (Incidence isn't decreased in cultures that practice circumcision at a later date.) Early circumcision seems to prevent penile cancer by allowing for better personal hygiene and minimizing inflammatory (and precancerous) lesions of the glans and prepuce. Such lesions include:
• leukoplakia—inflammation, with thickened patches that may fissure
• balanitis—inflammation of the penis associated with phimosis
• erythroplasia of Queyrat—squamous cell carcinoma in situ; velvety, erythematous lesion that becomes scaly and ulcerative
• penile horn—scaly, horn-shaped growth.

Signs and symptoms	In a circumcised man, early signs of penile cancer include a small circumscribed lesion, a pimple, or a sore on the penis. In an uncircumcised man, however, such early symptoms may go unnoticed, so penile cancer first becomes apparent when it causes late-stage symptoms, such as pain, hemorrhage, dysuria, purulent discharge, and obstruction of the urinary meatus. Rarely is metastasis the first sign of penile cancer.
Diagnosis	Positive diagnosis of penile cancer requires a tissue biopsy. Preoperative baseline studies include complete blood count, urinalysis, an electrocardiogram, and a chest X-ray. Enlarged inguinal lymph nodes resulting from infection (caused by the primary lesion) makes detection of nodal metastasis by a preoperative computed tomography scan difficult.
Treatment	Depending on the stage of the disease, treatment includes surgical resection of the primary tumor and, possibly, chemotherapy and radiation. Local tumors of the prepuce only require circumcision. Invasive tumors, however, require a partial penectomy if there is at least a 2-cm tumor-free margin; tumors of the base of the penile shaft require total penectomy and inguinal node dissection (done less often in the United States than in other countries where incidence is higher).

Radiation therapy may improve treatment effectiveness after resection of localized lesions without metastasis; it may also reduce the size of lymph nodes before nodal resection but is not adequate primary treatment for groin metastasis. Topical fluorouracil is used for precancerous lesions. A combination of bleomycin, methotrexate, and cisplatin is used for metastasis.

Special considerations	• Penile cancer calls for good patient teaching, psychological support, and comprehensive postoperative care. The patient with penile cancer fears disfigurement, pain, and loss of sexual function.

• Before penile surgery, spend time with the patient, and encourage him to talk about his fears.

• Supplement and reinforce patient teaching about the surgery and other treatment measures, and explain expected postoperative procedures, such as dressing changes and catheterization.

• Show the patient diagrams of the surgical procedure and pictures of the results of similar surgery to help him adapt to an altered body image.

• If the patient needs urinary diversion, refer him to the enterostomal therapist.

• After penectomy, constantly monitor the patient's vital signs and record his intake and output accurately.

• Provide comprehensive skin care to prevent skin breakdown from urinary diversion or suprapubic catheterization. Keep the skin dry and free from urine. If the patient has a suprapubic catheter, make sure the catheter is patent at all times.

• Administer analgesics as needed. Elevate the penile stump with a small towel or pillow to minimize edema.

• Check the surgical site often for signs of infection, such as foul odor or excessive drainage on dressing.

• If the patient has had inguinal node dissection, watch for signs of lymphedema, such as decreased circulation or disproportionate swelling of a leg.

• After partial penectomy, reassure the patient that the penile stump should be sufficient for urination and sexual function. New surgical reconstructive techniques are 90% successful. Refer him for psychological or sexual counseling.

Cervical cancer

The third most common cancer of the female reproductive system, cervical cancer is classified as either preinvasive or invasive.

Preinvasive cancer ranges from minimal cervical dysplasia, in which the lower third of the epithelia contains abnormal cells, to carcinoma in situ, in which the full thickness of epithelia contains abnormally proliferating cells (also known as cervical intraepithelial neoplasia). Preinvasive cancer is curable 75% to 90% of the time with early detection and proper treatment. If untreated, it may progress to invasive cervical cancer (depending on the form in which it appears).

In invasive carcinoma, cancer cells penetrate the basement membrane and can spread directly to contiguous pelvic structures or disseminate to distant sites by lymphatic routes. Invasive carcinoma of the uterine cervix is responsible for 4,500 deaths annually in the United States alone. In almost all cases (95%), the histologic type is squamous cell carcinoma, which varies from well-differentiated cells to highly anaplastic spindle cells. Only 5% are adenocarcinomas. Invasive carcinoma usually occurs between ages 30 and 50; it rarely occurs under age 20.

Causes

While the cause is unknown, several predisposing factors have been related to the development of cervical cancer: frequent intercourse at a young age (under age 16), multiple sexual partners, multiple pregnancies, and herpes virus II and other venereal infections.

Signs and symptoms

Preinvasive cervical cancer produces no symptoms or other clinically apparent changes. Early invasive cervical cancer causes abnormal vaginal bleeding, persistent vaginal discharge, and postcoital pain and bleeding. In advanced stages, it causes pelvic pain, vaginal leakage of urine and feces from a fistula, anorexia, weight loss, and anemia.

Diagnosis

A cytologic examination (Papanicolaou [Pap] test) can detect cervical cancer before clinical evidence appears. (Systems of Pap test classification may vary from hospital to hospital.) Abnormal cervical cytology routinely calls for colposcopy, which can detect the presence and extent of preclinical lesions requiring biopsy and histologic examination.

Staining with Lugol's solution (strong iodine) or Schiller's solution (iodine, potassium iodide, and purified water) may identify areas for biopsy when the results disclose abnormal cells but there's no obvious lesion. Although the tests are nonspecific, they do distinguish between normal and abnormal tissues: Normal tissues absorb the iodine and turn brown; abnormal tissues are devoid of glycogen and won't change color. Additional studies, such as lymphangiogra-

Staging cervical cancer

Treatment decisions depend on accurate staging. The International Federation of Gynecology and Obstetrics defines cervical cancer stages as follows.

Stage 0
Carcinoma in situ, intraepithelial carcinoma

Stage I
Cancer confined to the cervix (extension to the corpus should be disregarded)

Stage IA
Preclinical malignant lesions of the cervix (diagnosed only microscopically)

Stage IA1
Minimal microscopically evident stromal invasion

Stage IA2
Lesions detected microscopically, measuring 5 mm or less from the base of the epithelium, either surface or glandular, from which it originates; lesion width shouldn't exceed 7 mm

Stage IB
Lesions measuring more than 5 mm deep and 7 mm wide, whether seen clinically or not (preformed spatial involvement shouldn't alter the staging but should be recorded for future treatment decisions)

Stage II
Extension beyond the cervix but not to the pelvic wall; cancer involves the vagina but hasn't spread to the lower third

Stage IIA
No obvious parametrial involvement

Stage IIB
Obvious parametrial involvement

Stage III
Extension to the pelvic wall; on rectal examination, no cancer-free space exists between the tumor and the pelvic wall; tumor involves the lower third of the vagina; this includes all cases with hydronephrosis or nonfunctioning kidney

Stage IIIA
No extension to the pelvic wall

Stage IIIB
Extension to the pelvic wall and hydronephrosis or nonfunctioning kidney, or both

Stage IV
Extension beyond the true pelvis or involvement of the bladder or the rectal mucosa

Stage IVA
Spread to adjacent organs

Stage IVB
Spread to distant organs

---

phy, cystography, and major organ and bone scans, can detect metastasis. (See *Staging cervical cancer.*)

Treatment   Appropriate treatment depends on accurate clinical staging. Preinvasive lesions may be treated with total excisional biopsy, cryosurgery, laser destruction, ionization (and frequent Pap test follow-up), or, rarely, hysterectomy. Therapy for invasive squamous cell carcinoma may include radical hysterectomy and radiation therapy (internal, external, or both).

Special considerations

• Management of cervical cancer requires skilled preoperative and postoperative care, comprehensive patient teaching, and emotional and psychological support.

• If the patient is having a biopsy, drape and prepare her as for a routine Pap test and pelvic examination. Have a container of formaldehyde ready to preserve the specimen during transfer to the pathology lab. Explain to the patient that she may feel pressure, minor abdominal cramps, or a pinch from the punch forceps. Reassure her that pain will be minimal, because the cervix has few nerve endings.

• If the patient will undergo cryosurgery, drape and prepare her as for a routine Pap test and pelvic examination. Explain that the procedure takes approximately 15 minutes, during which time a refrigerant will be used to freeze the cervix. Warn the patient that she may experience abdominal cramps, headache, and sweating, but reassure her that she'll feel little, if any, pain.

• If the patient is having laser therapy, drape and prepare her as for a routine Pap test and pelvic examination. Explain that the procedure takes approximately 30 minutes and may cause abdominal cramps.

• After excisional biopsy, cryosurgery, and laser therapy, tell the patient to expect a discharge or spotting for about 1 week after these procedures, and advise her not to douche, use tampons, or engage in sexual intercourse during this time. Tell her to watch for and report signs of infection. Stress the need for a follow-up Pap test and a pelvic examination within 3 to 4 months after these procedures and periodically thereafter.

• Teach the patient what to expect postoperatively if a hysterectomy is necessary.

• After surgery, monitor vital signs every 4 hours.

• Watch for signs of complications after surgery, such as bleeding, abdominal distention, severe pain, and breathing difficulties.

• Administer analgesics, prophylactic antibiotics, and S.C. heparin as needed.

• Encourage deep breathing and coughing.

• Find out if the patient is to have internal or external therapy, or both. Usually, internal radiation therapy is the first procedure.

• Explain that external outpatient radiation therapy, when necessary, continues for 4 to 6 weeks. The patient may be hospitalized for a course of internal radiation treatment (an intracavitary implant of radium, cesium, or some other radioactive material).

• Explain the internal radiation procedure, and answer the patient's questions. Internal radiation requires a 2- to 3-day hospital stay, bowel preparation, a povidone-iodine vaginal douche, a clear liquid diet, and nothing by mouth the night before the implantation; it also requires an indwelling urinary catheter.

• Tell the patient that the procedure is performed in the operating room under general anesthesia and that a radium applicator is inserted.

• Remember that safety precautions — time, distance, and shielding — begin as soon as the radioactive source is in place. Inform the patient that she'll require a private room.

• Encourage the patient to lie flat and limit movement while the implant is in place. If she prefers, elevate the head of the bed slightly.

• Check vital signs every 4 hours; watch for skin reaction, vaginal bleeding, abdominal discomfort, or evidence of dehydration. Make sure the patient can reach everything she needs without stretching or straining.

• Assist the patient in range-of-motion *arm* exercises (leg exercises and other body movements could dislodge the implant).

• If necessary, administer a tranquilizer to help the patient relax and remain still.

• Organize the time you spend with the patient to minimize your exposure to radiation.

• Inform visitors of safety precautions, and hang a sign listing these precautions on the patient's door.

• Teach the patient to watch for and report uncomfortable adverse effects. Because radiation therapy may increase susceptibility to infection by lowering the white blood cell

count, warn the patient to avoid persons with obvious infections during therapy.
• Instruct the patient to use a vaginal dilator to prevent vaginal stenosis and to facilitate vaginal examinations and sexual intercourse.
• Reassure the patient that this disease and its treatment shouldn't radically alter her lifestyle or prohibit sexual intimacy.

Uterine cancer

The most common gynecologic cancer, uterine cancer (cancer of the endometrium) usually affects postmenopausal women between ages 50 and 60; it's uncommon between ages 30 and 40 and extremely rare before age 30. Most premenopausal women who develop uterine cancer have a history of anovulatory menstrual cycles or other hormonal imbalances. An average of 33,000 new cases of uterine cancer are reported annually; of these, 5,500 are eventually fatal.

Causes

Uterine cancer seems linked to several predisposing factors:
• low fertility index and anovulation
• abnormal uterine bleeding
• obesity, hypertension, or diabetes
• familial tendency
• history of uterine polyps or endometrial hyperplasia
• estrogen therapy (without progesterone).

Uterine cancer is typically an adenocarcinoma that metastasizes late, usually from the endometrium to the cervix, ovaries, fallopian tubes, and other peritoneal structures. It may spread to distant organs, such as the lungs and the brain, through the blood or the lymphatic system. Lymph node involvement can also occur. Less common uterine tumors include adenoacanthoma, endometrial stromal sarcoma, lymphosarcoma, mixed mesodermal tumors (including carcinosarcoma), and leiomyosarcoma.

Signs and
symptoms

Uterine enlargement and persistent and unusual premenopausal bleeding, or any postmenopausal bleeding, are the
most common indications of uterine cancer. The discharge
may at first be watery and blood-streaked but gradually becomes more bloody. Other symptoms, such as pain and
weight loss, don't appear until the cancer is well advanced.

Diagnosis

Unfortunately, a Papanicolaou test, so useful for detecting
cervical cancer, doesn't dependably predict early-stage
uterine cancer. Diagnosis of uterine cancer requires endometrial, cervical, and endocervical biopsies. Negative biopsies call for a fractional dilatation and curettage to determine
the diagnosis. Positive diagnosis requires the following tests
for baseline data and staging:
• *multiple cervical biopsies* and *endocervical curettage* to
pinpoint cervical involvement
• *Schiller's test,* staining the cervix and vagina with an iodine
solution that turns healthy tissues brown; cancerous tissues
resist the stain
• *complete physical examination*
• *chest X-ray* or *computed tomography scan*
• *excretory urography* and, possibly, *cystoscopy*
• *complete blood studies*
• *electrocardiogram*
• *proctoscopy* or *barium enema studies* if bladder and rectal
involvement are suspected. (See *Staging uterine cancer.*)

Treatment

Appropriate treatment varies, depending on the extent of the
disease. Surgery, rarely curative, generally involves total abdominal hysterectomy, bilateral salpingo-oophorectomy, or
possibly omentectomy with or without pelvic or preaortic
lymphadenectomy. Total exenteration involves removal of all
pelvic organs, including the vagina, and is done only when
the disease is sufficiently contained to allow surgical removal of diseased parts. (See *Managing pelvic exenteration,*
page 112.)
Radiation therapy may be used when the tumor isn't well
differentiated. Intracavitary or external radiation, or both,
given 6 weeks before surgery, may inhibit recurrence and
lengthen survival time.
Hormonal therapy, using synthetic progesterones – such
as megestrol or medroxyprogesterone – may be adminis-

Staging uterine cancer

The International Federation of Gynecology and Obstetrics defines uterine (endometrial) cancer stages as follows.

Stage 0
Carcinoma in situ

Stage I
Carcinoma confined to the corpus

Stage IA
Length of the uterine cavity 8 cm or less

Stage IB
Length of the uterine cavity more than 8 cm; stage I cases are subgrouped by the following histologic grades of the adenocarcinoma:

G1 — Highly differentiated adenomatous carcinoma

G2 — Moderately differentiated adenomatous carcinoma with partly solid areas

G3 — Predominantly solid or entirely undifferentiated carcinoma

Stage II
Carcinoma has involved the corpus and the cervix but has not extended outside the uterus

Stage III
Carcinoma has extended outside the uterus but not outside the true pelvis

Stage IV
Carcinoma has extended outside the true pelvis or has obviously involved the mucosa of the bladder or rectum

Stage IVA
Spread to adjacent organs

Stage IVB
Spread to distant organs

---

tered for systemic disease. Tamoxifen (which produces a 20% to 40% response rate) may be given as a second line of treatment.

Chemotherapy, using varying combinations of cisplatin, doxorubicin, etoposide, and dactinomycin is usually tried when other treatments have failed.

Special considerations

• Provide patients with uterine cancer with as much patient teaching as possible to help them cope with surgery, radiation, and chemotherapy. Also provide comprehensive postoperative care and psychological support.
• Before surgery, reinforce your patient teaching about the surgery, and explain the routine tests (repeated blood tests the morning after surgery) and postoperative care. If the patient is to have a lymphadenectomy *and* a total hysterec-

Managing pelvic exenteration

Before pelvic exenteration
• Teach the patient about ileal conduit and possible colostomy, and make sure the patient understands that her vagina will be removed.
• To minimize the risk of infection, supervise a rigorous bowel and skin preparation procedure. Decrease the residue in the patient's diet for 48 to 72 hours, then maintain a diet ranging from clear liquids to nothing by mouth. Administer oral or I.V. antibiotics, as ordered, and prepare skin daily with antibacterial soap.
• Instruct the patient about postoperative procedures and prepare her to have I.V. therapy, a central venous pressure catheter, a blood drainage system, and an unsutured perineal wound with gauze packing.

After pelvic exenteration
• Check the stoma, incision, and perineal wound for drainage. Be especially careful to check the perineal wound for bleeding after the packing is removed. Expect red or serosanguineous drainage, but suspect a complication if drainage is excessive, continuously bright red, foul-smelling, or purulent, or if there's bleeding from the conduit.
• Provide excellent skin care because of draining urine and feces. Use warm water and saline solution to clean the skin because soap may be too drying and may increase skin breakdown.

tomy, explain that she'll probably have a blood drainage system for about 5 days after surgery.
• Explain how to care for the indwelling urinary catheter.
• Fit the patient with antiembolism stockings for use during and after surgery.
• Make sure the patient's blood has been typed and cross-matched.
• If the patient is premenopausal, inform her that removal of her ovaries will induce menopause.
• After surgery, the fluid contents of the blood drainage system should not exceed 400 ml. Measure the fluid contents of the drainage system every shift.
• If the patient has received S.C. heparin, continue administration until the patient is fully ambulatory again. Give prophylactic antibiotics and provide good care of the indwelling urinary catheter.
• Check vital signs every 4 hours. Watch for any sign of complications, such as bleeding, abdominal distention, severe pain, and wheezing or other breathing difficulties. Provide analgesics as needed.

• Regularly encourage the patient to breathe deeply and cough to help prevent complications. Promote the use of an incentive spirometer once every waking hour to help keep the lungs expanded.

• Find out if the patient is to have internal or external radiation or both. Usually, internal radiation therapy is done first.

• Explain the internal radiation procedure, answer the patient's questions, and encourage her to express her fears and concerns.

• Explain that internal radiation usually requires a 2- to 3-day hospital stay, bowel preparation, a povidone-iodine vaginal douche, a clear liquid diet, and nothing taken by mouth the night before implantation.

• Mention that internal radiation also requires an indwelling urinary catheter.

• Tell the patient that if the procedure is performed in the operating room, she will receive a general anesthetic. She will be placed in a dorsal position, with her knees and hips flexed, and her heels resting in footrests. Explain further that the radiation source may be implanted in the vagina by the doctor, or by a member of the radiation team while the patient is in her room.

• Remember that safety precautions, including time, distance, and shielding, must be imposed immediately after the patient's radioactive source has been implanted. (See *Internal radiation safety precautions,* page 114.)

• Tell the patient that she'll require a private room.

• Encourage the patient to limit movement while the source is in place. If she prefers, elevate the head of the bed slightly. Make sure the patient can reach everything she needs (call bell, telephone, water) without stretching or straining.

• Assist the patient in range-of-motion arm exercises (leg exercises and other body movements could dislodge the source).

• If necessary, administer a tranquilizer to help the patient relax and remain still.

• Organize the time you spend with the patient to minimize your exposure to radiation.

• Check the patient's vital signs every 4 hours; watch for a skin reaction, vaginal bleeding, abdominal discomfort, or evidence of dehydration.

Internal radiation safety precautions

Keep in mind three cardinal safety requirements when caring for a patient undergoing internal radiation therapy.

Time
Wear a radiosensitive badge. Remember, your exposure increases with time, and the effects are cumulative. Therefore, carefully plan the time you spend with the patient to prevent overexposure. (However, don't rush procedures, ignore the patient's psychological needs, or give the impression that you can't get out of the room fast enough.)

Distance
Radiation loses its intensity with distance. Avoid standing at the foot of the patient's bed, where you're in line with the radiation.

Shield
Lead shields reduce radiation exposure. Use them whenever possible.

In internal radiation therapy, remember that the patient is radioactive while the radiation source is in place—usually 48 to 72 hours.
• Pregnant women should not be assigned to care for radiation patients.
• Check the position of the source applicator every 4 hours. If it appears dislodged, notify the doctor immediately. If it's completely dislodged, remove the patient from the bed; pick up the applicator with long forceps, place it on a lead-shielded transport cart, and notify the doctor immediately.
• *Never* pick up the source with your bare hands. Notify the radiation safety officer whenever there's an accident, and keep a lead-shielded transport cart on the unit as long as the patient has a source in place.

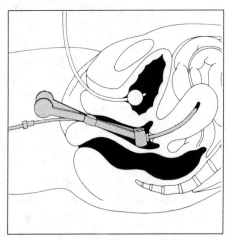

Positioning of internal radiation applicator for uterine cancer

• Inform visitors of safety precautions and hang a sign listing these precautions on the patient's door.
• If the patient receives external radiation, teach her and her family about the therapy before it begins. Tell them that treatment is usually given 5 days a week for 6 weeks. Warn the patient not to scrub body areas marked with indelible ink for treatment, because it's important to direct treatment to exactly the same area each time.

• Instruct the patient to maintain a high-protein, high-carbo hydrate, low-residue diet to reduce bulk and yet maintain calories.

• Administer diphenoxylate with atropine as needed to minimize diarrhea, a possible adverse effect of pelvic radiation.

• To minimize skin breakdown and reduce the risk of skin infection, tell the patient to keep the treatment area dry, to avoid wearing clothes that rub against the area, and to avoid using heating pads, alcohol rubs, or any skin creams.

• Teach the patient how to use a vaginal dilator to prevent vaginal stenosis and facilitate vaginal examinations and sexual intercourse.

• Remember, a uterine cancer patient needs special counseling and psychological support to help her cope with this disease and the necessary treatment. Fearful about her survival, she may also be concerned that treatment will alter her lifestyle and prevent sexual intimacy.

• Explain that except in total pelvic exenteration, the vagina remains intact and that once she recovers, sexual intercourse is possible.

• Your presence and interest alone will help the patient, even if you can't answer every question she may ask.

Vaginal cancer

A rare gynecologic cancer, vaginal cancer usually appears as squamous cell carcinoma, but occasionally as melanoma, sarcoma, or adenocarcinoma (clear cell adenocarcinoma has an increased incidence in young women whose mothers took diethylstilbestrol). Vaginal cancer generally occurs in women in their early to mid-50s, but some of the rarer types do occur in younger women, and rhabdomyosarcoma appears in children.

Causes

In most cases, the cause of vaginal cancer is unknown. The exception is with clear cell carcinoma, which has been linked to intrauterine exposure to diethylstilbestrol. Other suspected causes include the herpesviruses. Vaginal cancer varies in severity according to its location and effect on lymphatic drainage. (The vagina is a thin-walled structure with rich lymphatic drainage.) Vaginal cancer is similar to cervical cancer in that it may progress from an intraepithelial tumor to an invasive cancer. However, it spreads more slowly than cervical cancer.

A lesion in the upper third of the vagina (the most common site) usually metastasizes to the groin nodes; a lesion in the lower third (the second most common site) usually metastasizes to the hypogastric and iliac nodes; but a lesion in the middle third metastasizes erratically. A posterior lesion displaces and distends the vaginal posterior wall before spreading to deep layers. By contrast, an anterior lesion spreads more rapidly into other structures and deep layers, because unlike the posterior wall, the anterior vaginal wall is not flexible.

Signs and symptoms

Commonly, the patient with vaginal cancer has experienced abnormal bleeding and discharge. Also, she may have a small or large, often firm, ulcerated lesion in any part of the vagina. As the cancer progresses, it commonly spreads to the bladder (producing frequent voiding and bladder pain), the rectum (bleeding), vulva (lesion), pubic bone (pain), or other surrounding tissues.

Diagnosis

The diagnosis of vaginal cancer is based on the presence of abnormal cells on a vaginal Papanicolaou test. Careful examination and biopsy rule out the cervix and vulva as the primary sites of the lesion. In many cases, however, the cervix contains the primary lesion that has metastasized to the vagina. In such cases, a biopsy is performed on any visible lesion, and the specimen is evaluated histologically. (See *Staging vaginal cancer.*)

Visualization of the entire vagina is sometimes difficult because the speculum blades may hide a lesion, or the patient may be uncooperative because of discomfort. When lesions are not visible, colposcopy is used to search out abnormalities. Painting the suspected vaginal area with Lugol's solution also helps identify malignant areas by staining glycogen-containing normal tissue, while leaving abnormal tissue unstained.

Staging vaginal cancer

The International Federation of Gynecology and Obstetrics has established this staging system as a guide to the treatment and the prognosis of vaginal cancer.

Stage 0
Carcinoma in situ; intraepithelial carcinoma

Stage I
Carcinoma limited to the vaginal wall

Stage II
Carcinoma has involved the subvaginal tissue but has not extended to the pelvic wall

Stage III
Carcinoma has extended to the pelvic wall

Stage IV
Carcinoma has extended beyond the true pelvis or has involved the mucosa of the bladder or rectum

Treatment

In early stages, treatment aims to preserve the normal parts of the vagina. Topical chemotherapy with fluorouracil and laser surgery can be used for stages 0 and I. Radiation or surgery varies with the size, depth, and location of the lesion and the patient's desire to maintain a functional vagina. Preservation of a functional vagina is possible only in the early stages. Survival rates are the same for patients treated with radiation as for those with surgery.

Surgery is usually recommended only when the tumor is so extensive that exenteration is needed, because close proximity to the bladder and rectum permits only minimal tissue margins around resected vaginal tissue.

Radiation therapy is the preferred treatment for advanced vaginal cancer. Most patients need preliminary external radiation treatment to shrink the tumor before internal radiation can begin. Then, if the tumor is localized to the vault and the cervix is present, radiation (using radium or cesium) can be given with an intrautcrine tandem or ovoids; if the cervix is absent, a specially designed vaginal applicator is used instead.

To minimize complications, radioactive sources and filters are carefully placed away from radiosensitive tissues, such as the bladder and rectum. Internal radiation lasts 48 to 72 hours, depending on the dosage.

Special
considerations

• Explain the internal radiation procedure, answer the patient's questions, and encourage her to express her fears and concerns.
• Because the effects of radiation are cumulative, wear a radiosensitive badge and a lead shield (if available) when you enter the patient's room.
• Check with the radiation therapist concerning the maximum recommended time that you can safely spend with the patient when giving direct care.
• While the radiation source is in place, the patient must lie flat on her back. Insert an indwelling urinary catheter (usually done in the operating room), and do not change the patient's linens unless they are soiled. Give only partial bed baths, and make sure the patient has a call bell, phone, water, or anything else she needs within easy reach. The patient will need a clear liquid or low-residue diet and an antidiarrheal drug to prevent bowel movements.
• To compensate for immobility, encourage the patient to do active range-of-motion exercises with both arms.
• Before radiation treatment, explain the necessity of immobilization, and tell the patient what it entails (such as no linen changes and the use of an indwelling urinary catheter). Throughout therapy, encourage her to express her anxieties.
• Instruct the patient to use a stent or do prescribed exercises to prevent vaginal stenosis. Coitus is also helpful in preventing stenosis.

Ovarian cancer

After cancer of the lung, breast, and colon, primary ovarian cancer ranks as the most common cause of cancer deaths among American women. In women with previously treated breast cancer, metastatic ovarian cancer is more common than cancer at any other site.

Prognosis varies with the histologic type and stage of the disease but is generally poor because ovarian tumors produce few early signs and are usually advanced at diagnosis. Although about 40% of women with ovarian cancer survive for 5 years, the overall survival rate has not improved significantly.

Three main types of ovarian cancer exist:

• Primary epithelial tumors account for 90% of all ovarian cancers and include serous cystadenocarcinoma, mucinous cystadenocarcinoma, and endometrioid and mesonephric malignancies. Serous cystadenocarcinoma is the most common type and accounts for 50% of all cases.

• Germ cell tumors include endodermal sinus malignancies, embryonal carcinoma (a rare ovarian cancer that appears in children), immature teratomas, and dysgerminoma.

• Sex cord (stromal) tumors include granulosa cell tumors (which produce estrogen and may have feminizing effects), granulosa-theca cell tumors, and rare arrhenoblastomas (which produce androgen and have virilizing effects).

Causes

Exactly what causes ovarian cancer isn't known. Its incidence is noticeably higher in women of an upper socioeconomic level between ages 20 and 54. However, it can occur during childhood. Other contributing factors include age at menopause; infertility; celibacy; high-fat diet; exposure to asbestos, talc, and industrial pollutants; nulliparity; familial tendency; and a history of breast or uterine cancer.

Primary epithelial tumors arise in the müllerian epithelia; germ cell tumors, in the ovum itself; and sex cord tumors, in the ovarian stroma. Ovarian tumors spread rapidly intraperitoneally by local extension or surface seeding and, occasionally, through the lymph and blood circulatory systems. Generally, extraperitoneal spread is through the diaphragm into the chest cavity, which may cause pleural effusion. Other types of metastasis are rare.

Signs and symptoms

Typically, symptoms vary with the size of the tumor. An ovary may grow to considerable size before it produces overt symptoms. Occasionally, in the early stages, ovarian cancer causes vague abdominal discomfort, dyspepsia, and other mild GI disturbances.

As the cancer progresses, it causes urinary frequency, constipation, pelvic discomfort, distention, and weight loss. Tumor rupture, torsion, or infection may cause pain, which, in young patients, may mimic appendicitis.

Granulosa cell tumors have feminizing effects (such as bleeding between periods in premenopausal women); conversely, arrhenoblastomas have virilizing effects. Advanced ovarian cancer causes ascites, postmenopausal bleeding and pain (rarely), and symptoms relating to metastatic sites (most often pleural effusion).

Diagnosis

Positive diagnosis of ovarian cancer requires clinical evaluation, complete patient history, surgical exploration, and histologic studies. (See *Staging ovarian cancer.*) Preoperative evaluation includes a complete physical examination, including a pelvic examination with Papanicolaou test (positive in only a small number of women with ovarian cancer) and the following special tests:

• *abdominal ultrasonography, computed tomography scan,* or *X-ray* (which may delineate tumor size)
• *complete blood count, blood chemistry testing,* and *electrocardiography*
• *excretory urography* for information on renal function and possible urinary trait anomalies or obstruction
• *chest X-ray* for distant metastasis and pleural effusion
• *barium enema* (especially in patients with GI symptoms) to reveal obstruction and size of tumor
• *lymphangiography* to show lymph node involvement
• *mammography* to rule out primary breast cancer
• *liver function studies* or a *liver scan* in patients with ascites
• *ascites fluid aspiration* for identification of typical cells by cytology
• *laboratory tumor marker studies,* such as the CA-125 study to detect cancer antigen 125, carcinoembryonic antigen, and serum human chorionic gonadotropin.

Despite extensive testing, accurate diagnosis and staging are impossible without exploratory laparotomy, including lymph node evaluation and tumor resection.

Treatment

According to the staging of the disease and the patient's age, treatment of ovarian cancer requires varying combinations of surgery, chemotherapy and, in some cases, radiation.

Occasionally, in girls or young women with a unilateral encapsulated tumor who wish to maintain fertility, the following conservative approach may be appropriate:
• resection of the involved ovary

Staging ovarian cancer

The International Federation of Gynecology and Obstetrics has established this staging system, which is based on findings at clinical examination, surgical exploration, or both. Histology is taken into consideration, as is cytology in effusions. Ideally, biopsies should be obtained from any suspicious areas outside of the pelvis.

To evaluate the impact on the prognosis of the different criteria for allotting cases to stage IC or IIC, consider whether rupture of the capsule was spontaneous or caused by the surgeon or if the source of malignant cells detected was peritoneal washings or ascites.

Stage I
Growth limited to the ovaries

Stage IA
Growth limited to one ovary; no ascites. No tumor on the external surface; capsule intact

Stage IB
Growth limited to both ovaries; no ascites. No tumor on the external surfaces; capsules intact

Stage IC
Tumor either stage IA or IB but with tumor on surface of one or both ovaries; or with capsule ruptured; or with ascites present containing malignant cells or with positive peritoneal washings

Stage II
Growth involving one or both ovaries with pelvic extension

Stage IIA
Extension or metastasis, or both, to the uterus or tubes (or both)

Stage IIB
Extension to other pelvic tissues

Stage IIC
Tumor either stage IIA or IIB but with tumor on surface of one or both ovaries; or with capsule (or capsules) ruptured; or with ascites present containing malignant cells or with positive peritoneal washings

Stage III
Tumor involving one or both ovaries with peritoneal implants outside the pelvis or positive retroperitoneal or inguinal nodes; superficial liver metastasis equals stage III; or tumor limited to the true pelvis but with histologically proved malignant extension to small bowel or omentum

Stage IIIA
Tumor grossly limited to the true pelvis with negative nodes but with histologically confirmed microscopic seeding of abdominal peritoneal surfaces

Stage IIIB
Tumor of one or both ovaries with histologically confirmed implants of abdominal peritoneal surfaces, none exceeding 2 cm in greatest dimension; nodes are negative

Stage IIIC
Abdominal implants greater than 2 cm in greatest dimension or positive retroperitoneal or inguinal nodes, or both

Stage IV
Growth involving one or both ovaries with distant metastasis; if pleural effusion is present, there must be positive cytology to suggest stage IV; parenchymal liver metastasis equals stage IV

ıopsies of the momentum and the uninvolved ovary
ıeritoneal washings for cytologic examination of pelvic fluid
careful follow-up, including periodic chest X-rays to rule out
ıng metastasis.

Ovarian cancer usually requires more aggressive treatment, including total abdominal hysterectomy and bilateral
salpingo-oophorectomy with tumor resection, omentectomy, appendectomy, lymph node biopsies with lymphadenectomy, tissue biopsies, and peritoneal washings. Complete
tumor resection is impossible if the tumor has surrounded
other organs or if it involves organs that can't be resected.
Bilateral salpingo-oophorectomy in a prepubertal girl necessitates hormone replacement therapy, beginning at puberty,
to induce the development of secondary sex characteristics.

Chemotherapy extends survival time in most ovarian
cancer patients. It is largely palliative in advanced disease.
However, prolonged remissions are being achieved in some
patients.

Chemotherapeutic drugs useful in ovarian cancer include melphalan, chlorambucil, thiotepa, methotrexate, cyclophosphamide, doxorubicin, vincristine, vinblastine,
dactinomycin, bleomycin, paclitaxel, and cisplatin.

These drugs are usually given in combination and they
may be administered intraperitoneally as well.

Radiation therapy is generally not used for ovarian cancer because the resulting myelosuppression would limit the
effectiveness of chemotherapy.

Radioisotopes have been used as adjuvant therapy, but
they cause small-bowel obstructions and stenosis.

Administration of I.V. biological response modifiers – in-
terleukin-2, interferons, and monoclonal antibodies – is currently being investigated.

**Special
considerations**

• Tailor your care to the patient's individual treatment regimen.
• Before surgery, thoroughly explain all preoperative tests, the
course of treatment, and surgical and postoperative procedures.
• Reinforce what the surgeon has told the patient about the
procedures listed in the consent form. Explain that this form
lists multiple procedures because the extent of the surgery
can be determined only after the surgery has begun.

• Explain to premenopausal women that bilateral oo-
tomy artificially induces menopause, so they may exp-
ence hot flashes, headaches, palpitations, insomnia,
depression, and excessive perspiration.
• After surgery, monitor vital signs, I.V. fluids, and intake and
output. Maintain good catheter care. Check the dressing
regularly for excessive drainage or bleeding, and watch for
signs of infection.
• Provide abdominal support and watch for abdominal distention. Encourage coughing and deep breathing. Reposition the patient often and encourage her to walk shortly after
surgery.
• Monitor and treat adverse effects of radiation and chemotherapy.
• If the patient is receiving immunotherapy, watch for flulike
symptoms that may last 12 to 24 hours after drug administration. Give aspirin or acetaminophen for fever. Keep the patient well covered with blankets, and provide warm liquids
to relieve chills. Administer an antiemetic as needed.
• Provide psychological support for the patient and her family. Encourage open communication, while discouraging
"smothering" of the patient by her family.
• If the patient is a young woman who grieves for her lost
ability to bear children, try to help her (and her family)
overcome feelings that "there's nothing else to live for."
• If the patient is a child, find out whether or not her parents
have told her she has cancer, and deal with her questions
accordingly.
• Enlist the help of a social worker, chaplain, and other
members of the health care team for additional supportive
care.

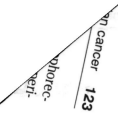

the vulva

Accounting for approximately 4% of all gynecologic malignancies, cancer of the vulva can occur at any age, even in
infants, but its peak incidence is in the mid-60s. The most
common cancer of the vulva is squamous cell carcinoma.
Early diagnosis increases the chance of effective treatment
and survival. Lymph node dissection allows a 5-year survival
rate in 85% of patients if it reveals no positive nodes; otherwise, the survival rate falls to less than 75%.

Causes

Although the cause of cancer of the vulva is unknown, several factors seem to predispose women to this disease:
• leukoplakia (white epithelial hyperplasia) — in about 25% of
patients
• chronic vulva granulomatous disease
• chronic pruritus of the vulva, with friction, swelling, and
dryness
• pigmented moles that are constantly irritated by clothing or
perineal pads
• irradiation of the skin, such as nonspecific treatment for
pelvic cancer
• sexually transmitted diseases (herpes simplex, condyloma
acuminatum)
• obesity
• hypertension
• diabetes
• nulliparity.

**Signs and
symptoms**

In 50% of patients, cancer of the vulva begins with vulval
pruritus, bleeding, or a small vulval mass (which may start
as a small ulcer on the surface; eventually, it becomes infected and painful), so such symptoms call for immediate
diagnostic evaluation. Less common signs include a mass in
the groin and abnormal urination or defecation.

Diagnosis

A Papanicolaou test that reveals abnormal cells, pruritus,
bleeding, or a small vulval mass strongly suggests cancer of
the vulva. Firm diagnosis requires histologic examination.
Abnormal tissues for biopsy are identified by colposcopic

Staging cancer of the vulva

Stage 0
Carcinoma in situ

Stage I
Tumor confined to skin surface of vulva, 2 cm or less in diameter; nodes not palpable or are palpable in either groin, not enlarged, and mobile (not clinically suspicious of neoplasm)

Stage II
Tumor confined to the vulva or the perineum, or both, more than 2 cm in diameter, nodes not palpable or are palpable in either groin, not enlarged, and mobile (not clinically suspicious of neoplasm)

Stage III
Tumor of any size with (1) adjacent spread to the urethra and any or all of the vagina, the perineum, and the anus or (2) nodes palpable in either or both groins (enlarged, firm, and mobile, but clinically suspicious of neoplasm)

Stage IV
Tumor of any size (1) infiltrating the bladder mucosa or the rectal mucosa, or both, including the upper part of the urethral mucosa or (2) fixed to the bone or other distant metastasis; fixed or ulcerated nodes in either or both groins

---

examination to pinpoint vulval lesions or abnormal skin changes and by staining with toluidine blue O dye, which, after rinsing with diluted acetic acid, is retained by diseased tissues.

Other diagnostic measures include a complete blood count, an X-ray, an electrocardiogram, and a thorough physical (including pelvic) examination. Occasionally, a computed tomography scan may pinpoint lymph node involvement.

Treatment

Depending on the stage of the disease, cancer of the vulva usually calls for radical or simple vulvectomy (or laser therapy for some small lesions). (See *Staging cancer of the vulva.*) Radical vulvectomy requires bilateral dissection of superficial and deep inguinal lymph nodes. Resection may include the urethra, vagina, and bowel, increasing the risk of postoperative complications. Plastic surgery, including mucocutaneous graft to reconstruct pelvic structures, may be done later.

Small, confined lesions with no lymph node involvement may require a simple vulvectomy or hemivulvectomy (without pelvic node dissection). Personal considerations (young age, active sexual life) may also mandate such conservative management. However, a simple vulvectomy requires careful postoperative surveillance because it leaves the patient at higher risk for developing a new lesion. Local cryosurgery, laser surgery, or systemic chemotherapy with cisplatin and bleomycin may be used.

If extensive metastasis, advanced age, or fragile health rules out surgery, irradiation of the primary lesion offers palliative treatment.

Special considerations

• Provide good patient teaching, preoperative and postoperative care, and psychological support to help prevent complications and speed recovery.
• Before surgery, instruct the patient about the surgery and postoperative procedures, such as the use of an indwelling urinary catheter, preventive respiratory care, and exercises to prevent venous stasis.
• Encourage the patient to ask questions, and answer them honestly.
• After surgery, provide scrupulous routine gynecologic care and special care to reduce pressure at the operative site, reduce tension on suture lines, and promote healing through better air circulation.
• Place the patient on an air mattress or a convoluted foam mattress, and use a cradle to support the top bedcovers.
• Periodically reposition the patient with pillows. Make sure her bed has a trapeze bar to help her move.
• For several days after surgery, the patient will be maintained on I.V. fluids or a clear liquid diet. As needed, give her an antidiarrheal drug three times daily to reduce the discomfort and possible infection caused by defecation. Later, as needed, give stool softeners and a low-residue diet to combat constipation.
• Teach the patient how to thoroughly clean the surgical site.
• Check the operative site regularly for bleeding, foul-smelling discharge, or other signs of infection. The wound area will look lumpy, bruised, and battered, making it difficult to detect occult bleeding. This situation calls for a doctor or a primary nurse, who can more easily detect subtle changes in appearance. Within 5 to 10 days after surgery, help the patient to walk. Encourage and assist her in coughing and range-of-motion exercises.

• To prevent urine contamination, the patient will have an indwelling urinary catheter in place for 2 weeks. Record fluid intake and output, and provide standard catheter care.

• Counsel the patient and her partner. Explain that sensation in the vulva will eventually return after the nerve endings heal, and they will probably be able to have sexual intercourse 6 to 8 weeks following surgery. Explain that they may want to try different sexual techniques, especially if surgery has removed the clitoris. Help the patient adjust to the drastic change in her body image.

Fallopian tube cancer

Primary fallopian tube cancer is extremely rare. When it does occur, it usually affects postmenopausal women in their 50s and 60s, but occasionally it affects younger women. Because this disease is generally well advanced before diagnosis (up to 30% of such cancers are bilateral with extratubal spread), the prognosis is poor.

Causes

The causes of fallopian tube cancer aren't clear, but this disease appears to be linked with nulliparity. In fact, over half the women with this disease have never had children.

Signs and symptoms

Generally, early-stage fallopian tube cancer produces no symptoms. Late-stage disease is characterized by an enlarged abdomen with a palpable mass, amber-colored vaginal discharge, excessive bleeding during menstruation, or, at other times, abdominal cramps, frequent urination, bladder pressure, persistent constipation, weight loss, and unilateral colicky pain produced by hydrops tubae profluens. (This last symptom occurs when the abdominal end of the fallopian tube closes, causing the tube to become greatly distended until its accumulated secretions suddenly overflow into the uterus.)

Metastasis develops by local extension or by lymphatic spread to the abdominal organs or to the pelvic, aortic, and inguinal lymph nodes. Extra-abdominal metastasis is rare.

Unexplained postmenopausal bleeding and an abnormal Papanicolaou test (suspicious or positive in up to 50% of all cases) suggest this diagnosis, but laparotomy is usually necessary to confirm fallopian tube cancer. When such cancer involves both the ovary and fallopian tube, the primary site is very difficult to identify. Preoperative workup includes:
• an *ultrasound* or *plain film* of the abdomen to help delineate tumor mass
• *excretory urography* to evaluate renal function and to identify any urinary tract anomalies and ureteral obstruction
• *chest X-ray* to rule out metastasis
• *barium enema* to rule out intestinal obstruction
• *routine blood studies*
• *electrocardiogram.*

Treatment

In fallopian tube cancer, treatment consists of total abdominal hysterectomy, bilateral salpingo-oophorectomy, and omentectomy; chemotherapy with progestogens, cyclophosphamide, and cisplatin; and external radiation for 5 to 6 weeks. All patients should receive some form of adjunctive therapy (radiation or chemotherapy), even when surgery has removed all evidence of the disease.

Special considerations

• Provide ample preoperative patient preparation and postoperative care, patient teaching, psychological support, and symptomatic measures to relieve adverse effects of radiation and chemotherapy and to promote a successful recovery and minimize complications.
• Before surgery, reinforce the explanation of the diagnostic and treatment procedures. Explain the need for preoperative studies, and tell the patient what to expect: fasting from the evening before surgery, an enema to clear the bowel, insertion of an indwelling urinary catheter attached to a drainage bag, an abdominal and possibly a pelvic preparation, placement of an I.V. line, and possibly a sedative.
• Describe the tubes and dressings the patient can expect to have in place when she returns from surgery.
• Teach the patient deep-breathing and coughing techniques to prepare for postoperative exercises.
• After surgery, check vital signs every 4 hours. Be alert for fever, tachycardia, and hypotension.

• Monitor I.V. fluids.
• Change dressings regularly, and check for excessive drainage and bleeding and signs of infection.
• Provide antiembolism stockings.
• Encourage regular deep breathing and coughing.
• If necessary, institute incentive spirometry.
• Turn the patient often, and help her reposition herself, using pillows for support.
• Auscultate for bowel sounds. When the patient's bowel function returns, ask the dietitian to provide a clear liquid diet initially, then, when tolerated, a regular diet.
• Encourage the patient to walk within 24 hours after surgery. Reassure her that she won't harm herself or cause wound dehiscence by sitting up or walking.
• Provide psychological support. Encourage the patient to express anxieties and fears. If she seems worried about the effect of surgery on her sexual activity, reassure her that this surgery will not inhibit sexual intimacy.
• Before radiation therapy begins, explain that the area to be irradiated will be marked with ink to precisely locate the treatment field. Explain that radiation may cause a skin reaction, bladder irritation, myelosuppression, and other systemic reactions.
• During and after treatment, watch for and treat adverse effects of radiation and chemotherapy.
• Before discharge, to minimize adverse effects during outpatient radiation and chemotherapy, advise the patient to maintain a high-carbohydrate, high-protein, low-fat, low-bulk diet to maintain caloric intake but reduce bulk. Suggest that she eat several small meals a day instead of three large ones.
• Include the patient's spouse or other close relatives in patient care and teaching as much as possible.
• To help detect fallopian tube and other gynecologic cancers early, stress the importance of a regular pelvic examination to all patients. Tell them to contact a doctor promptly about any gynecologic symptom.

Self-test questions

You can quickly review your comprehension of this chapter on genital neoplasms by answering the following questions. The answers to these questions and their rationales appear on pages 191 to 193.

Case history
questions

The doctor has discovered a small, hard nodule while performing a digital rectal examination on Mr. Schwartz. He orders follow-up diagnostic studies including blood tests for serum acid phosphatase and prostate-specific antigen, ultrasonography, and a biopsy of the lesion to rule out prostate cancer. Test results reveal the nodule to be a prostate carcinoma.

1. Which of the following statements is true regarding prostate cancer?
   a. It is the second most common neoplasm in men over age 50.
   b. It is the third leading cause of death in men.
   c. Sarcoma is its most common form.
   d. Most prostate cancers originate in the posterior of the prostate gland.

2. After undergoing a prostatectomy, Mr. Schwartz should be monitored for which possible adverse effects?
   a. Increased libido
   b. Incontinence
   c. Priapism
   d. Gynecomastia

3. After having a suprapubic prostatectomy, Mr. Schwartz should begin perineal exercises in:
   a. 6 to 12 hours.
   b. 24 to 48 hours.
   c. 72 hours.
   d. 1 week.

Kathryn Jillson visits her gynecologist because of postmenopausal bleeding. She expresses concern about a watery, blood-streaked discharge. During the physical examination, the doctor palpates an enlarged uterus. Later in the week, he performs a fractional dilatation and curettage to determine the cause. The biopsy report indicates uterine cancer. Ms. Jillson is admitted to the hospital for a total hysterectomy.

4. A predisposing factor for uterine cancer is:
   a. multiple pregnancies.
   b. a history of anorexia.
   c. hypoglycemia.
   d. estrogen therapy without progesterone.

5. Ms. Jillson also requires a lymphadenectomy and returns to her room postoperatively with a blood drainage system in place. The nurse measures the fluid level during every shift. She should notify the doctor immediately when the drainage exceeds:
   a. 50 ml/shift.
   b. 125 ml/shift.
   c. 250 ml/shift.
   d. 400 ml/shift.

Additional questions

6. A patient with testicular cancer undergoes chemotherapy, which includes the drug vinblastine. Which adverse reaction does this drug cause?
   a. Ototoxicity
   b. Nephrotoxicity
   c. Neurotoxicity
   d. Cardiotoxicity

7. Precancerous penile lesions are treated with:
   a. fluorouracil.
   b. bleomycin.
   c. methotrexate.
   d. cisplatin.

8. Invasive cervical carcinoma occurs between ages:
   a. 12 and 18.
   b. 20 and 25.
   c. 30 and 50.
   d. 55 and 70.

9. The preferred treatment for advanced vaginal cancer is:
   a. laser surgery.
   b. topical chemotherapy.
   c. systemic chemotherapy.
   d. radiation therapy.

10. In women with previously treated breast cancer, which is the most common site of metastasis?
   a. Cervix
   b. Ovaries
   c. Vulva
   d. Fallopian tubes

CHAPTER 6

Bone, Skin, and Soft-Tissue Neoplasms

Cancer of the bone, skin, and soft tissue can be just as serious as cancer in other major organs. Both primary malignant tumors and metastatic lesions may target these structures.

Primary malignant bone tumors

A rare form of cancer, primary malignant bone tumors constitute less than 1% of all malignant tumors. Most bone tumors are secondary, caused by seeding from a primary site. Primary malignant bone tumors are more common in males, especially in children and adolescents, although some types do occur in persons between ages 35 and 60.

Primary malignant bone tumors may originate in osseous or nonosseous tissue. (See *Comparing primary malignant bone tumors,* page 134.) Osseous bone tumors arise from the bony structure itself and include osteogenic sarcoma (the most common), parosteal osteogenic sarcoma, chondrosarcoma, and malignant giant cell tumor. Together they make up 60% of all malignant bone tumors. Nonosseous tumors arise from hematopoietic, vascular, and neural tissues and include Ewing's sarcoma, fibrosarcoma, and chordoma. Osteogenic and Ewing's sarcomas are the most common bone tumors in children.

Comparing primary malignant bone tumors

TYPE	CLINICAL FEATURES	TREATMENT
Osseous origin		
Osteogenic sarcoma	• Osteoid tumor present in specimen • Tumor arises from bone-forming osteoblast and bone-digesting osteoclast • Occurs most often in femur, but also tibia and humerus; occasionally, in fibula, ileum, vertebra, or mandible • Usually in males ages 10 to 30	• Surgery (tumor resection, high thigh amputation, hemipelvectomy, interscapulothoracic surgery) • Chemotherapy
Parosteal osteogenic sarcoma	• Develops on surface of bone instead of interior • Progresses slowly • Occurs most often in distal femur, but also in tibia, humerus, and ulna • Usually in females ages 30 to 40	• Surgery (tumor resection, possible amputation, interscapulothoracic surgery, hemipelvectomy) • Chemotherapy • Combination of above
Chondrosarcoma	• Develops from cartilage • Painless; grows slowly, but is locally recurrent and invasive • Occurs most often in pelvis, proximal femur, ribs, and shoulder girdle • Usually in males ages 30 to 50	• Hemipelvectomy, surgical resection (ribs) • Radiation (palliative) • Chemotherapy
Malignant giant cell tumor	• Arises from benign giant cell tumor • Found most often in long bones, especially in knee area • Usually in females ages 18 to 50	• Curettage • Total excision • Radiation for recurrent disease
Nonosseous origin		
Ewing's sarcoma	• Originates in bone marrow and invades shafts of long and flat bones • Usually affects lower extremities, most often femur, innominate bones, ribs, tibia, humerus, vertebra, and fibula; may metastasize to lungs • Pain increasingly severe and persistent • Usually in males ages 10 to 20 • Prognosis poor	• High-voltage radiation (tumor is very radiosensitive) • Chemotherapy to slow growth • Amputation only if there's no evidence of metastases
Fibrosarcoma	• Relatively rare • Originates in fibrous tissue of bone • Invades long or flat bones (femur, tibia, mandible) but also involves periosteum and overlying muscle • Usually in males ages 30 to 40	• Amputation • Radiation • Chemotherapy • Bone grafts (with low-grade fibrosarcoma)
Chordoma	• Derived from embryonic remnants of notochord • Progresses slowly • Usually found at end of spinal column and in spheno-occipital, sacrococcygeal, and vertebral areas • Characterized by constipation and visual disturbances • Usually in males ages 50 to 60	• Surgical resection (often resulting in neural defects) • Radiation (palliative, or when surgery not applicable, as in occipital area)

Causes	The causes of primary malignant bone tumors are unknown. Some researchers suggest that primary malignant bone tumors arise in areas of rapid growth, because children and young adults with such tumors seem to be much taller than average. Additional theories point to heredity, trauma, and excessive radiotherapy.
Signs and symptoms	Bone pain is the most common indication of primary malignant bone tumors. It's often more intense at night and is not usually associated with mobility. The pain is dull and is usually localized, although it may be referred from the hip or spine and result in weakness or a limp. Another common sign is the presence of a mass or tumor. The tumor site may be tender and may swell; the tumor itself is often palpable. Pathologic fractures are common. In late stages, the patient may be cachectic, with fever and impaired mobility.
Diagnosis	Various studies may be performed to detect and stage bone cancer: • *Biopsy (by incision or by aspiration)* is essential for confirming primary malignant bone tumors. • *Bone X-rays, radioisotope bone scans,* and *computed tomography scans* show tumor size. • *Serum alkaline phosphatase* levels are usually elevated in patients with sarcoma.
Treatment	Excision of the tumor with a 3″ (7.6 cm) margin is the treatment of choice. It may be combined with preoperative chemotherapy. In some patients, radical surgery (such as hemipelvectomy or interscapulothoracic amputation) is necessary. However, surgical resection of the tumor (often with preoperative *and* postoperative chemotherapy) has saved limbs from amputation. Intensive chemotherapy includes administration of combinations of doxorubicin, vincristine, cyclophosphamide, cisplatin, and dacarbazine. Chemotherapy may be infused intra-arterially into the long bones of the legs.

Special
considerations

• Be sensitive to the emotional strain caused by the threat of amputation. Encourage communication and help the patient set realistic goals.

• If the surgery will affect the patient's legs, have a physical therapist teach him how to use assistive devices (such as a walker) preoperatively.

• Also teach the patient how to readjust his body weight so that he can get in and out of the bed and wheelchair.

• Before surgery, start I.V. infusions to maintain fluid and electrolyte balance and to have an open vein available if blood or plasma is needed during surgery.

• After surgery, check vital signs every hour for the first 4 hours, every 2 hours for the next 4 hours, and then every 4 hours if the patient is stable.

• Check the dressing periodically for oozing.

• Elevate the foot of the bed or place the stump on a pillow for the first 24 hours. (Be careful not to leave the stump elevated for more than 48 hours, because this may lead to contractures.)

• To ease the patient's anxiety, administer analgesics for pain before morning care. If necessary, brace the patient with pillows, keeping the affected part at rest.

• Urge the patient to eat foods high in protein, vitamins, and folic acid and to get plenty of rest and sleep to promote recovery.

• Encourage physical exercise.

• Administer laxatives, if necessary, to maintain proper elimination.

• Encourage fluids to prevent dehydration. Record intake and output accurately. After a hemipelvectomy, insert a nasogastric tube to prevent abdominal distention. Continue low gastric suction for 2 days after surgery or until the patient can tolerate a liquid diet.

• Administer antibiotics to prevent infection. Give transfusions, if necessary, and administer medication to control pain. Keep drains in place to facilitate wound drainage and prevent infection. Use an indwelling urinary catheter until the patient can void voluntarily.

• Keep in mind that rehabilitation programs after limb salvage surgery will vary, depending on the patient, the body part affected, and the type of surgery performed. For example, one patient may have a surgically implanted prosthesis (for example, after joint surgery), whereas another may have reconstructive surgery requiring an allograft (such as bone from a bone bank) or an autograft (bone from the patient's own body).

• Encourage early rehabilitation for amputees. Start physical therapy 24 hours postoperatively. Pain is usually not severe after amputation. If it is, watch for various wound complications, such as hematoma, excessive stump edema, or infection.

• Be aware of "phantom limb" syndrome, in which the patient "feels" an itch or tingling in an amputated extremity. This can last for several hours or persist for years. Explain that this sensation is normal and usually subsides.

• To avoid contractures and ensure the best conditions for wound healing, warn the patient not to hang the stump over the edge of the bed; sit in a wheelchair with the stump flexed; place a pillow under his hip, knee, or back, or between his thighs; lie with knees flexed; rest an above-the-knee stump on the crutch handle; or abduct an above-the-knee stump.

• Wash the stump, massage it gently, and keep it dry until it heals. Make sure the bandage is firm and is worn day and night. Know how to reapply the bandage to shape the stump for a prosthesis.

• To help the patient select a prosthesis, consider his needs and the types of prostheses available. The rehabilitation staff will help him make the final decision, but because most patients are uninformed about choosing a prosthesis, give some guidelines. Keep in mind the patient's age and possible vision problems. Generally, children need relatively simple devices, whereas elderly patients may need prostheses that provide more stability. Consider finances too. Children outgrow prostheses, so advise parents to plan accordingly.

• The same points are applicable for an interscapulothoracic amputee, but losing an arm causes a greater cosmetic problem. Consult an occupational therapist, who can teach the patient how to perform daily activities with one arm.

• Try to instill a positive attitude toward recovery. Urge the patient to resume an independent lifestyle. Refer elderly patients to community health services, if necessary. Suggest tutoring for children to help them keep up with schoolwork.

Multiple myeloma

Also known as malignant plasmacytoma, plasma cell myeloma, and myelomatosis, multiple myeloma is a disseminated neoplasm of marrow plasma cells that infiltrates bone to produce osteolytic lesions throughout the skeleton (flat bones, vertebrae, skull, pelvis, and ribs). In late stages, it infiltrates the body organs (liver, spleen, lymph nodes, lungs, adrenal glands, kidneys, skin, and GI tract). Multiple myeloma strikes about 9,600 people yearly—mostly men over age 40.

The prognosis is usually poor because the disease is often diagnosed after it has already infiltrated the vertebrae, pelvis, skull, ribs, clavicle, and sternum. By then, skeletal destruction is widespread and, without treatment, leads to vertebral collapse; 52% of patients die within 3 months of diagnosis, 90% within 2 years. Early diagnosis and treatment prolong the lives of many patients by 3 to 5 years. Death usually follows complications, such as infection, renal failure, hematologic imbalance, fractures, hypercalcemia, hyperuricemia, or dehydration.

Causes

Although the exact cause of multiple myeloma is unknown, the impaired normal immunoglobulin production that occurs with the disease may result from a monocyte or macrophage related to immaturity in B lymphocytes (which normally become antibody-secreting plasma cells).

Signs and symptoms

The earliest indication of multiple myeloma is severe, constant back pain that increases with exercise. Arthritic symptoms may also occur, such as achiness, joint swelling, and tenderness, possibly from vertebral compression. Other effects include fever, malaise, slight evidence of peripheral neuropathy (such as peripheral paresthesia), and pathologic fractures.

As multiple myeloma progresses, symptoms of vertebral compression may become acute, accompanied by anemia, weight loss, thoracic deformities (ballooning), and loss of body height—5" (12.7 cm) or more—due to vertebral collapse. Renal complications such as pyelonephritis (caused

All about Bence Jones protein

The hallmark of multiple myeloma, this protein (a light chain of gamma globulin) was named for Henry Bence Jones, an English doctor who in 1848 noticed that patients with a curious bone disease excreted a unique protein—unique in that it coagulated at 113° to 131° F (45° to 55° C), then redissolved when heated to boiling.

In 1889, Otto Kahler, an Austrian, demonstrated that Bence Jones protein was related to myeloma. Bence Jones protein is not found in the urine of *all* multiple myeloma patients, but it is almost never found in patients without this disease.

by tubular damage from large amounts of Bence Jones protein, hypercalcemia, and hyperuricemia) may occur. Severe, recurrent infection, such as pneumonia, may follow damage to nerves associated with respiratory function.

Diagnosis

After a physical examination and a careful medical history, the following diagnostic tests and nonspecific laboratory abnormalities confirm the presence of multiple myeloma:
• *Complete blood count* shows moderate or severe anemia. The differential may show 40% to 50% lymphocytes but seldom more than 3% plasma cells. Rouleaux formations (often the first clue) seen on the differential smear result from elevation of the erythrocyte sedimentation rate.
• *Urine studies* may show Bence Jones protein and hypercalciuria. (See *All about Bence Jones protein.*) Absence of Bence Jones protein doesn't rule out multiple myeloma; however, its presence almost invariably confirms the disease.
• *Bone marrow aspiration* detects myelomatous cells (this is indicated by an abnormal number of immature plasma cells).
• *Serum electrophoresis* shows elevated globulin spike that is electrophoretically and immunologically abnormal.
• *X-rays* during early stages may show only diffuse osteoporosis. Eventually, they show multiple, sharply circumscribed osteolytic (punched-out) lesions, particularly on the skull, pelvis, and spine—the characteristic lesions of multiple myeloma.
• *Excretory urography* can assess renal involvement. To avoid precipitation of Bence Jones protein, iothalamate or diatri-

zoate is used instead of the usual contrast medium. And although oral fluid restriction is usually the standard procedure before excretory urography, patients with multiple myeloma receive large quantities of fluid, generally orally but sometimes I.V., before this procedure.

Treatment

Long-term treatment of multiple myeloma consists mainly of chemotherapy to suppress plasma cell growth and control pain. Some combinations include cyclophosphamide, doxorubicin, and prednisone; and carmustine, doxorubicin, and prednisone. Also, adjuvant local radiation reduces acute lesions, such as collapsed vertebrae, and relieves localized pain.

Other treatment usually includes a combination of melphalan and prednisone in high intermittent doses or low continuous daily doses, and analgesics for pain. For spinal cord compression, the patient may require a laminectomy; for renal complications, dialysis.

Because the patient may have bone demineralization and may lose large amounts of calcium into blood and urine, he is a prime candidate for renal stones, nephrocalcinosis, and, eventually, renal failure due to the hypercalcemia. Hypercalcemia is managed with hydration, diuretics, corticosteroids, oral phosphate, and mithramycin I.V. to decrease serum calcium levels.

Special considerations

• Encourage fluid intake; tell the patient to drink 3,000 to 4,000 ml fluids daily, particularly before his excretory urography. Monitor fluid intake and output (daily output should not be less than 1,500 ml).
• Encourage the patient to walk (immobilization increases bone demineralization and vulnerability to pneumonia), and give analgesics as needed to lessen pain. Never allow the patient to walk unaccompanied; be sure that he uses a walker or other supportive aid to prevent falls. Because the patient is particularly vulnerable to pathologic fractures, he may be fearful. Give reassurance and allow him to move at his own pace.
• Prevent complications by watching for fever or malaise, which may signal the onset of infection, and for signs of other problems, such as severe anemia and fractures.

• If the patient is bedridden, change his position every 2 hours. Perform passive range-of-motion exercises, and encourage deep-breathing exercises. Promote active exercises when the patient can tolerate them.

• If the patient is taking melphalan (a phenylalanine derivative of nitrogen mustard that depresses bone marrow), make sure to check his blood count (platelet and white blood cell) before each treatment. If he is taking prednisone, watch closely for infection because this drug often masks it.

• Whenever possible, get the patient out of bed within 24 hours after laminectomy. Check for hemorrhage, motor or sensory deficits, and loss of bowel or bladder function. Position the patient as necessary, maintain alignment, and logroll him when turning.

• Provide much-needed emotional support for the patient and his family because they are likely to be very anxious. Help relieve their anxiety by truthfully informing them about diagnostic tests (including painful procedures, such as bone marrow aspiration and biopsy), treatment, and the prognosis. If needed, refer them to an appropriate community resource for additional support.

Basal cell epithelioma

A slow-growing, destructive skin tumor, basal cell epithelioma (basal cell carcinoma) usually occurs in persons over age 40; it's more prevalent in blond, fair-skinned men and is the most common malignant tumor affecting whites.

Causes

Prolonged sun exposure is the most common cause of basal cell epithelioma, but arsenic ingestion, radiation exposure, burns, immunosuppression, and, rarely, vaccinations are other possible causes.

Although the pathogenesis of basal cell epithelioma is uncertain, some experts now hypothesize that it originates when, under certain conditions, undifferentiated basal cells become carcinomatous instead of differentiating into sweat glands, serum, and hair.

Signs and
symptoms

Three types of basal cell epithelioma occur:
• Noduloulcerative lesions occur most often on the face, particularly the forehead, eyelid margins, and nasolabial folds. In early stages, these lesions are small, smooth, pinkish, and translucent papules. Telangiectatic vessels cross the surface, and the lesions are occasionally pigmented. As the lesions enlarge, their centers become depressed and their borders become firm and elevated. Ulceration and local invasion eventually occur. These ulcerated tumors, known as "rodent ulcers," rarely metastasize; however, if untreated, they can spread to vital areas and become infected or cause massive hemorrhage if they invade large blood vessels.
• Superficial basal cell epitheliomas commonly appear on the chest and back, often several at a time. They're oval or irregularly shaped, lightly pigmented plaques, with sharply defined, slightly elevated, threadlike borders. Because of superficial erosion, these lesions appear scaly and have small, atrophic areas in the center that resemble psoriasis or eczema. They're usually chronic and don't tend to invade other areas. Superficial basal cell epitheliomas are related to ingestion of or exposure to arsenic-containing compounds.
• Sclerosing basal cell epitheliomas (morphea-like epitheliomas) are waxy, sclerotic, yellow to white plaques without distinct borders. Occurring on the head and neck, sclerosing basal cell epitheliomas often look like small patches of scleroderma.

Diagnosis

All types of basal cell epitheliomas are diagnosed by clinical appearance. Incisional or excisional biopsy, and histologic study may help to determine the tumor type and histologic subtype.

Treatment

Depending on the size, location, and depth of the lesion, treatment may include curettage and electrodesiccation, chemotherapy, surgical excision, radiation, or chemosurgery, as follows:
• Curettage and electrodesiccation offer good cosmetic results for small lesions.
• Topical fluorouracil is often used for superficial lesions. This medication produces marked local irritation or inflammation in the involved tissue but no systemic effects.

• Microscopically controlled surgical excision carefully removes recurrent lesions until a tumor-free plane is achieved. After removal of large lesions, skin grafting may be required.
• Radiation is used if the tumor location requires it, and for elderly or debilitated patients who might not withstand surgery.
• Cryotherapy with liquid nitrogen freezes and kills the cells.
• Chemosurgery is often necessary for persistent or recurrent lesions, it consists of periodic applications of a fixative paste (such as zinc chloride) and subsequent removal of fixed pathologic tissue. Treatment continues until tumor removal is complete.

Special considerations

• Instruct the patient to eat frequent small meals that are high in protein. Suggest egg nog, pureed foods, or liquid protein supplements if the lesion has invaded the oral cavity and caused eating problems.
• Tell the patient that to prevent disease recurrence, he needs to avoid excessive sun exposure and use a strong sunscreen or sunshade to protect his skin from damage by ultraviolet rays.
• Advise the patient to relieve local inflammation from topical fluorouracil with cool compresses or corticosteroid ointment.
• Instruct the patient with noduloulcerative basal cell epithelioma to wash his face gently when ulcerations and crusting occur; scrubbing too vigorously may cause bleeding.

Squamous cell carcinoma

An invasive tumor with metastatic potential that arises from the keratinizing epidermal cells, squamous cell carcinoma occurs most often in fair-skinned, white men over age 60. Outdoor employment and residence in a sunny, warm climate (the southwestern United States and Australia, for example) greatly increase the risk of developing squamous cell carcinoma.

Causes

Predisposing factors associated with squamous cell carcinoma include overexposure to the sun's ultraviolet rays, the presence of premalignant lesions (such as actinic keratosis or Bowen's disease), X-ray therapy, ingestion of herbicides containing arsenic, chronic skin irritation and inflammation, exposure to local carcinogens (such as tar and oil), and hereditary diseases (such as xeroderma pigmentosum and albinism). In rare cases, squamous cell carcinoma may develop on the site of smallpox vaccination, psoriasis, or chronic discoid lupus erythematosus. (See *Premalignant skin lesions.*)

Signs and symptoms

Squamous cell carcinoma commonly develops on the skin of the face, the ears, the dorsa of the hands and forearms, and other sun-damaged areas. Lesions on sun-damaged skin tend not to be as invasive, with less tendency to metastasize than lesions on unexposed skin. Notable exceptions to this tendency are squamous cell lesions on the lower lip and the ears. These are almost invariably markedly invasive metastatic lesions, with a generally poor prognosis.

Transformation from a premalignant lesion to squamous cell carcinoma may begin with induration and inflammation of the preexisting lesion. When squamous cell carcinoma arises from normal skin, the nodule grows slowly on a firm, indurated base. If untreated, this nodule eventually ulcerates and invades underlying tissues. Metastasis can occur to the regional lymph nodes, producing characteristic systemic symptoms of pain, malaise, fatigue, weakness, and anorexia.

Diagnosis

An excisional biopsy provides definitive diagnosis of squamous cell carcinoma. Other appropriate laboratory tests depend on systemic symptoms. (See *Staging squamous cell carcinoma,* page 146.)

Treatment

The size, shape, location, and invasiveness of a squamous cell tumor and the condition of the underlying tissue determine the treatment method used; a deeply invasive tumor may require a combination of techniques. All the major treatment methods have excellent rates of cure; generally, the prognosis is better with a well-differentiated lesion than with a

Premalignant skin lesions

DISEASE	CAUSE	PATIENT	LESION	TREATMENT
Actinic keratosis	Solar radiation	White men with fair skin (middle-aged to elderly)	Reddish-brown lesions 1 mm to 1 cm in size (may enlarge if untreated) on face, ears, lower lip, bald scalp, dorsa of hands and forearms	Topical fluorouracil, cryosurgery using liquid nitrogen, or curettage by electrodesiccation
Bowen's disease	Unknown	White men with fair skin (middle-aged to elderly)	Brown to reddish-brown lesions, with scaly surface on exposed and unexposed areas	Surgical excision, topical fluorouracil
Erythroplasia of Queyrat	Bowen's disease of the mucous membranes	Men (middle-aged to elderly)	Red lesions, with a glistening or granular appearance on mucous membranes, particularly the glans penis in uncircumcised men	Surgical excision
Leukoplakia	Smoking, alcohol, chronic cheek-biting, ill-fitting dentures, misaligned teeth	Men (middle-aged to elderly)	Lesions on oral, anal, and genital mucous membranes vary in appearance from smooth and white to rough and gray	Elimination of irritating factors, surgical excision, or curettage by electrodesiccation (if lesion is still premalignant)

poorly differentiated one in an unusual location. Depending on the type of lesion, treatment may consist of:
• wide surgical excision
• electrodesiccation and curettage, which offer good cosmetic results for smaller lesions
• radiation therapy, which generally is used for older or debilitated patients
• chemosurgery, which is reserved for resistant or recurrent lesions. (See *Treating actinic keratosis with topical fluorouracil*, page 147.)

Staging squamous cell carcinoma

The American Joint Committee on Cancer uses the following TNM (*t*umor, *n*ode, *me*tastasis) system for staging squamous cell carcinoma.

Primary tumor
TX—primary tumor can't be assessed
T0—no evidence of primary tumor
Tis—carcinoma in situ
T1—tumor 2 cm or less in greatest dimension
T2—tumor between 2 and 5 cm in greatest dimension
T3—tumor more than 5 cm in greatest dimension
T4—tumor invades deep extradermal structures (such as cartilage, skeletal muscle, or bone)

Regional lymph nodes
NX—regional lymph nodes can't be assessed

N0—no evidence of regional lymph node involvement
N1—regional lymph node involvement

Distant metastasis
MX—distant metastasis can't be assessed
M0—no known distant metastasis
M1—distant metastasis

Staging categories
Squamous cell carcinoma progresses from mild to severe as follows:
Stage 0—Tis, N0, M0
Stage I—T1, N0, M0
Stage II—T2, N0, M0; T3, N0, M0
Stage III—T4, N0, M0; any T, N1, M0
Stage IV—any T, any N, M1

Special considerations

• Emphasize meticulous wound care, emotional support, and thorough patient instruction when caring for a patient with squamous cell carcinoma.
• Coordinate a consistent plan for changing the patient's dressings. Establishing a standard routine helps the patient and family learn how to care for the wound.
• Keep the wound dry and clean.
• Try to control odor with balsam of Peru, yogurt flakes, oil of cloves, or other odor-masking substances, even though they are often ineffective for long-term use. Topical or systemic antibiotics also temporarily control odor and eventually alter the lesion's bacterial flora.
• Be prepared for other problems that accompany a metastatic disease (pain, fatigue, weakness, and anorexia).
• Help the patient and family set realistic goals and expectations.
• Disfiguring lesions are distressing to both the patient and you. Try to accept the patient as he is and help increase his self-esteem through a strong, caring relationship.

Treating actinic keratosis with topical fluorouracil

Fluorouracil is available in different strengths (1%, 2%, and 5%) as a cream or solution. Local application causes immediate stinging and burning, followed later by erythema, vesiculation, erosion, superficial ulceration, necrosis, and re-epithelialization. The 5% solution induces the most severe inflammatory response, but provides complete involution of the lesions with little recurrence.

Be careful to keep fluorouracil away from eyes, scrotum, or mucous membranes. Warn the patient to avoid exces- sive exposure to the sun during the course of treatment because it intensi- fies the inflammatory reaction.

Continue application of fluorouracil until the lesions reach the ulcerative and necrotic stages (usually 2 to 4 weeks); then consider application of a corticosteroid preparation as an anti- inflammatory agent. Possible adverse ef- fects of treatment include postinflamma- tory hyperpigmentation. Complete healing occurs within 1 to 2 months, with excellent results.

• To prevent squamous cell carcinoma, tell the patient to avoid excessive sun exposure, wear protective clothing (hats and long sleeves), periodically examine the skin for precan- cerous lesions and have any removed promptly.
• Instruct the patient to use strong sunscreening agents con- taining para-aminobenzoic acid, benzophenone derivatives, and zinc oxide. He should apply these agents 30 to 60 min- utes before sun exposure.
• Tell the patient to use lip sunscreens to protect the lips from sun damage.

Malignant melanoma

A neoplasm that arises from melanocytes, malignant mela- noma is relatively rare and accounts for only 1% to 2% of all malignancies. The three types of melanomas are superficial spreading melanoma, nodular malignant melanoma, and lentigo maligna melanoma. Melanoma is slightly more com- mon in women than in men and is rare in children. Inci- dence peaks between ages 50 and 70 but is increasing in younger age-groups.

Melanoma spreads through the lymphatic and vascular systems and metastasizes to the regional lymph nodes, skin, liver, lungs, and central nervous system. Recurrence is unpredictable, however, and metastasis may not appear for more than 5 years after resection of the primary lesion.

The prognosis varies with tumor thickness. Generally, superficial lesions are curable, whereas deeper lesions tend to metastasize. The prognosis is better for a tumor on an extremity (which is drained by one lymphatic network) than for one on the head, neck, or trunk (which is drained by several networks).

Causes

Several factors seem to influence the development of melanoma:

• Excessive exposure to sunlight. Melanoma is most common in sunny, warm areas and often develops on parts of the body that are exposed to the sun.

• Skin type. Most persons who develop melanoma have blond or red hair, fair skin, and blue eyes; are prone to sunburn; and are of Celtic or Nordic ancestry. Melanoma is rare among blacks; when it does develop, it usually arises in lightly pigmented areas (such as the palms, plantar surface, or mucous membranes).

• Hormonal factors. Pregnancy may increase risk and exacerbate growth.

• Family history. Melanoma occurs slightly more often within families.

• Past history of melanoma. A person who has had one melanoma is at greater risk for developing a second.

Signs and symptoms

Common sites for melanoma are the head and neck in men, the legs in women, and the backs of persons exposed to excessive sunlight. Up to 70% arise from a preexisting nevus. (See *Recognizing potentially malignant nevi*.) Melanoma rarely appears in the conjunctiva, choroid, pharynx, mouth, vagina, or anus.

Suspect melanoma when any skin lesion or nevus enlarges, changes color, becomes inflamed or sore, itches, ulcerates, bleeds, undergoes textural changes, or shows signs of surrounding pigment regression (halo nevus or vitiligo).

Each type of melanoma has special characteristics:

Recognizing potentially malignant nevi

Nevi (moles) are skin lesions that are often pigmented and may be hereditary. They begin to grow in childhood (occasionally they're congenital) and become more numerous in young adults. Up to 70% of patients with melanoma have a history of a preexisting nevus at the tumor site. Of these, approximately one-third are reported to be congenital; the remainder develop later in life.

Changes in nevi (color, size, shape, texture, ulceration, bleeding, or itching) suggest possible malignant transformation. The presence or absence of hair within a nevus has no significance.

Types of nevi

• *Junctional nevi* are flat or slightly raised and light to dark brown, with melanocytes confined to the epidermis. Usually, they appear before age 40. These nevi may change into compound nevi if junctional nevus cells proliferate and penetrate into the dermis.

• *Compound nevi* are usually tan to dark brown and slightly raised, although size and color vary. They contain melanocytes in both the dermis and epidermis, and they rarely undergo malignant transformation. Excision is necessary only to rule out malignant transformation or for cosmetic reasons.

• *Dermal nevi* are elevated lesions from 2 to 10 mm in diameter, and vary in color from flesh to brown. They usually develop in older adults and generally arise on the upper part of the body. Excision is necessary only to rule out malignant transformation.

• *Blue nevi* are flat or slightly elevated lesions from 0.5 to 1 cm in diameter. They appear on the head, neck, arms, and dorsa of the hands and are twice as common in women as in men. Their blue color results from pigment and collagen in the dermis, which reflect blue light but absorb other wavelengths. Excision is necessary to rule out pigmented basal cell epithelioma or melanoma, or for cosmetic reasons.

• *Dysplastic nevi* are generally greater than 5 mm in diameter, with irregularly notched or indistinct borders. Coloration is usually a variable mixture of tan and brown, sometimes with red, pink, and black pigmentation. No two lesions are exactly alike. They occur in great numbers (typically over 100 at a time), never singly, usually appearing on the back, scalp, chest, and buttocks. Dysplastic nevi are potentially malignant, especially in patients with a personal or familial history of melanoma. Skin biopsy confirms diagnosis; treatment is by surgical excision, followed by regular physical examinations (every 6 months) to detect any new lesions or changes in existing lesions.

• *Lentigo maligna* (melanotic freckle of Hutchinson) is a precursor to malignant melanoma. (In fact, about one-third of them eventually give rise to malignant melanoma.) Usually, they occur in persons over age 40, especially on exposed skin areas such as the face. At first, these lesions are flat, tan spots, but they gradually enlarge and darken and develop black speckled areas against their tan or brown background. Each lesion may simultaneously enlarge in one area and regress in another. Histologic examination shows typical and atypical melanocytes along the epidermal basement membrane. Removal by simple excision (not electrodesiccation and curettage) is recommended.

• Superficial spreading melanoma, the most common type, usually develops between ages 40 and 50. Such a lesion arises on an area of chronic irritation. In women, it's most common between the knees and ankles; in blacks and Asians, on the toe webs and soles (lightly pigmented areas subject to trauma).

Characteristically, this melanoma is red, white, and blue over a brown or black background and has an irregular, notched margin. Its surface is irregular, with small elevated tumor nodules that may ulcerate and bleed. Horizontal growth may continue for many years; when vertical growth begins, the prognosis worsens.

• Nodular malignant melanoma usually develops between ages 40 and 50, grows vertically, invades the dermis, and metastasizes early. Such a lesion is usually a polypoidal nodule, with uniformly dark discoloration (it may be grayish), and looks like a blackberry. Occasionally, this melanoma is flesh-colored, with flecks of pigment around its base (possibly inflamed).

• Lentigo maligna melanoma is relatively rare. It arises from a lentigo maligna on an exposed skin surface and usually occurs between ages 60 and 70. This lesion looks like a large (3- to 6-cm) flat freckle of tan, brown, black, whitish, or slate color, and has irregularly scattered black nodules on the surface. It develops slowly, usually over many years, and eventually may ulcerate. This melanoma commonly develops under the fingernails, on the face, and on the back of the hands.

Diagnosis

A skin biopsy with histologic examination can distinguish malignant melanoma from a benign nevus, seborrheic keratosis, and pigmented basal cell epithelioma; a skin biopsy can also determine tumor thickness. (See *Staging malignant melanoma.*) A physical examination, paying particular attention to lymph nodes, can point to metastatic involvement.

Baseline laboratory studies include complete blood count with differential, erythrocyte sedimentation rate, platelet count, liver function studies, and urinalysis. Depending on the depth of tumor invasion and metastatic spread, baseline diagnostic studies may also include chest X-ray and a computed tomography (CT) scan of the chest and abdomen.

Staging malignant melanoma

Several systems exist for staging malignant melanoma, including the TNM (*tumor, node, metastasis*) system, developed by the American Joint Committee on Cancer, and Clark's system, which classifies tumor progression according to skin layer penetration.

Primary tumor

TX—primary tumor can't be assessed
T0—no evidence of primary tumor
Tis—melanoma in situ (atypical melanotic hyperplasia, severe melanotic dysplasia), not an invasive lesion (Clark's Level I)
T1—tumor 0.75 mm in thickness or less invades the papillary dermis (Clark's Level II)
T2—tumor between 0.75 and 1.5 mm thick, or tumor invades the interface between the papillary and reticular dermis (Clark's Level III), or both
T3—tumor between 1.5 and 4 mm thick, or tumor invades the reticular dermis (Clark's Level IV), or both
T3a—tumor between 1.5 and 3 mm thick
T3b—tumor between 3 and 4 mm thick
T4—tumor more than 4 mm thick, or tumor invades subcutaneous tissue (Clark's Level V), or tumor has one or more satellites within 2 cm of the primary tumor
T4a—tumor more than 4 mm thick, or invades subcutaneous tissue, or both
T4b—one or more satellites exist within 2 cm of the primary tumor

Regional lymph nodes

NX—regional lymph nodes can't be assessed
N0—no evidence of regional lymph node involvement
N1—metastasis 3 cm or less in greatest dimension in any regional lymph node
N2—metastasis greater than 3 cm in greatest dimension in any regional lymph node, or in-transit metastasis, or both

Distant metastasis

MX—distant metastasis can't be assessed
M0—no evidence of distant metastasis
M1—distant metastasis
M1a—metastasis in skin, subcutaneous tissue, or lymph nodes beyond the regional nodes
M1b—visceral metastasis

Staging categories

Malignant melanoma progresses from mild to severe as follows:
Stage I—T1, N0, M0; T2, N0, M0
Stage II—T3, N0, M0
Stage III—T4, N0, M0; any T, N1, M0; any T, N2, M0
Stage IV—any T, any N, M1

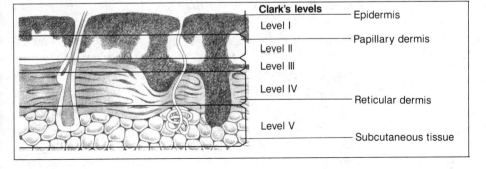

Clark's levels
Level I ——— Epidermis
Level II ——— Papillary dermis
Level III
Level IV ——— Reticular dermis
Level V ——— Subcutaneous tissue

Signs of bone metastasis may call for a bone scan; central nervous system metastasis, a CT scan of the brain.

Treatment

A patient with malignant melanoma requires surgical resection to remove the tumor. The extent of resection depends on the size and location of the primary lesion. Closure of a wide resection may require a skin graft. Surgical treatment may also include regional lymphadenectomy.

Deep primary lesions may merit adjuvant chemotherapy and biotherapy to eliminate or reduce the number of tumor cells. Radiation therapy is usually reserved for metastatic disease. It doesn't prolong survival but may reduce tumor size and relieve pain.

Regardless of treatment, melanomas require close long-term follow-up to detect metastasis and recurrences. Statistics show that 13% of recurrences develop more than 5 years after primary surgery.

Special considerations

• Perform a careful physical, psychological, and social evaluation and provide preoperative teaching, meticulous postoperative care, and psychological support. Doing so can make the patient more comfortable, speed recovery, and prevent complications.
• After diagnosis, review treatment alternatives. Tell the patient what to expect before and after surgery, what the wound will look like, and what type of dressing he'll have. Warn him that the donor site for a skin graft may be as painful if not more painful than the tumor excision site itself. Honestly answer any questions he may have regarding surgery, chemotherapy, and radiation.
• After surgery, be careful to prevent infection. Check dressings often for excessive drainage, foul odor, redness, or swelling. If surgery included lymphadenectomy, minimize lymphedema by applying a compression stocking and instructing the patient to keep the extremity elevated.
• During chemotherapy, know which adverse effects to expect and take measures to minimize them. For instance, give an antiemetic as ordered to reduce nausea and vomiting.
• To prepare the patient for discharge, emphasize the need for close follow-up to detect recurrences early. Explain that recurrences and metastasis, if they occur, are often delayed,

so follow-up must continue for years. Tell the patient how to recognize signs of recurrence.

• Provide psychological support. Encourage the patient to verbalize his fears.

• In advanced metastatic disease, control and prevent pain with consistent, regularly scheduled administration of analgesics. *Don't* wait to relieve pain until after it occurs.

• Make referrals for home care, social services, and spiritual and financial assistance as needed.

• If the patient is dying, identify the needs of the patient and his family and friends, and provide appropriate support and care.

• To help prevent malignant melanoma, stress the detrimental effects of overexposure to solar radiation, especially to fair-skinned, blue-eyed patients. Recommend that they use a sunblock or sunscreen. In all physical examinations, especially in fair-skinned persons, look for unusual nevi or other skin lesions.

Kaposi's sarcoma

Initially, this cancer of the lymphatic cell wall was described as a rare blood vessel sarcoma, occurring mostly in elderly Italian and Jewish men. In recent years, the incidence of Kaposi's sarcoma has risen dramatically along with the incidence of acquired immunodeficiency syndrome (AIDS). Currently, it's the most common AIDS-related cancer.

Kaposi's sarcoma causes structural and functional damage. When associated with AIDS, it progresses aggressively, involving the lymph nodes, the viscera, and possibly GI structures.

Causes

The exact cause of Kaposi's sarcoma is unknown, but the disease may be related to immunosuppression. Genetic or hereditary predisposition is also suspected.

Signs and symptoms

The initial sign of Kaposi's sarcoma is one or more obvious lesions in various shapes, sizes, and colors (ranging from red-

Laubenstein's stages in Kaposi's sarcoma

The following staging system was proposed by L.J. Laubenstein for use in evaluating and treating patients who have acquired immunodeficiency syndrome and Kaposi's sarcoma.

Stage I
Locally indolent cutaneous lesions

Stage II
Locally aggressive cutaneous lesions

Stage III
Mucocutaneous and lymph node involvement

Stage IV
Visceral involvement.

Within each stage, a patient may have different symptoms classified as a stage subtype—A or B—as follows:

Subtype A—no systemic signs or symptoms

Subtype B—one or more systemic signs and symptoms, including 10% or more weight loss, fever of unknown origin that exceeds 100° F (37.7° C) for more than 2 weeks, chills, lethargy, night sweats, anorexia, and diarrhea.

brown to dark purple) appearing most commonly on the skin, buccal mucosa, hard and soft palates, lips, gums, tongue, tonsils, conjunctiva, and sclera. In advanced disease, the lesions may join, becoming one large plaque. Untreated lesions may appear as large, ulcerative masses.

Other signs and symptoms include:
• a health history of AIDS
• pain (if the sarcoma advances beyond the early stages or if a lesion breaks down or impinges on nerves or organs)
• edema from lymphatic obstruction
• dyspnea (in pulmonary involvement), wheezing, hypoventilation, and respiratory distress from bronchial blockage.

The most common extracutaneous sites are the lungs and GI tract (esophagus, oropharynx, and epiglottis). Signs and symptoms of disease progression and metastasis include severe pulmonary involvement and GI involvement leading to digestive problems.

Diagnosis

The diagnosis of Kaposi's sarcoma is made following a tissue biopsy that identifies the lesion's type and stage. (See *Laubenstein's stages in Kaposi's sarcoma.*) Then a computed tomography scan may be performed to detect and evaluate possible metastasis.

Treatment

Although treatment isn't indicated for all patients, indications include cosmetically offensive, painful, or obstructive lesions of rapidly progressing disease.

Radiation therapy, chemotherapy, and biotherapy with biological response modifiers are treatment options. Radiation therapy palliates symptoms, including pain from obstructing lesions in the oral cavity or extremities and edema caused by lymphatic blockage. It may also be used for cosmetic improvement.

Chemotherapy includes combinations of doxorubicin, vinblastine, vincristine, and etoposide.

Biotherapy with interferon alfa-2b may be used for AIDS-related Kaposi's sarcoma. The treatment reduces the number of skin lesions but is ineffective in advanced disease.

Special considerations

• Listen to the patient's fears and concerns and answer his questions honestly. Stay with him during periods of severe stress and anxiety.
• The patient who is coping poorly may need a referral for psychological counseling. Family members may also need help in coping with the patient's disease and with any associated demands that the disorder places upon them.
• As appropriate, allow the patient to participate in care decisions whenever possible, and encourage him to participate in self-care measures as much as he can.
• Inspect the patient's skin routinely. Look for new lesions and skin breakdown. If the patient has painful lesions, help him into a more comfortable position.
• Follow universal precautions when caring for the patient.
• Give pain medications. Suggest distractions and relaxation techniques.
• To help the patient adjust to changes in his appearance, provide encouragement and urge him to share his feelings.
• Monitor the patient's weight daily.
• Supply the patient with high-calorie, high-protein meals. If he can't tolerate regular meals, provide him with frequent smaller meals. Consult with the dietitian and plan meals around the patient's treatment.
• If the patient can't take food by mouth, administer I.V. fluids. Also provide antiemetics and sedatives as needed.

• Be alert for adverse effects of radiation therapy or chemotherapy—such as anorexia, nausea, vomiting, and diarrhea—and take steps to prevent or alleviate them.

• Teach the patient about treatments. Make sure he understands how to manage adverse reactions. For example, during radiation therapy, instruct him to keep irradiated skin dry to avoid breakdown and subsequent infection.

• Explain all prescribed medications, including any possible adverse effects and drug interactions.

• Explain infection prevention techniques and demonstrate measures to prevent infection. Advise the patient not to share his toothbrush or other items that may be contaminated with blood, especially if he also has AIDS.

• Help the patient plan alternating activity and rest. Teach energy-conservation techniques. Encourage him to set priorities, accept others' help, and delegate nonessential tasks.

• Explain the proper use of assistive devices, when appropriate, to ease ambulation and promote independence.

• Stress the need for ongoing treatment and care.

• Refer the patient to support groups. If his prognosis is poor (less than 6 months to live), suggest immediate hospice care. Explain the benefits of initiating and executing advance directives and a durable power of attorney.

Self-test questions

You can quickly review your comprehension of this chapter on bone, skin, and soft-tissue neoplasms by answering the following questions. The answers to these questions and their rationales appear on pages 193 to 195.

Case history questions

John Knowles, age 45 and physically fit, develops a severe, constant back pain that increases with exercise. Worried that he might have pulled a muscle or a ligament during a workout, he makes an appointment to see his doctor.

Mr. Knowles reports a generalized malaise over the past several weeks and tells the doctor that he suspects a lingering virus because he has had a low-grade fever off and on for several weeks. Slight evidence of peripheral neuropathy

*is noted during the physical examination. Routine X-rays and
blood and urine studies are ordered to detect abnormalities.*

1. When you evaluate a complete blood count, your first
clue that the patient may have multiple myeloma may be:
   a. decreased hemoglobin levels.
   b. elevated hematocrit.
   c. rouleaux formation seen on differential smear.
   d. elevated white blood cell count.

2. Which urine abnormality confirms multiple myeloma?
   a. Glycosuria
   b. Acid urine pH
   c. High specific gravity
   d. Presence of Bence Jones protein

3. After a complete diagnostic workup, Mr. Knowles is diagnosed with multiple myeloma. The doctor tells him that he
will need chemotherapy. Antineoplastic agents commonly
used to treat multiple myeloma include:
   a. cisplatin and fluorouracil.
   b. cytarabine and doxorubicin.
   c. doxorubicin and carmustine.
   d. carboplatin and cyclophosphamide.

*After noticing a change in a long-standing, nonmalignant skin
lesion on his forehead, Karl Benson makes an appointment
with a dermatologist. A biopsy of the lesion reveals squamous cell carcinoma.*

4. Which of the following statements regarding this type of
skin cancer is true?
   a. It occurs most often in dark-skinned people.
   b. It is invasive.
   c. It predominantly affects men ages 30 to 40.
   d. An increased risk of squamous cell carcinoma is as-
       sociated with hormonal factors.

5. Squamous cell skin lesions generally carry a poor prognosis when found on the:
   a. lower lip and ears.
   b. cheeks and upper lip.

c. fingers and hands.

d. neck and forehead.

6. To prevent further incidences of squamous cell carcinoma of the skin, Mr. Benson should avoid excessive sun exposure. When sun exposure is unavoidable, he should apply a strong sunscreen:

a. immediately before sun exposure.

b. within 5 minutes of sun exposure.

c. within 10 to 20 minutes of sun exposure.

d. within 30 to 60 minutes of sun exposure.

Additional questions

7. Which of the following primary malignant bone tumors occurs most often in children?

a. Fibrosarcoma

b. Chordoma

c. Giant cell

d. Ewing's sarcoma

8. In primary malignant bone tumors, bone pain is:

a. more intense at night.

b. associated with mobility.

c. usually described as "pins and needles".

d. usually generalized.

9. Superficial basal cell epitheliomas may be described as:

a. small, smooth, pinkish, and translucent papules with depressed centers and firm, elevated borders when the lesions enlarge.

b. oval or irregularly shaped, lightly pigmented plaques with sharply defined borders.

c. waxy, sclerotic, yellow to white plaques without distinct borders.

d. scaly-surfaced, brownish to reddish-brown lesions.

10. Kaposi's sarcoma is characterized by which of the following signs or symptoms?

a. Hyperventilation

b. Severe pain

c. Obvious, colorful lesions

d. Obesity

CHAPTER 7

Blood and Lymph Neoplasms

When cancer affects the circulatory or lymphatic systems, the entire body may become affected quickly.

Hodgkin's disease

This disease is characterized by painless, progressive enlargement of the lymph nodes, spleen, and other lymphoid tissue resulting from proliferation of lymphocytes, histiocytes, eosinophils, and Reed-Sternberg cells. The latter cells are the disease's special histologic feature. (See *Reed-Sternberg cells*, page 160.)

Untreated, Hodgkin's disease follows a variable but relentlessly progressive and ultimately fatal course. However, recent advances in therapy have made Hodgkin's disease potentially curable, even in advanced stages, and appropriate treatment now yields a 5-year survival rate for approximately 90% of patients.

Causes

The cause of Hodgkin's disease is unknown. The disease is most common in young adults, with a higher incidence in men than in women. It occurs in all races but is slightly more common in whites. Its incidence peaks in two age-groups: ages 15 to 38 and after age 50 — except in Japan, where it occurs exclusively among people over age 50.

Signs and symptoms

The first sign of Hodgkin's disease is usually a painless swelling of one of the cervical lymph nodes (but sometimes the maxillary, mediastinal, or inguinal lymph nodes), occasionally in a patient who has a history of recent upper respiratory

Reed-Sternberg cells

These enlarged, abnormal histiocytes (Reed-Sternberg cells) from an excised lymph node suggest Hodgkin's disease. Note the large, distinct nucleoli.

Reed-Sternberg cells indicate Hodgkin's disease when they coexist with one of these four histologic patterns:
• lymphocyte predominance
• mixed cellularity
• lymphocyte depletion
• nodular sclerosis.

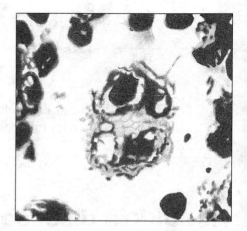

infection. In older patients, the first symptoms may be non-specific—persistent fever, night sweats, fatigue, weight loss, and malaise. Rarely, if the mediastinum is initially involved, Hodgkin's disease may produce early respiratory symptoms.

Another early and characteristic indication of Hodgkin's disease is pruritus, which, while mild at first, becomes acute as the disease progresses. Other symptoms depend on the degree and location of systemic involvement.

Lymph nodes may enlarge rapidly, producing pain and obstruction, or enlarge slowly and painlessly for months or years. It's not unusual to see the lymph nodes "wax and wane" but they usually don't return to normal. Sooner or later, most patients develop systemic manifestations, including enlargement of retroperitoneal nodes and nodular infiltrations of the spleen, the liver, and bones. At this late stage, other symptoms include edema of the face and neck, progressive anemia, possible jaundice, nerve pain, and increased susceptibility to infection.

Diagnosis

Measures for confirming Hodgkin's disease include a thorough medical history and a complete physical examination, followed by a lymph node biopsy checking for the presence of Reed-Sternberg cells, abnormal histiocyte proliferation, and nodular fibrosis and necrosis.

Other appropriate diagnostic tests include bone marrow, liver, mediastinal, lymph node, and spleen biopsies, and routine chest X-ray, abdominal computed tomography scan, lung scan, bone scan, and lymphangiography, to detect lymph node or organ involvement. Laparoscopy and lymph node biopsy are performed to complete staging.

Hematologic tests show mild to severe normocytic anemia; normochromic anemia (in 50%); elevated, normal, or reduced white blood cell count and differential showing any combination of neutrophilia, lymphocytopenia, monocytosis, and eosinophilia. Elevated serum alkaline phosphatase levels indicate liver or bone involvement.

The same diagnostic tests are also used for staging. A staging laparotomy is necessary for patients under age 55 or without obvious stage III or stage IV disease, lymphocyte predominance, or medical contraindications. (See *Staging Hodgkin's disease*, page 162.) Diagnosis must rule out other disorders that also enlarge the lymph nodes.

Treatment

Appropriate therapy (chemotherapy or radiation, or both, varying with the stage of the disease) depends on careful physical examination with accurate histologic interpretation and proper clinical staging. Correct and timely treatment allows longer survival and even induces an apparent cure in many patients.

Radiation therapy is used alone for stage I and stage II and in combination with chemotherapy for stage III. Chemotherapy is used for stage IV, sometimes inducing a complete remission. The well-known MOPP protocol (mechlorethamine, vincristine [Oncovin], procarbazine, and prednisone) was the first to provide significant cures to patients with generalized Hodgkin's disease; another useful combination is ABVI (doxorubicin [Adriamycin], bleomycin, vinblastine, and dacarbazine). Treatment with these antineoplastic drugs may require concomitant antiemetics, sedatives, or antidiarrheals to combat adverse GI effects.

New treatments include high-dose chemotherapeutic agents with autologous bone marrow transplantation or autologous peripheral stem cell transfusions. Biotherapy alone has not proved effective.

Staging Hodgkin's disease

Treatment of Hodgkin's disease depends on the stage it has reached—that is, the number, location, and degree of involved lymph nodes. The Ann Arbor classification system, adopted in 1971, divides Hodgkin's disease into four stages.

Doctors subdivide each stage into categories. Category A includes patients without defined signs and symptoms, and category B includes patients who experience such defined signs as recent unexplained weight loss, fever, and night sweats.

Stage I	**Stage II**	**Stage III**	**Stage IV**
Hodgkin's disease appears in a single lymph node region (I) or a single extralymphatic organ (IE).	The disease appears in two or more nodes on the same side of the diaphragm (II) and in an extralymphatic organ (IIE).	Hodgkin's disease spreads to both sides of the diaphragm (III) and to an extralymphatic organ (IIIE), the spleen (IIIS), or both (IIIES).	The disease disseminates, involving one or more extralymphatic organs or tissues, with or without lymph node involvement.

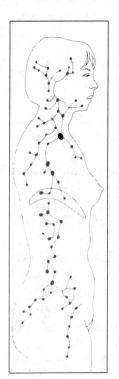 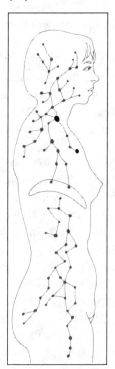 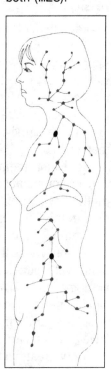 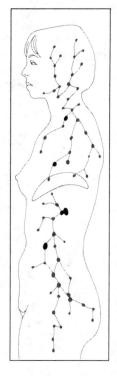

Special
considerations

- Because many patients with Hodgkin's disease receive radiation or chemotherapy as outpatients, tell the patient to watch for and promptly report adverse effects of radiation and chemotherapy (particularly anorexia, nausea, vomiting, diarrhea, fever, and bleeding).
- Inform the patient that he can minimize adverse effects of radiation therapy by maintaining good nutrition (aided by eating small, frequent meals of his favorite foods); drinking plenty of fluids; pacing his activities to counteract therapy-induced fatigue; and keeping the skin in irradiated areas dry.
- Instruct the patient to control pain and bleeding of stomatitis by using a soft toothbrush, cotton swab, or anesthetic mouthwash such as viscous lidocaine (as prescribed); by applying petroleum jelly to his lips; and by avoiding astringent mouthwashes.
- If a female patient is of childbearing age, advise her to delay pregnancy until prolonged remission, because radiation and chemotherapy can cause genetic mutations and spontaneous abortions.
- Because the patient with Hodgkin's disease has usually been healthy up to this point, he is likely to be especially distressed. Provide emotional support and offer appropriate reassurance. Ease the patient's anxiety by sharing your optimism about his prognosis.
- Make sure the patient and his family know that the local chapter of the American Cancer Society is available for information, financial assistance, and supportive counseling.

Malignant lymphomas

Also called non-Hodgkin's lymphomas or lymphosarcomas, malignant lymphomas are a heterogeneous group of malignant diseases originating in lymph glands and other lymphoid tissue. Lymphomas usually are defined by histologic, anatomic, and immunomorphic characteristics by the National Cancer Institute. However, the Rappaport histologic and Lukes-Collins classification are also used in some settings. (See *Classifying malignant lymphomas,* page 164.)

Classifying malignant lymphomas

Staging and classifying systems for malignant lymphomas include the National Cancer Institute's (NCI) system (named the "Working formulation for classification of non-Hodgkin's lymphomas for clinical usage"), the Rappaport histologic classification, and Lukes-Collins classification. (*Note:* The NCI also cites a "miscellaneous" category, which includes these lymphomas: composite, mycosis fungoides, histiocytic, extramedullary plasmacytoma, and unclassifiable.)

N.C.I.	RAPPAPORT	LUKES-COLLINS
Low grade		
• Small lymphocytic cell	• Diffuse, well-differentiated lymphocytic	• Small lymphocytic and B-cell or T-cell type
• Follicular, predominantly small cleaved cell	• Nodular, poorly differentiated lymphocytic	• Small cleaved follicular center cell, follicular only or follicular and diffuse
• Follicular, mixed small and large cell	• Nodular, mixed lymphoma	• Small cleaved follicular center cell, follicular; large cleaved follicular center cell, follicular
Intermediate grade		
• Follicular, predominantly large cell	• Nodular, histiocytic lymphoma	• Large cleaved or noncleaved follicular center cell, or both, follicular
• Diffuse, small cleaved cell	• Diffuse, poorly differentiated lymphoma	• Small cleaved follicular center cell, diffuse
• Diffuse, mixed small cleaved and large cell	• Diffuse, mixed lymphocytic-histiocytic	• Small cleaved, large cleaved, or large noncleaved follicular center cell, diffuse
• Diffuse, large cell cleaved and noncleaved	• Diffuse, histiocytic lymphoma	• Large cleaved or noncleaved follicular center cell, diffuse
High grade		
• Diffuse, large cell immunoblastic	• Diffuse, histiocytic lymphoma	• Immunoblastic sarcoma, T-cell or B-cell type
• Small noncleaved cell	• Lymphoblastic, convoluted or nonconvoluted	• Convoluted T cell
• Large cell, lymphoblastic	• Undifferentiated, Burkitt's and non-Burkitt's diffuse, undifferentiated lymphoma	• Small noncleaved follicular center cell

Nodular lymphomas have a better prognosis than the diffuse form of the disease, but in both, the prognosis is worse than in Hodgkin's disease.

Causes

The cause of malignant lymphomas is unknown, although some theories suggest a viral source. Up to 35,000 new cases appear annually in the United States alone. Malignant lymphomas are two to three times more common in men than in women and occur in all age-groups. Although rare in children, they occur about one to three times more often and cause twice as many deaths as Hodgkin's disease in children under age 15. Incidence rises with age; median age is 50. These lymphomas seem linked to race or ethnic group, with increased incidence in whites and people of Jewish ancestry.

Signs and symptoms

Usually, the first indication of malignant lymphoma is swelling of the lymph glands, enlarged tonsils and adenoids, and painless, rubbery nodes in the cervical supraclavicular areas. In children, these nodes are usually in the cervical region, and the disease causes dyspnea and coughing. As the lymphoma progresses, the patient develops symptoms specific to the area involved and systemic complaints of fatigue, malaise, weight loss, fever, and night sweats.

Diagnosis

Confirmation requires histologic evaluation of biopsied lymph nodes; of tonsils, bone marrow, liver, bowel, or skin; or of tissue removed during exploratory laparotomy. (Biopsy differentiates malignant lymphoma from Hodgkin's disease.) Other tests include bone and chest X-rays, lymphangiography, liver and spleen scan, computed tomography scan of the abdomen, and excretory urography.

Laboratory tests include a complete blood count (may show anemia), uric acid (elevated or normal), serum calcium (elevated if bone lesions are present), serum protein (normal), and liver function studies.

Treatment

Appropriate treatment of malignant lymphomas may include radiation therapy or chemotherapy. Radiation therapy is used mainly in the early localized stage of the disease. Total nodal irradiation is often effective for both nodular and diffuse histologies.

Chemotherapy is most effective with combinations of multiple antineoplastic agents. For example, cyclophosphamide, doxorubicin (Adriamycin), vincristine (Oncovin), and prednisone (CHOP) can induce a complete remission in 70%

to 80% of patients with nodular histology and in 20% to 55% of patients with diffuse histology. Other combinations – such as methotrexate, bleomycin, Adriamycin, Cytoxan, vincristine (Oncovin), and prednisone (M-BACOP) – induce prolonged remission and a possible cure for the diffuse form of the disease.

Special considerations

• Observe the patient who's receiving radiation or chemotherapy for anorexia, nausea, vomiting, and diarrhea. Plan small, frequent meals scheduled around treatment.
• If the patient can't tolerate oral feedings, administer I.V. fluids and as needed give antiemetics and sedatives.
• Instruct the patient to keep irradiated skin dry.
• Provide emotional support by informing the patient and family about the prognosis and diagnosis and by listening to their concerns. If needed, refer them to the local chapter of the American Cancer Society for information and counseling. Stress the need for continued treatment and follow-up care.

Mycosis fungoides

In the United States, mycosis fungoides (MF) strikes more than 1,000 persons of all races annually; most are between ages 40 and 60. Unlike other lymphomas, MF allows an average life expectancy of 7 to 10 years after diagnosis. If correctly treated, particularly before it has spread beyond the skin, MF may go into remission for many years. However, after MF has reached the tumor stage, progression to severe disability or death is rapid. (Other names for MF include malignant cutaneous reticulosis and granuloma fungoides.)

Causes

A rare, chronic malignant T-cell lymphoma of unknown cause, MF originates in the reticuloendothelial system of the skin, eventually affecting lymph nodes and internal organs.

Signs and symptoms

The first sign of MF may be generalized erythroderma, possibly associated with itching. Eventually, MF evolves into varied combinations of infiltrated, thickened, or scaly patches, tumors, or ulcerations.

Diagnosis

A definitive diagnosis of MF depends on a history of multiple, varied, and progressively severe skin lesions associated with characteristic histologic evidence of lymphoma cell infiltration of the skin, with or without involvement of the lymph nodes or visceral organs. Consequently, this diagnosis is often missed during the early stages until lymphoma cells are sufficiently numerous in the skin to show up in biopsy.

Other diagnostic tests help confirm MF: a complete blood count and differential; a fingerstick smear for Sézary cells (abnormal circulating lymphocytes), which may be present in the erythrodermic variants of MF (Sézary syndrome); blood chemistry studies to screen for visceral dysfunction; a chest X-ray; liver-spleen isotopic scanning; lymphangiography; and a lymph node biopsy to assess lymph node involvement. These tests also help to stage the disease—a necessary prerequisite to treatment.

Treatment

Depending on the stage of the disease and its rate of progression, past treatment and results, the patient's age and overall clinical status, the treatment facilities available, and other factors, treatment of MF may include topical, intralesional, or systemic corticosteroid therapy; phototherapy; methoxsalen photochemotherapy; radiation; topical, intralesional, or systemic treatment with mechlorethamine hydrochloride; and other systemic chemotherapy.

Application of topical mechlorethamine hydrochloride (nitrogen mustard) is the preferred treatment for inducing remission in pretumorous stages. Mycotic plaques may also be treated with sunlight and topical steroids.

Total body electron beam radiation, which is less toxic to internal organs than standard photon beam radiation, has induced remission in some patients with early-stage MF.

Chemotherapy is employed primarily for patients with advanced MF. Systemic treatment with chemotherapeutic agents (cyclophosphamide, methotrexate, doxorubicin, bleomycin, etoposide, and steroids) and interferon alfa produces transient regression.

Special
considerations

• If the patient has difficulty applying nitrogen mustard to all involved skin surfaces, provide assistance. But wear gloves to prevent contact sensitization and to protect yourself from exposure to chemotherapeutic agents.

• If the patient is receiving drug treatment, watch for adverse effects and infection.

• The patient who is receiving radiation therapy will probably develop alopecia and erythema. Suggest that he wear a wig to improve his self-image and protect his scalp until hair regrowth begins, and suggest or give medicated oil baths to ease erythema.

• Because pruritus is often worse at night, the patient may need larger bedtime doses of antipruritics or sedatives as ordered to ensure adequate sleep. When the patient's symptoms have interrupted sleep, postpone early morning care to allow him more sleep.

• The patient with intense pruritus has an overwhelming need to scratch—often to the point of removing epidermis and replacing pruritus with pain, which some patients find easier to endure. Realize that you can't keep such a patient from scratching; the best you can do is help minimize the damage. Advise the patient to keep his fingernails short and clean and to wear a pair of soft, white cotton gloves when itching is unbearable.

• The malignant skin lesions are likely to make the patient depressed, fearful, and self-conscious. Fully explain the disease and its stages to help the patient and family understand and accept the disease.

• Provide reassurance and support by demonstrating a positive but realistic attitude. Reinforce your verbal support by touching the patient without any hint of anxiety or distaste.

Acute leukemia

A malignant proliferation of white blood cell (WBC) precursors (blasts) in bone marrow or lymph tissue and their accumulation in peripheral blood, bone marrow, and body tissues results in acute leukemia. The most common forms are acute lymphoblastic (lymphocytic) leukemia (ALL), in which there is abnormal growth of lymphocytic precursors (lymphoblasts); acute myeloblastic (myelogenous) leukemia (AML), characterized by rapid accumulation of myeloid precursors (myeloblasts); and acute monoblastic (monocytic) leukemia, or Schilling's type, distinguished by a marked increase in monocyte precursors (monoblasts). Acute myelomonocytic leukemia is another variant.

Untreated, acute leukemia is invariably fatal, usually because of complications that result from leukemia cells' infiltration of bone marrow or vital organs. With treatment, the prognosis varies. In ALL, treatment induces remission in 90% of children (average survival time: 5 years) and in 65% of adults (average survival time: 1 to 2 years). Children between ages 2 and 8 have the best survival rate – about 50% – with intensive therapy. In AML, the average survival time is only 1 year after diagnosis, even with aggressive treatment. In acute monoblastic leukemia, treatment induces remissions lasting 2 to 10 months in 50% of children; adults survive only about 1 year after diagosis, even with treatment.

Causes

Research on predisposing factors isn't conclusive but points to some combination of viruses (viral remnants have been found in leukemia cells), genetic and immunologic factors, and exposure to radiation and certain chemicals. (See *Predisposing factors in acute leukemia,* page 170.)

Pathogenesis isn't clearly understood, but immature, nonfunctioning WBCs appear to accumulate first in the tissue where they originate (lymphocytes in lymph tissue, granulocytes in bone marrow). (See *What happens in leukemia,* page 171.) These immature WBCs then spill into the bloodstream and from there infiltrate other tissues, eventually causing organ malfunction because of encroachment or hemorrhage.

Acute leukemia is more common in males than in females, in whites (especially people of Jewish descent), in children between ages 2 and 5 (ALL accounts for 80% of leukemia incidence in this age-group), and in persons who live in urban and industrialized areas. Acute leukemia ranks 20th in causes of cancer-related deaths among people of all age-groups. Among children, it's the most common form of

Predisposing factors in acute leukemia

Although the exact causes of most leukemias remain unknown, increasing evidence suggests a combination of contributing factors.

Acute lymphoblastic leukemia
• Familial tendency
• Monozygotic twins
• Congenital disorders, such as Down's syndrome, Bloom syndrome, Fanconi's anemia, ataxia-telangiectasia, and congenital agammaglobulinemia
• Viruses

Acute myeloblastic leukemia
• Familial tendency

• Monozygotic twins
• Congenital disorders, such as Down's syndrome, Bloom syndrome, Fanconi's anemia, ataxia-telangiectasia, and congenital agammaglobulinemia
• Ionizing radiation
• Exposure to the chemical benzene and cytotoxins such as alkylating agents
• Viruses

Acute monoblastic leukemia
• Unknown (radiation therapy, exposure to chemicals, heredity, and infections show little correlation to this disease)

---

cancer. In the United States, an estimated 11,000 persons develop acute leukemia annually.

Signs and symptoms

Acute leukemia's signs and symptoms are a sudden onset of high fever accompanied by thrombocytopenia and abnormal bleeding, such as nosebleeds, gingival bleeding, purpura, ecchymoses, petechiae, easy bruising after minor trauma, and prolonged menses. Nonspecific symptoms, such as low-grade fever, weakness, and lassitude, may persist for days or months before visible symptoms appear.

Other insidious signs include pallor, chills, and recurrent infections. In addition, ALL, AML, and acute monoblastic leukemia may cause dyspnea, anemia, fatigue, malaise, tachycardia, palpitations, systolic ejection murmur, and abdominal or bone pain.

When leukemia cells cross the blood-brain barrier and thereby escape the effects of systemic chemotherapy, the patient may develop signs of meningeal leukemia (confusion, lethargy, headache).

Diagnosis

Typical clinical findings and bone marrow aspirate showing a proliferation of immature WBCs confirm acute leukemia. An aspirate that's dry or free of leukemia cells in a patient

What happens in leukemia

This illustration shows how white blood cells (agranulocytes and granulocytes) proliferate in the bloodstream in leukemia, overwhelming red blood cells (RBCs) and platelets.

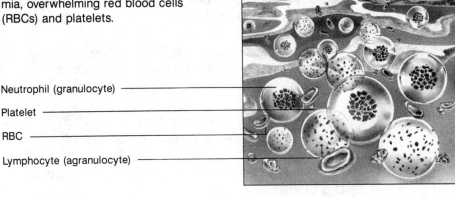

Neutrophil (granulocyte)

Platelet

RBC

Lymphocyte (agranulocyte)

with typical clinical findings requires bone marrow biopsy, usually of the posterior superior iliac spine. Blood counts show thrombocytopenia and neutropenia. A differential leukocyte count determines the leukemia cell type, and lumbar puncture detects meningeal involvement.

Treatment

Systemic chemotherapy aims to eradicate leukemia cells and induce remission (fewer than 5% of blast cells in the marrow and peripheral blood are normal). Chemotherapy varies according to the form of leukemia:
• meningeal infiltration — intrathecal instillation of methotrexate or cytarabine with cranial radiation
• ALL — vincristine, prednisone, high-dose cytarabine, L-asparaginase, AMSA, and daunorubicin. Because of the 40% risk of meningeal leukemia in ALL, intrathecal methotrexate or cytarabine is given. Radiation therapy is given for testicular infiltration.
• AML — a combination of I.V. daunorubicin and cytarabine or, if these fail to induce remission, a combination of cyclophosphamide, vincristine, prednisone, or methotrexate; high-dose cytarabine alone or with other drugs; amsacrine; etoposide; and 5-azacytidine and mitoxantrone

• Acute monoblastic leukemia—cytarabine and thioguanine with daunorubicin or doxorubicin.

Bone marrow transplant may be possible. Treatment also may include antibiotic, antifungal, and antiviral drugs and granulocyte injections to control infection, transfusions of platelets to prevent bleeding, and transfusions of red blood cells to prevent anemia.

Special considerations

• For the leukemia patient, emphasize comfort, minimize the adverse effects of chemotherapy, promote preservation of veins, manage complications, and provide teaching and psychological support.

• Because so many of these patients are children, be especially sensitive to their emotional needs and those of their families.

• Before treatment, explain the disease course, treatment, and adverse effects.

• Teach the patient and his family how to recognize infection (fever, chills, cough, or sore throat) and abnormal bleeding (bruising or petechiae), and how to stop such bleeding (applying pressure or ice to the area).

• Promote good nutrition. Explain that chemotherapy may cause weight loss and anorexia, so encourage the patient to eat and drink high-calorie, high-protein foods and beverages. However, chemotherapy and adjunctive prednisone may cause weight gain, so dietary counseling and teaching are helpful.

• Help establish an appropriate rehabilitation program for the patient during remission.

• Watch for signs of meningeal infiltration (confusion, lethargy, or headache). After intrathecal chemotherapy, place the patient in the Trendelenburg position for 30 minutes. Force fluids, and keep the patient supine for 4 to 6 hours. Check the lumbar puncture site often for bleeding.

• If the patient receives cranial radiation, teach him about potential adverse effects, and do what you can to minimize them.

• Prevent hyperuricemia, a possible result of rapid lysis of leukemia cells induced by chemotherapy. Give the patient about 2 liters of fluid daily, and give acetazolamide, sodium bicarbonate tablets, and allopurinol. Check urine pH often—

it should be above 7.5. Watch for a rash or another hypersensitivity reaction to allopurinol.

• Watch for early signs of cardiotoxicity, such as arrhythmia, and signs of heart failure if the patient receives daunorubicin or doxorubicin.

• Control infection by placing the patient in a private room and imposing reverse isolation, if necessary. (The benefits of reverse isolation are controversial.)

• Coordinate patient care so the leukemia patient doesn't come in contact with staff who also care for patients with infections or infectious diseases. Avoid using indwelling urinary catheters and giving I.M. injections because they provide an avenue for infection. Screen staff and visitors for contagious diseases, and be sure to watch for any signs of infection.

• Provide thorough skin care by keeping the patient's skin and perianal area clean, applying mild lotions or creams to keep the skin from drying and cracking, and thoroughly cleaning it before all invasive skin procedures.

• Change I.V. tubing according to your hospital's policy. Use strict aseptic technique and a metal scalp-vein needle (metal butterfly needle) when starting I.V.s. If the patient receives total parenteral nutrition, give scrupulous subclavian catheter care.

• Monitor temperature every 4 hours; patients with fever over 101° F (38.3°) and decreased WBC counts should receive prompt antibiotic therapy.

• Watch for bleeding; if it occurs, apply ice compresses and pressure, and elevate the extremity. Avoid giving I.M. injections, aspirin, and aspirin-containing drugs. Also avoid taking rectal temperatures, giving rectal suppositories, and doing digital examinations.

• Prevent constipation by providing adequate hydration, a high-residue diet, stool softeners, and mild laxatives, and by encouraging walking.

• Control mouth ulceration by checking often for obvious ulcers and gum swelling and by providing frequent mouth care and saline rinses. Tell the patient to use a soft toothbrush and to avoid hot, spicy foods and overuse of commercial mouthwashes.

• Also check the rectal area daily for induration, swelling, erythema, skin discoloration, or drainage.

- Provide psychological support by establishing a trusting relationship to promote communication. Allow the patient and his family to verbalize their anger and depression. Let the family participate in his care as much as possible.
- Minimize stress by providing a calm, quiet atmosphere that's conducive to rest and relaxation. For children particularly, be flexible with patient care and visiting hours to promote maximum interaction with family and friends and to allow time for schoolwork and play.
- For those patients who fail to respond to chemotherapy, and in the terminal phase of the disease, supportive care is directed toward maintaining comfort; managing pain, fever, and bleeding; and providing support for the patient and family. Provide the opportunity for religious counseling, and discuss the option of home or hospice care.

Chronic granulocytic leukemia

Also known as chronic myelogenous or myelocytic leukemia, chronic granulocytic leukemia (CGL) is characterized by the abnormal overgrowth of granulocytic precursors (myeloblasts, promyelocytes, metamyelocytes, and myelocytes) in bone marrow, peripheral blood, and body tissues. CGL is most common in young and middle-aged adults and is slightly more common in men than in women; it is rare in children. In the United States, approximately 3,000 to 4,000 cases of CGL develop annually, accounting for roughly 20% of all cases of leukemia.

CGL's clinical course proceeds in two distinct phases: the insidious chronic phase, with anemia and bleeding abnormalities and, eventually, the acute phase (plastic crisis), in which myeloblasts, the most primitive granulocytic precursors, proliferate rapidly.

This disease is invariably fatal. Average survival time is 3 to 4 years after onset of the chronic phase and 3 to 6 months after onset of the acute phase.

Causes

Almost 90% of patients with CGL have the Philadelphia (Ph[1]) chromosome, an abnormality discovered in 1960 in which the long arm of chromosome 22 is translocated, usually to chromosome 9. Radiation and carcinogenic chemicals may induce this chromosome abnormality. Myeloproliferative diseases also seem to increase the incidence of CGL, and some clinicians suspect that an unidentified virus causes this disease.

Signs and symptoms

Typically, CGL induces the following clinical effects:
• anemia (fatigue, weakness, decreased exercise tolerance, pallor, dyspnea, tachycardia, and headache)
• thrombocytopenia, with resulting bleeding and clotting disorders (retinal hemorrhage, ecchymoses, hematuria, melena, bleeding gums, nosebleeds, and easy bruising)
• hepatosplenomegaly, with abdominal discomfort and pain in splenic infarction from leukemia cell infiltration.

Other symptoms include sternal and rib tenderness from leukemia infiltrations of the periosteum; low-grade fever; weight loss; anorexia; renal calculi or gout arthritis from increased uric acid excretion; occasionally, prolonged infection and ankle edema; and, rarely, priapism and vascular insufficiency.

Diagnosis

In patients with typical changes, chromosomal analysis of peripheral blood or bone marrow showing the Ph[1] chromosome and low leukocyte alkaline phosphatase levels confirm CGL. Other relevant diagnostic tests include:
• *white blood cell count* – leukocytosis (leukocytes more than 50,000/mm^3, ranging as high as 250,000/mm^3), occasional leukopenia (leukocytes less than 5,000/mm^3), neutropenia (neutrophils less than 1,500/mm^3) despite a high leukocyte count, and increased circulating myeloblasts
• *hemoglobin* – often less than 10 g/dl
• *hematocrit* – low (less than 30%)
• *platelet count* – thrombocytosis (greater than 1 million/mm^3) common
• *serum uric acid* – possibly greater than 8 mg/dl
• *bone marrow aspirate* or *biopsy* – hypercellular; characteristically shows bone marrow infiltration by significantly increased number of myeloid elements (biopsy is done only if

aspirate is dry); in the acute phase, myeloblasts predominate
• *computed tomography scan* — may identify the organs affected by leukemia.

Treatment

Aggressive chemotherapy has so far failed to produce remission in CGL. Consequently in the chronic phase, the goal of treatment is to control leukocytosis and thrombocytosis. The most commonly used oral agents are busulfan and hydroxyurea. Aspirin is commonly given to prevent stroke if the patient's platelet count is over 1 million/mm³.

Ancillary CGL treatments include:
• local splenic radiation or splenectomy to increase platelet count and decrease adverse effects related to splenomegaly
• leukapheresis (selective leukocyte removal) to reduce leukocyte count
• allopurinol to prevent secondary hyperuricemia or colchicine to relieve gout caused by elevated serum uric acid levels
• prompt treatment of infections that may result from chemotherapy-induced bone marrow suppression.

During the acute phase of CGL, lymphoblastic or myeloblastic leukemia may develop. Treatment is similar to that for acute lymphoblastic leukemia. Remission, if achieved, is commonly short lived. Bone marrow transplant may produce long asymptomatic periods in the early phase of illness, but has been less successful in the accelerated phase. Despite vigorous treatment, CGL usually progresses after onset of the acute phase.

Special considerations

• Provide meticulous supportive care, psychological support, and careful patient teaching to help the patient make the most of remissions and to minimize complications.
• When the disease is diagnosed, repeat and reinforce the explanation of the disease and its treatment to the patient and his family.
• Throughout the chronic phase of CGL when the patient is hospitalized, plan your care to help avoid exhaustion if the patient has persistent anemia. Schedule laboratory tests and physical care with frequent rest periods in between, and assist the patient with walking if necessary. Regularly check the patient's skin and mucous membranes for pallor, petechiae, and bruising.

• To minimize bleeding, suggest a soft-bristle toothbrush, ‹ electric razor, and other safety precautions.
• To minimize the abdominal discomfort of splenomegaly, provide small, frequent meals. For the same reason, prevent constipation with a stool softener or laxative as needed. Ask the dietary department to provide a high-bulk diet, and maintain adequate fluid intake.
• To prevent atelectasis, stress the need for coughing and deep-breathing exercises.
• Because the patient with CGL often receives outpatient chemotherapy throughout the chronic phase, sound patient teaching is essential.
• Explain the expected adverse effects of chemotherapy; pay particular attention to dangerous adverse effects such as bone marrow suppression.
• Tell the patient to watch for and immediately report signs and symptoms of infection: any fever over 100° F (37.7° C), chills, redness or swelling, sore throat, and cough.
• Instruct the patient to watch for signs of thrombocytopenia, to immediately apply ice and pressure to any external bleeding site, and to avoid aspirin and aspirin-containing compounds because of the risk of increased bleeding.
• Emphasize the importance of adequate rest to minimize the fatigue of anemia. To minimize the toxic effects of chemotherapy, stress the importance of a high-calorie, high-protein diet. (For more information on treatment during the acute phase, see "Acute leukemia," pages 168 to 174.)

Chronic lymphocytic leukemia

A generalized, progressive disease that is common in older people, chronic lymphocytic leukemia is marked by an uncontrollable spread of abnormal, small lymphocytes in lymphoid tissue, blood, and bone marrow. Nearly all patients with chronic lymphocytic leukemia are men over age 50. According to the American Cancer Society, chronic lymphocytic leukemia accounts for almost one-third of new leukemia cases annually.

Although the cause of chronic lymphocytic leukemia is unknown, researchers suspect hereditary factors (higher incidence has been recorded within families), still-undefined chromosomal abnormalities, and certain immunologic defects (such as ataxia-telangiectasia or acquired agammaglobulinemia). The disease does not seem to be associated with radiation exposure.

Signs and symptoms

Chronic lymphocytic leukemia is the most benign and the most slowly progressive form of leukemia. Clinical signs derive from the infiltration of leukemia cells in bone marrow, lymphoid tissue, and organ systems.

In early stages, patients usually complain of fatigue, malaise, fever, and nodal enlargement. They're particularly susceptible to infection.

In advanced stages, patients may experience severe fatigue and weight loss, with liver or spleen enlargement, bone tenderness, and edema from lymph node obstruction. Pulmonary infiltrates may appear when lung parenchyma is involved. Skin infiltrations, manifested by macular to nodular eruptions, occur in about half the cases of chronic lymphocytic leukemia.

As the disease progresses, bone marrow involvement may lead to anemia, pallor, weakness, dyspnea, tachycardia, palpitations, bleeding, and infection. Opportunistic fungal, viral, and bacterial infections commonly occur in late stages.

Diagnosis

Typically, chronic lymphocytic leukemia is an incidental finding during a routine blood test that reveals numerous abnormal lymphocytes. In early stages, the white blood cell (WBC) count is mildly but persistently elevated. Granulocytopenia is the rule, but the WBC count climbs as the disease progresses. Blood studies also show a hemoglobin count less than 11 g/dl, hypogammaglobulinemia, and depressed serum globulins. Other common developments include neutropenia (less than 1,500/mm^3), lymphocytosis (greater than 10,000/mm^3), and thrombocytopenia (less than 150,000/mm^3). Bone marrow aspiration and biopsy show lymphocytic invasion.

Treatment

Systemic chemotherapy includes alkylating agents, usually chlorambucil or cyclophosphamide, and sometimes steroids (prednisone) when autoimmune hemolytic anemia or thrombocytopenia occurs.

When chronic lymphocytic leukemia causes obstruction or organ impairment or enlargement, local radiation treatment can be used to reduce organ size. Allopurinol can be given to prevent hyperuricemia, a relatively uncommon finding.

Prognosis is poor if anemia, thrombocytopenia, neutropenia, bulk lymphadenopathy, and severe lymphocytosis are present.

Special considerations

• Plan patient care to relieve symptoms and prevent infection. Clean the patient's skin daily with mild soap and water. Frequent soaks may be ordered. Watch for signs of infection: temperature over 100° F (37.7° C), chills, redness, or swelling of any body part.

• Watch for signs of thrombocytopenia (black, tarry stools; easy bruising; nosebleeds; and bleeding gums) and anemia (pale skin, weakness, fatigue, dizziness, and palpitations).

• Advise the patient to avoid aspirin and products containing aspirin. Explain that many medications contain aspirin, even though their names don't make this clear. Teach him how to recognize aspirin variants on medication labels.

• Explain chemotherapy and its possible adverse effects. If the patient is to be discharged, tell him to avoid coming in contact with obviously ill people, especially children with common contagious childhood diseases. Urge him to eat high-protein foods and drink high-calorie beverages.

• Stress the importance of follow-up care, frequent blood tests, and taking all medications exactly as prescribed.

• Teach the patient the signs of recurrence (swollen lymph nodes in the neck, axilla, and groin and increased abdominal size or discomfort), and tell him to notify his doctor immediately if he detects any of these signs.

• Provide emotional support and be a good listener. Most patients with chronic lymphocytic leukemia are elderly; some are frightened. Try to keep their spirits up by concentrating on pleasantries such as improving their personal appearance, providing a soothing environment, and asking questions about their families. If possible, provide opportunities for their favorite activities.

Self-test questions

You can quickly review your comprehension of this chapter on blood and lymph neoplasms by answering the following questions. The answers to these questions and their rationales appear on pages 195 to 197.

Case history
questions

Kenneth Howard discovers a lump in his left inguinal area while taking a shower one morning. Frightened, he makes an appointment to see his doctor.

Information obtained during the history reveals that Mr. Howard had not noticed the enlarged lymph node before and has had a recent onset of pruritus, which he attributes to dry skin that sometimes occurs in the winter months. However, he does admit that this winter the pruritus has been much worse. He also reports having had a number of minor but annoying upper respiratory infections over the past several months.

On physical examination, Mr. Howard states that he feels no pain when the enlarged lymph node is palpated. Two days later, the lymph node is biopsied, and a diagnosis of Hodgkin's disease is made.

1. With appropriate treatment for Hodgkin's disease, the 5-year survival rate is approximately:
    a. 40%.
    b. 50%.
    c. 75%.
    d. 90%.

2. Which of the following statements is true regarding Hodgkin's disease?
    a. Lymph nodes may enlarge slowly over months or years or they may enlarge rapidly.
    b. Hodgkin's disease is slightly more common in blacks.

c. Decreased serum alkaline phosphatase indicates liver or bone involvement.

d. Radiation is ineffective in the treatment of Hodgkin's disease.

3. Which of the following abnormalities helps confirm the diagnosis of Hodgkin's disease?

a. Heinz bodies

b. Reed-Sternberg cells

c. Hexosaminidase A

d. Bence Jones protein

Sara Donne is diagnosed with acute lymphoblastic leukemia (ALL) following the sudden onset of high fever accompanied by thrombocytopenia and abnormal bleeding. Nonspecific symptoms noted on her history include weakness and lassitude present for several months, pallor, chills, and a history of recurrent infections. In addition, she complains of dyspnea, palpitations, and mild abdominal pain.

4. Which of the following predisposing factors may be present in the history of both ALL and acute myeloblastic leukemia patients?

a. Being a monozygotic twin

b. Exposure to ionizing radiation

c. Exposure to the chemical benzene

d. Use of alkylating agents

5. When auscultating the heart of a patient with ALL, you may detect what type of murmur?

a. Blowing holosystolic murmur

b. Mid-diastolic murmur

c. Systolic ejection murmur

d. Holosystolic decrescendo murmur

6. The patient with acute leukemia should avoid which of the following drugs?

a. Aspirin

b. Allopurinol

c. Acetazolamide

d. Acetaminophen

7. One of the first indications of malignant lymphoma is usually:
    a. fatigue.
    b. weight loss.
    c. night sweats.
    d. swelling of the lymph glands.

8. The preferred treatment for inducing remission in pretumerous mycosis fungoides is:
    a. total body electron beam radiation.
    b. chemotherapy.
    c. topical mechlorethamine hydrochloride.
    d. site-specific radiation therapy.

9. The Philadelphia chromosome is found in nearly 90% of patients with which of the following neoplasms?
    a. Acute lymphoblastic leukemia
    b. Chronic granulocytic leukemia
    c. Malignant lymphoma
    d. Hodgkin's disease

10. Chronic lymphocytic leukemia typically occurs in:
    a. men over age 50.
    b. children between ages 2 and 5.
    c. adults between ages 40 and 60.
    d. young and middle-aged adults.

Selected References
and Self-Test Answers and Rationales

Selected References 184

Self-Test Answers and Rationales 186

Selected References

Ashburn, M.A., et al. "Management of Pain in the Cancer Patient," *Anesthesia and Analgesia* 76(2):402-16, February 1993.

Austoker, J. "Diet and Cancer," *BMJ* 308(6944):1610-14, June 18, 1994.

Austoker, J., et al. "Smoking and Cancer: Smoking Cessation," 308(6942):1478-82, June 4, 1994.

"The Best Colon Cancer Tests," *Johns Hopkins Medical Letter Health After 50,* 5(9):1-2, November 1993.

Byrne, B. "Small Cell Lung Cancer," *Nursing Standard* 8(9):23-28, November 17-23, 1993.

Camp-Sorrell, D., and Wujcik, D. "Intravenous Immunoglobulin Administration: An Evaluation of Vital Sign Monitoring," *Oncology Nursing Forum* 21(3):531-35, April 1994.

Carney, P.A., et al. "The Periodic Health Examination Provided to Asymptomatic Older Women: An Assessment Using Standardized Patients," *Annals of Internal Medicine* 119(2):129-35, July 15, 1993.

Charnsangavej, C. "New Imaging Modalities for Follow-up of Colorectal Carcinoma," *Cancer* 71(12 Suppl):4236-40, June 15, 1993.

Davis, C.L., et al. "Palliative Care," *BMJ* 308(6940):1359-62, May 21, 1994.

DeVita, V., et al. *Cancer: Principles and Practice of Oncology,* 4th ed. Philadelphia: J.B. Lippincott Co., 1993.

Engelking, C. "New Approaches: Innovations in Cancer Prevention, Diagnosis, Treatment, and Support," *Oncology Nursing Forum* 21(1):62-71, January-February, 1994.

Erickson, J.H. *Oncologic Nursing,* 2nd ed. Springhouse, Pa.: Springhouse Corp., 1994.

"Examinations for Oral Cancer—United States, 1992," *JAMA* 271(16):1232, April 1994.

Finley, R.S. "Clinical Practice Guidelines for the Management of Cancer Pain," *Cancer Practice* 2(3):236-38, May-June 1994.

Goldenberg, D.M. "Monoclonal Antibodies in Cancer Detection and Therapy," *American Journal of Medicine* 94(3):297-312, March 1993.

Granda, C. "Nursing Management of Patients with Lymphedema Associated with Breast Cancer Therapy," *Cancer Nursing* 17(3):229-35, June 1994.

Groenwald, S.L., et al. *Cancer Nursing: Principles and Practice,* 3rd ed. Boston: Jones & Bartlett Publishers, 1993.

Jacox, A., et al. *Management of Cancer Pain: Clinical Practice Guideline, No. 9.* Rockville, Md.: Department of Health and Human Services, 1994.

Kumar, P.P., et al. "Role of Brachytherapy in the Management of the Skull Base Meningioma," *Cancer* 71(11):3726-31, June 1, 1993.

Lippman, S.M., et al. "Chemoprevention: Strategies for the Control of Cancer," *Cancer* 72(3 Suppl):984-90, August 1, 1993.

Meadows, A.T, et al. "Long-term Survival: Clinical Care, Research, and Education," *Cancer* 71(10 Suppl):3213-15, May 15, 1993.

McCorkle, R., and Grant, M. *Pocket Companion for Cancer Nursing.* Philadelphia: W.B. Saunders Co., 1994.

Mulshine, J.L., et al. "Scientific Basis for Cancer Prevention: Intermediate Cancer Markers," *Cancer* 72(3 Suppl):978-83, August 1, 1993.

Perez, C.A., et al. "Irradiation in Relapsing Carcinoma of the Prostate," *Cancer* 71(3 Suppl):1110-22, February 1, 1993.

Rogers, B.B. "Taxol: A Promising New Drug of the '90s," *Oncology Nursing Forum* 20(10):1483-89, November-December 1993.

Roye, C.F. "Pap Smear Screening for Adolescents: Rationale, Technique, and Follow-up," *Journal of Pediatric Health Care* 7(5):199-206, September-October 1993.

Stitik, F.P. "The New Staging of Lung Cancer," *Radiologic Clinics of North America* 32(4):635-47, July 1994.

Self-Test Answers and Rationales

Chapter 1:
Introduction

1. a Cancer is second only to cardiovascular disease as the leading cause of death in North America. Some epidemiologists predict it will be the leading cause of death by the year 2010. More than 1 million cancer cases are diagnosed yearly; the disease kills about 500,000 Americans annually. Cancer occurs predominantly in elderly adults with the incidence increasing geometrically with age. It generally is more common in men. Although cancer isn't very common in children, only accidental death exceeds it as the leading cause of death in this age-group.

2. a Researchers have now discovered about 100 cancer genes (many more may exist). Some are oncogenes, which activate cell division and play an important role in embryonic development. Others are tumor suppressor genes, which halt cell division.

3. d Benign tumors rarely cause cachexia whereas cachexia is typical with malignant tumors. Benign tumors are frequently encapsulated and well differentiated whereas malignant are often poorly delineated and differentiation is variable. Benign tumors rarely recur after surgical removal; malignant tumors frequently recur after surgical excision.

4. d Plant alkaloids prevent cellular reproduction of cancer cells by disrupting cell mitosis. Alkylating agents and nitrosoureas inhibit cell growth and division by reacting with deoxyribonucleic acid (DNA). Antimetabolites prevent cell growth by competing with metabolites in the production of nucleic acid. Antitumor antibiotics block cell growth by binding with DNA and interfering with DNA-dependent ribonucleic acid synthesis.

5. c A patient receiving external radiation therapy in areas of bone marrow production will need frequent blood counts (with particular attention to white blood cells and platelets) to detect adverse hematologic effects. External radiation therapy does not cause pain nor does it make the patient radioactive. Radiation therapy is not a substitute for chemotherapy; in fact, it may be combined with chemotherapy in the treatment of selected neoplasms.

Chapter 2: Head, neck, and spinal neoplasms

1. b Generally, clinical features of a brain tumor result from increased intracranial pressure from the pressure exerted by the tumor within the rigid cranial cavity. Such features vary with the type of tumor, its location, and the degree of invasion. Lumbar puncture results reveal increased protein in the cerebrospinal fluid (CSF) rather than a decreased level that would be present in a progressive loss of protein. Compression of a vertebral artery is a secondary factor only if the tumor is located nearby and severe compression seriously impedes cerebral flow. Likewise, pyramidal tract destruction is a secondary factor only if the tumor is located near a pyramidal tract and the destruction impedes message transmission along the involved pyramidal tract.

2. a An oligodendroglioma is a slow-growing brain tumor. It is the third most common glioma; an astrocytoma is the second most common malignant glioma (about 30% of all gliomas). An oligodendroglioma is more common in women than in men and more common in middle-aged adults than in young adults.

3. c Laryngeal cancer is classified by its location as supraglottal (false vocal cords), glottal (true vocal cords), or subglottal (downward extension from vocal cords). Cell type, symptom severity, and tumor size are used to determine treatment rather than classification of laryngeal cancer.

4. d After a partial laryngectomy, the patient must not use his voice for 2 to 3 days. After that, caution him to whisper until healing is complete. Using his voice earlier can lead to complications such as bleeding and laryngeal edema.

5. a Papillary carcinoma is the least virulent form of thyroid cancer and accounts for half of all thyroid cancers in adults. It metastasizes slowly into regional nodes of the neck, mediastinum, lungs, and other distant organs. Follicular, medullary, and spindle cell carcinomas are more virulent. Less common than papillary carcinoma, follicular carcinoma is more likely to recur and metastasize to the regional nodes and through blood vessels into the bones, liver, and lungs. Untreated medullary carcinoma grows rapidly and frequently metastasizes to bones, the liver, and kidneys. Spindle cell carcinoma metastasizes rapidly and causes death by tracheal invasion and compression of adjacent structures.

6. c Predisposing factors for thyroid cancer include radiation exposure (especially to the neck), prolonged thyroid-stimulating hormone secretion, familial predisposition, or chronic goiter. Subacute granulomatous thyroiditis, age over 65 (thyroid cancer can occur at any age), and excessive ingestion of iodized salt have not been identified as predisposing factors for thyroid cancer.

7. a Typical neurologic symptoms associated with a pituitary tumor include frontal headaches, visual disturbances, personality changes, seizures, and rhinorrhea. Lateral extension of a pituitary tumor involves cranial nerves III, IV, and VI (all dealing with eye movement) but not cranial nerve VII and IX (taste) and VIII (hearing).
   Balance is regulated by the cerebellum, which lies close to the brainstem, and not by the pituitary gland, which is located in the sella turcica below the hypothalamus and third ventricle of the brain.

8. c After transsphenoidal surgery in pituitary cancer, the patient will lose his sense of smell. The pituitary gland does not control bladder or bowel function. The patient may experience total visual loss (not just night vision), and it is usually regained following surgery.

9. b Meningiomas occur most often in women. Schwannomas, astrocytomas, and ependymomas occur with equal frequency in both men and women.

10. b A spinal tap shows clear yellow CSF from increased protein levels if CSF flow is completely blocked. If the flow is partially blocked, protein levels rise, but the fluid is only slightly yellow in proportion to the CSF protein level. CSF can be aspirated during a spinal tap even when the flow of CSF is blocked. Cloudy CSF suggests infection rather than blockage. CSF pressure can be measured even with complete blockage of CSF flow.

Chapter 3: Thoracic neoplasms

1. d Eighty percent of lung cancer patients are smokers. The risk is highest in smokers over age 40, especially if they began to smoke before age 15, have smoked a whole pack or more per day for 20 years, or work with or near asbestos.

2. c Hypercalcemia and hypophosphatemia result from ectopic parathyroid hormone (PTH) or PTH-related peptide production by epidermoid lung cancer. Gynecomastia most commonly results from large-cell lung cancer; Cushing's and carcinoid syndromes from small-cell carcinoma; and hyponatremia with the syndrome of inappropriate secretion of antidiuretic hormone or possibly atrial natriuretic factor from small-cell carcinoma.

3. a Fluorouracil and cisplatin may be used to treat non-small cell lung cancer. Along with these agents, leucovorin calcium may be given. This folic acid substance is used to prevent or decrease the toxicity caused by the antineoplastic agents. Other chemotherapy combinations (carboplatin and cyclophosphamide; doxorubicin, cisplatin, and etoposide; and doxorubicin, bleomycin, vinblastine, and dacarbazine) are not used to treat lung cancer. Instead, the combination of carboplatin and cyclophosphamide is used to treat ovarian cancer and epithelial cancer; doxorubicin, cisplatin, and etoposide to treat gastric cancer; and doxorubicin, bleomycin, vinblastine, and dacarbazine to treat Hodgkin's lymphoma.

4. c Following thoracic surgery, position the patient on the surgical side to promote drainage and lung reexpansion. Placing the patient in a prone or supine position or on the nonsurgical side does not promote drainage and lung reexpansion.

5. a Breast cancer occurs more often in the upper outer quadrant of the breast. It also occurs more often in the left breast than the right. Women at high risk for breast cancer include those who have long menstrual cycles or began menses early or menopause late. Asian and Indian women have a lower risk for breast cancer than Hispanic women.

6. d The most important factor in predicting survival time in breast cancer is the number of involved lymph nodes. Important but less significant factors in predicting survival time are tumor size, type of breast cancer, and history of breast cancer in the other breast.

7. b Following a modified radical mastectomy, drainage from the incision should be serous after the first 4 hours postoperatively. Bloody drainage is abnormal 24 hours postoperatively and reflects a bleeding problem. Milky white to gray and yellowish drainage are also abnormal and may indicate an infection.

8. c Lymphedema may be prevented after a mastectomy by having the patient exercise her hand and arm regularly and avoid activities that might cause infection in the hand or arm (infection increases the chance of developing lymphedema). Such prevention is important because lymphedema can't be treated effectively. Advise the patient to wear loose (not tightly fitting) rubber gloves when washing dishes to prevent constricting the circulation. Tell her that daily use of lanolin hand cream helps prevent dry skin from cracking, which could lead to infection. Dangling the affected arm every 3 to 4 hours daily would increase (not decrease) the risk of lymphedema.

Chapter 4:
Abdominal
and pelvic
neoplasms

1. a. The pylorus and antrum of the stomach are the most common sites of gastric carcinoma. Other stomach parts affected (in order of decreasing frequency) are the lesser curvature, the cardia, the body of the stomach, and the greater curvature.

2. d In a Billroth II procedure, the lower stomach and duodenum are removed. The remaining part of the stomach is then anastomosed to the jejunum. A subtotal gastrectomy involves partial removal of the stomach; a total gastrectomy involves resection of the entire stomach. The gallbladder is not routinely removed during gastric surgery.

3. b In gastric cancer, radiation therapy is most effective if given on an empty stomach. It's less effective if the patient eats immediately before the treatment or drinks a glass of milk 1 hour before the treatment. Taking an antacid 30 minutes immediately after the treatment will not minimize or prevent gastric upset that may occur as an adverse effect of radiation therapy.

4. b Stasis-induced inflammation, as in achalasia or stricture is a prediposing factor for esophageal cancer. Other predisposing factors include chronic irritation, as in heavy smoking and excessive use of alcohol; previous head and neck tumors; and nutritional deficiency, as in untreated sprue and Plummer-Vinson syndrome. Hypoglycemia, ulcerative colitis, and anorexia nervosa have not been identified as predisposing factors for esophageal cancer.

5. a Over 90% of pancreatic tumors are duct cell adenocarcinomas and arise most frequently (67% of cases) in the head of the pancreas. Insulinomas are relatively uncommon islet cell tumors that may be benign or malignant. Less common types of pancreatic exocrine cancer include acinar cell carcinoma and cystadenocarcinoma.

6. c If the patient has a sigmoid colostomy, instruct him to irrigate it every 1 to 3 days (twice daily is unnecessary) to achieve regularity. Irrigating only when constipation occurs will not help the patient become regular and may be harmful because a bowel obstruction can occur if constipation is severe.

7. b Kidney cancer is twice as common in men as in women. This disease accounts for about 2% of all adult cancers and usually strikes after age 40 (but not after age 60) with peak incidence between ages 50 and 60. The 5-year survival rate is approximately 50%; the 10-year survival rate, 18% to 23%.

8. a Instruct a patient with liver cancer to restrict sodium and fluids (to minimize edema) and protein (to reduce blood ammonia buildup). No alcohol is allowed. Restriction of potassium, polyunsaturated fats, and fat-soluble vitamins is unnecessary.

9. d Commonly, the first sign of bladder cancer is gross, painless, intermittent hematuria (often with clots in the urine). Invasive lesions often cause suprapubic pain, which occurs after voiding (not with a full bladder). Urinary tract infection and incontinence are not typical signs of bladder cancer. Urinary tract infection may be a secondary effect if urinary retention results from the lesion causing obstruction or from invasive procedures used to diagnose and treat bladder cancer. Incontinence may occur as a secondary effect if the urinary sphincter is involved.

10. d Gallbladder cancer may metastasize to local lymph nodes, the liver, lungs (especially lower lobes), and the peritoneum. Because of spread to the peritoneum, the ovaries in females (not the testes in males) may be involved. The usual metastatic sites for gallbladder cancer do not include the brain or kidneys.

Chapter 5: Genital neoplasms

1. d About 85% of prostate carcinomas originate in the posterior part of the prostate gland; the rest near the urethra. Malignant prostate tumors seldom result from the benign hyperplastic enlargement that commonly develops around the prostatic urethra in elderly men. Prostate cancer is the most common (not second most common) neoplasm in men over age 50 and the second leading cause of death in men (not the third). Adenocarcinoma is its most common form; only rarely does it occur as a sarcoma.

2. b Urinary incontinence may result from a prostatectomy, usually occurring after postoperative removal of the catheter, but leakage generally subsides within 6 months in 85% to 90% of men. Refractory urinary incontinence may be treated by a surgically implanted artifical urinary sphincter. Increased libido, priapism, and gynecomastia are not adverse effects of a prostatectomy.

3. b Encourage the patient to begin perineal exercises within 24 to 48 hours after surgery to minimize incontinence. The patient is usually not fully recovered from the effects of anesthesia within 6 to 12 hours after surgery and would not be physically able to perform perineal exercises. Waiting longer than 48 hours to start the exercise may prolong the incontinence.

4. d The use of estrogen therapy without progesterone is a predisposing factor for uterine cancer. A low fertility index and anovulation (not multiple pregnancies) is also a predisposing factor. Obesity (rather than anorexia) and a history of diabetes (rather than hypoglycemia) have also been identified as predisposing factors. Other such factors include previous abnormal uterine bleeding, hypertension, a familial tendency, and a history of uterine polyps, or endometrial hyperplasia.

5. d If the patient has a blood drainage system in place, notify the surgeon immediately if drainage exceeds 400 ml because this may indicate hemorrhaging. Amounts less than this do not constitute an emergency. However, if the patient suddenly drains more than during previous shifts (even if less than 400 ml), alert the surgeon because this may indicate abnormal bleeding or an infection.

6. c Vinblastine may cause neurotoxicity, including such symptoms as peripheral paresthesias, jaw pain, and muscle cramps. Ototoxicity, nephrotoxicity, and cardiotoxicity are not associated with vinblastine therapy.

7. a Topical fluorouracil is used to treat precancerous penile lesions. Don plastic gloves before applying this medication, and wash your hands immediately afterwards. A combination of bleomycin, methotrexate, and cisplatin is used for metastatic lesions stemming from penile cancer.

8. c Cervical cancer is the third most common cancer of the female reproductive system. The invasive form usually occurs between ages 30 and 50. It rarely occurs under age 20 and isn't common in women between ages 20 and 30 or over age 50.

9. d Radiation therapy is the preferred treatment for advanced vaginal cancer. Most patients need preliminary external radiation treatment to shrink the tumor before internal radiation can begin. Surgery is usually recommended only when the tumor is so extensive that exenteration is needed because close proximity to the bladder and rectum permits only minimal tissue margins around resected vaginal tissue. Laser surgery combined with topical fluorouracil is reserved for early stages of vaginal cancer to preserve the normal parts of the vagina. Systemic chemotherapy has not proved effective in vaginal cancer.

10. b In women with previously treated breast cancer, metastatic ovarian cancer is more common than cancer at any other site, including the cervix, vulva, and fallopian tubes.

Chapter 6: Bone, skin, and soft-tissue neoplasms

1. c In multiple myeloma, rouleaux formations (often the first clue) are seen on differential smear of the complete blood count. They result from elevation of the erythrocyte sedimentation rate. A decreased hemoglobin is also present showing moderate to severe anemia. However, anemia alone may stem from many causes and alone does not suggest multiple myeloma as the first clue. An elevated hematocrit and elevated white blood cell count are not diagnostic findings in this disease.

2. d The presence of Bence Jones protein almost always confirms multiple myeloma. But its absence doesn't rule out this disease. Glycosuria may occur in diabetes mellitus but bears no relationship to multiple myeloma. An acid urine pH is associated with renal tuberculosis (not renal involvement caused by multiple myeloma). Multiple myeloma may cause a low (rather than high) urine specific gravity if it involves the kidneys resulting in pyelonephritis.

3. c In multiple myeloma, a combination of doxorubicin and carmustine is used. Other treatment combinations include carmustine, cyclophosphamide, and prednisone; vincristine, carmustine, cyclophosphamide, melphalan, and prednisone; vincristine, doxorubicin, and dexamethasone; vincristine, carmustine, doxorubicin, and prednisone; or vincristine, cyclophosphamide, doxorubicin, and prednisone. The chemotherapy combination of cisplatin and fluorouracil is used to treat head and neck cancer; cytarabine and doxorubicin to treat leukemia; and doxorubicin and cisplatin to treat bony sarcoma.

4. b An invasive tumor with metastatic potential, squamous cell carcinoma of the skin arises from the keratinizing epidermal cells. It occurs most often in fair-skinned (not dark-skinned) white males over age 60. Although hormonal factors may play a role in the development of malignant melanoma, it is not considered a predisposing factor in squamous cell carcinoma of the skin.

5. a Lesions on sun-damaged skin, such as the face and the dorsa of the hands and forearms, tend to be less invasive and less likely to metastasize than lesions on unexposed skin. Notable exceptions are squamous cell lesions on the lower lip and ears, which are almost invariably markedly invasive metastatic lesions with a generally poor prognosis.

6. d Tell patients to apply a strong sunscreening agent 30 to 60 minutes before sun exposure. Applying the sunscreen less than 30 minutes before sun exposure may result in less effective initial blocking of the sun's harmful rays.

7. d Ewing's sarcomas and osteogenic bone tumors are the most common primary malignant bone tumors in children. Fibrosarcoma, chordoma, and malignant giant cell bone tumors also occur in children.

8. a Bone pain is the most common indication of primary malignant bone tumors. It is often more intense at night and isn't usually associated with mobility. The pain is usually described as dull (not "pins and needles") and is usually localized (not generalized), although it may be referred from the hip or spine and result in weakness or a limp.

9. b Superficial basal cell epitheliomas are oval or irregularly shaped, lightly pigmented plaques, with sharply defined, slightly elevated, threadlike borders. Due to superficial erosion, they appear scaly and have small, atrophic central areas that resemble psoriasis or eczema.

Noduloulcerative basal cell epitheliomas are small, smooth, pinkish, and translucent. As the lesions enlarge, their centers become depressed and their borders become firm and elevated. Sclerosing basal cell epitheliomas are waxy, sclerotic, yellow to white plaques without distinct borders and often look like small patches of scleroderma. The pre-malignant skin lesions of Bowen's disease are brown to reddish brown with a scaly surface.

10. c Kaposi's sarcoma is characterized by obvious colorful lesions. They vary in shape, size, and color (ranging from red-brown to dark purple) and occur most commonly on the skin, buccal mucosa, hard and soft palates, lips, gums, tongue, tonsils, conjunctiva, and sclera. Auscultation may uncover wheezing and hypoventilation in the patient with Kaposi's sarcoma rather than hyperventilation. If the sarcoma advances beyond the early stages or if a lesion breaks down, the patient may report pain. Usually, however, the lesions remain pain-free unless they impinge on nerves or organs. The patient with Kaposi's sarcoma is usually thin because he has acquired immunodeficiency syndrome.

**Chapter 7:
Blood and
lymph
neoplasms**

1. d Recent advances in therapy make Hodgkin's disease potentially curable, even in advanced stages. Appropriate treatment yields a 5-year survival rate of approximately 90%.

2. a In Hodgkin's disease, lymph nodes may enlarge rapidly, producing pain and obstruction, or enlarge slowly and painlessly for months or years. The lymph nodes may "wax and wane," but usually don't return to normal. The disease occurs in all races but is slightly more common in whites (not blacks). An elevated (not decreased) serum alkaline phosphatase level indicates liver or bone involvement. Radiation therapy may effectively treat Hodgkin's disease and is used alone or in combination with chemotherapy.

3. b Hodgkin's disease is characterized by a special histologic feature—the presence of Reed-Sternberg giant cells in lymph node tissue. Reed-Sternberg cells are enlarged, abnormal histiocytes.

Heinz bodies do not form in Hodgkin's disease. They are particles of denatured hemoglobin that have precipitated out of the cytoplasm of red blood cells (RBCs) and that have collected in small masses and attached to the cell membranes. They form as a result of drug injury to RBCs, the presence of unstable hemoglobins, unbalanced globin chain synthesis caused by thalassemia, or an RBC enzyme deficiency.

Hexosaminidase is a group of enzymes normally found in serum samples. These enzymes are necessary for the metabolism of gangliosides (water-soluble glycolipids found primarily in brain tissue). An absence of hexosaminidase A indicates Tay-Sachs disease, and has nothing to do with Hodgkin's disease.

The presence of Bence Jones protein in the urine is the hallmark of multiple myeloma not Hodgkin's disease. Bence Jones protein isn't found in all multiple myeloma patients, but it's almost never found in patients without this disease.

4. a A predisposing factor common to both acute lymphoblastic leukemia (ALL) and acute myeloblastic leukemia (AML) is being a monozygotic twin. Other shared predisposing factors include a familial tendency, selected congenital disorders, and viruses. Predisposing factors for AML and not ALL include exposure to ionizing radiation or to the chemical benzene or the use of alkylating agents.

5. c ALL, AML, and acute monoblastic leukemia may cause a systolic ejection murmur as well as dyspnea, anemia, fatigue, malaise, tachycardia, palpitations, and abdominal or bone pain. A blowing holosystolic murmur, a mid-diastolic murmur, and a holosystolic decrescendo murmur are not typical murmurs in leukemia; instead they reflect valvular disorders.

6. a Aspirin and aspirin-containing drugs should not be given to a patient with acute leukemia because aspirin increases the risk of bleeding. However, a patient with acute leukemia may require acetazolamide and allopurinol to prevent hyperuricemia, a possible result of rapid chemotherapy-induced leukemic cell lysis. Acetaminophen may be used as needed to treat a fever or relieve minor aches and pains.

7. d Usually the first indications of malignant lymphoma are swelling of the lymph glands, enlarged tonsils and adenoids, and painless, rubbery nodes in the cervical supraclavicular areas. As the lymphoma progresses, the patient develops symptoms specific to the area involved and systemic complaints of fatigue, malaise, weight loss, fever, and night sweats.

8. c Application of topical mechlorethamine hydrochloride (nitrogen mustard) is the preferred treatment for inducing remission in pretumerous stages of mycosis fungoides. Radiation therapy is used mainly in the early localized stage of malignant lymphomas. Total body electron beam radiation has induced remission in some patients with early mycosis fungoides. Chemotherapy is used primarily in advanced disease.

9. b Almost 90% of patients with chronic granulocytic leukemia have the Philadelphia (Ph[1]) chromosome, in which the long arm of chromosome 22 is translocated, usually to chromosome 9. In ALL, malignant lymphoma, and Hodgkin's disease, patients do not exhibit the Ph[1] chromosome.

10. a Nearly all patients with chronic lymphocytic leukemia are men over age 50. Acute leukemia is most common in children between ages 2 and 5; mycosis fungoides in adults between ages 40 and 60; and chronic granulocytic leukemia in young and middle-aged adults.

Appendices and Index

Appendix A—Chemotherapeutic Drugs 200

Appendix B—Chemotherapy Acronyms and
                  Protocols 239

Appendix C—*ICD-9-CM* Classification of
                  Neoplastic Disorders 263

Index 289

Chemotherapeutic Drugs

In this appendix, you'll find the indications and pharmacologic classification of each chemotherapeutic drug, along with adverse reactions and drug interactions, drug incompatibilities for the patient on a multiple-drug regimen, and important administration guidelines.

Aldesleukin
Proleukin

Pharmacologic classification
Aldesleukin is a human recombinant interleukin-2 derivative that exhibits antitumor activity.

Indications
Metastastic renal cell carcinoma

Adverse reactions
• Blood: *anemia, thrombocytopenia, leukopenia,* coagulation disorders, leukocytosis, eosinophilia.
• CNS: mental status changes, headache, dizziness, sensory dysfunction, special senses disorders, syncope, motor dysfunction, coma.
• CV: *hypotension, sinus tachycardia,* **arrhythmias,** bradycardia, **premature ventricular contractions,** premature atrial contractions, *myocardial ischemia, MI, CHF, cardiac arrest, myocarditis, endocarditis, CVA,* pericardial effusion, thrombosis.
• GI: *nausea, vomiting, diarrhea, stomatitis, anorexia,* **bleeding,** *dyspepsia, constipation.*
• GU: *oliguria,* **anuria,** *proteinuria, hematuria, dysuria, urine retention, urinary frequency, elevated BUN* and serum creatinine levels.
• Hepatic: *jaundice, ascites, hepatomegaly, elevated bilirubin, transaminase, and alkaline phosphate levels.*
• Respiratory: **pulmonary congestion,** dyspnea, **pulmonary edema, respiratory failure, pleural effusion, apnea, pneumothorax,** tachypnea.
• Skin: rash, *pruritus, erythema, dry skin,*

exfoliative dermatitis, purpura, alopecia, petechiae.
• Other: *hypomagnesemia, acidosis, hypocalcemia, hypophosphatemia, hypokalemia, hyperuricemia, hypoalbuminemia, hypoproteinemia, hyponatremia, hyperkalemia,* arthralgia, myalgia, fever, chills, abdominal pain, chest pain, back pain, fatigue, weakness, malaise, edema, phlebitis, sepsis, weight gain or loss, conjunctivitis.

Interactions
Antihypertensive agents: may potentiate aldesleukin's hypotensive effects.
Cardiotoxic, hepatotoxic, myelotoxic, nephrotoxic drugs: cause enhanced toxicity. Avoid when possible.
Glucocorticoids: may reduce aldesleukin's antitumor effects and should be avoided.
Psychotropic drugs, analgesics, antiemetics, narcotics, sedatives, tranquilizers: may produce additive CNS effects.

Incompatibility
Is incompatible with albumin and may be incompatible with some drugs. Do not administer with albumin and check with the pharmacist before administering with any other drug. Do not use bacteriostatic water or 0.9% sodium chloride injection when reconstituting the drug because these diluents cause increased aggregation of the drug.

Administration guidelines
• Perform standard hematologic tests, including CBC, differential, and platelet counts; serum electrolyte levels; and renal and hepatic function tests, before therapy. Also obtain chest X-ray before therapy. Repeat tests daily during drug administration.
• To avoid altering the pharmacologic properties of the drug, reconstitute and dilute carefully, and follow manufacturer's recommendations.
• Reconstitute the vial containing 22 million IU (1.3 mg/ml) with 1.2 ml sterile water for injection. Direct the stream at the sides of the

Common reactions are in *italics;* life-threatening reactions in **bold italics.**

vial and gently swirl to reconstitute. Do not shake.
• Add the ordered dose of reconstituted drug to 50 ml D₅W and infuse over 15 minutes. Do not use an in-line filter. Plastic infusion bags are preferred because they provided consistent drug delivery in early clinical trials.
• The reconstituted solution will have a concentration of 18 million IU (1.1 mg/ml). The reconstituted drug should be particle-free and colorless to slightly yellow.
• Vials are for single-use only and contain no preservatives. Discard unused drug.
• Store powder for injection or reconstituted solutions in the refrigerator. After reconstitution and dilution, administer drug within 48 hours. Return the solution to room temperature before administering drug.
• Hold dose and notify doctor if patient develops moderate to severe lethargy or somnolence because continued administration can result in coma.
• If toxicity occurs, modify dosage by holding a dose or interrupting therapy rather than by reducing the dose.
• Besides its use to treat metastatic renal cell carcinoma, the drug has been investigated for a number of other cancers, including Kaposi's sarcoma, metastatic melanoma, colorectal cancer, and malignant lymphoma.

Altretamine (hexamethylmelamine, HMM)
Hexalen

Pharmacologic classification
Altretamine is an alkylating agent.

Indications
Palliative treatment for persistent or recurrent ovarian cancer, following first-line therapy with a cisplatin or alkylating agent-based combination

Adverse reactions
• Blood: mild to severe anemia, leukopenia, thrombocytopenia.
• CNS: mild to moderate neurotoxicity, peripheral neuropathy, mood disorders, ataxia,

dizziness, vertigo, consciousness disorders, fatigue, seizures.
• GI: mild to severe dose-related nausea and vomiting, increased alkaline phosphatase, anorexia.
• Other: hepatic toxicity, rash, pruritus, alopecia.

Interactions
Cimetidine: increases altretamine's half-life and potential for toxicity through inhibition of microsomal drug metabolism.
MAO inhibitors: may cause severe orthostatic hypotension.

Incompatibility
None.

Administration guidelines
• Premedication with antiemetics may decrease incidence or severity of nausea and vomiting.
• Monitor peripheral blood counts at least monthly and before each course of therapy.
• Perform neurologic examinations regularly during administration to check for neurotoxicities. Concomitant administration of 100 mg pyridoxine may diminish neurotoxicity.
• Tolerance to GI effects may develop after several weeks of therapy. If severity is uncontrolled with antiemetics, dosage reduction may be required.

Asparaginase
Elspar, Kidrolase

Pharmacologic classification
Asparaginase is an enzyme (L-asparagine amidohydrolase) that hydrolyzes the amino acid, asparagine, thereby depriving tumor cells of this required substance.

Indications
Acute lymphocytic leukemia

Adverse reactions
• Blood: *hypofibrinogenemia* and depression of clotting factors, *thrombocytopenia, leukopenia,* depression of serum albumin.

Common reactions are in *italics;* life-threatening reactions in *bold italics.*

• CNS: lethargy, somnolence, headache, confusion, agitation, tremor.
• Skin: *rash, urticaria*
• GI: *vomiting* (may last up to 24 hours), *anorexia, nausea,* cramps, weight loss, stomatitis.
• GU: *azotemia,* **renal failure,** uric acid nephropathy, glucosuria, polyuria.
• Hepatic: elevated AST and ALT levels; elevated alkaline phosphatase and bilirubin (direct and indirect) levels; **hepatotoxicity.**
• Metabolic: *hyperglycemia;* increased or decreased levels of total lipids; *increased blood ammonia.*
• Other: **hypersensitivity reaction** such as **anaphylaxis** (relatively common), **hemorrhagic pancreatitis.**

Interactions
Methotrexate: may have decreased effectiveness because asparaginase destroys the actively replicating cells that methotrexate requires for its cytotoxic action.
Prednisone: may result in hyperglycemia from an additive effect on the pancreas.
Vincristine: can cause additive neuropathy and disturbances of erythropoiesis.

Incompatibility
Is not incompatible with other drugs, but reconstituted solutions may occasionally develop gelatinous fibers on standing. Filtration through a 5-micron filter will remove the fibers with no loss of potency, but filtration through a 0.2-micron filter may result in some potency loss.

Administration guidelines
• Conduct skin test before initial dose and when 1 week has elapsed between doses. Observe site for 1 hour. Erythema and wheal formation indicate a positive reaction.
• Reconstitute drug for I.M. administration with 2 ml unpreserved 0.9% sodium chloride or sterile water for injection. Do not use if precipitate forms.
• Expect I.M. injections to contain no more than 2 ml per injection. Multiple injections may be used for each dose.
• I.V. administration: Reconstitute with 5 ml of sterile water for injection, sodium chloride injection, or D₅W and administer I.V. over 30

minutes. Filtration through a 5-micron in-line filter during administration will remove particulate matter that may develop on standing; filtration through a 0.2-micron filter will result in a loss of potency. Do not use if precipitate forms.
• Shake vial gently when reconstituting. Vigorous shaking will result in a decrease in potency.
• Refrigerate unopened dry powder. Reconstituted solution is stable 8 hours at room temperature, 24 hours refrigerated.
• I.V. administration of asparaginase with or immediately before vincristine or prednisone may increase toxicity reactions.
• Don't use a sole agent to induce remission unless combination therapy is inappropriate. Not recommended for maintenance therapy.
• Keep epinephrine, diphenhydramine, and I.V. corticosteroids available for treatment of anaphylaxis.
• Discontinue drug at the first sign of renal failure or pancreatitis.

Bleomycin sulfate
Blenoxane

Pharmacologic classification
Bleomycin sulfate is an antibiotic antineoplastic agent that is cell cycle–specific in the G₂ and M phases.

Indications
Squamous cell carcinoma of the head and neck, skin, penis, cervix, and vulva; lymphomas such as Hodgkin's disease, reticulum cell sarcoma, and lymphosarcoma; and testicular carcinoma classified as embryonal cell, choriocarcinoma, or teratocarcinoma

Adverse reactions
• GI: nausea, *vomiting, stomatitis, prolonged anorexia in 13% of patients,* diarrhea.
• Respiratory: pneumonitis; dose-limiting **pulmonary fibrosis** in 10% of patients.
• Skin: rash, *erythema, vesiculation and hardening and discoloration of palmar and plantar skin in 8% of patients;* desquamation of

Common reactions are in *italics;* life-threatening reactions in **bold italics.**

hands, feet, and pressure areas; *hyperpigmentation; acne.*
• Other: *alopecia,* phlebitis, fever, chills, *leukocytosis, allergic reaction* **(anaphylaxis).**

Interactions
Digoxin: decreased serum digoxin levels.
Phenytoin: decreased serum phenytoin levels. Monitor closely.

Incompatibility
Is incompatible with many drugs. Additive drugs that cause some or total loss of bleomycin activity include aminophylline, ascorbic acid injection, carbenicillin disodium, cefazolin sodium, cephalothin sodium, hydrocortisone sodium succinate, methotrexate, mitomycin, nafcillin sodium, penicillin G sodium, and terbutaline sulfate. Diazepam is physically incompatible with bleomycin.

Administration guidelines
• Premedication with aspirin, steroids, and diphenhydramine may reduce drug fever and risk of anaphylaxis.
• Reduce dosage in patients with renal or pulmonary impairment.
• Administer a 1-unit test dose before therapy to assess hypersensitivity to bleomycin. The test dose can be incorporated as part of the total dose for the regimen.
• To prepare solution for I.M. administration, reconstitute the drug with 1 to 5 ml of 0.9% sodium chloride solution for injection, sterile water for injection, D₅W, or bacteriostatic water for injection.
• For I.V. administration, dilute with a minimum of 5 ml of diluent and administer over 10 minutes as I.V. push.
• Prepare infusions of bleomycin in glass bottles, as absorption of drug to plastic occurs with time. Plastic syringes do not interfere with bleomycin activity.
• Prepare and handle drug cautiously; wear gloves and wash hands after preparing and administering.
• Administer drug by intracavitary, intra-arterial, or intratumoral injection.
• Cumulative lifetime dosage should not exceed 400 units.
• Bleomycin is stable for 24 hours at room temperature and 48 hours under refrigera-

tion. Refrigerate unopened vials containing dry powder.
• Have epinephrine, diphenhydramine, I.V. corticosteroids, and oxygen available in case of anaphylactic reaction.
• Discontinue drug if patient develops signs of pulmonary fibrosis or mucocutaneous toxicity. Pulmonary function tests may predict fibrosis.

Busulfan
Myleran

Pharmacologic classification
Busulfan is an alkylating agent that is cell cycle–nonspecific.

Indications
Palliative treatment of chronic myelogenous (myeloid, myelocytic, granulocytic) leukemia

Adverse reactions
• Blood: WBC count falling after about 10 days and continuing to fall for 2 weeks after stopping drug; *thrombocytopenia; leukopenia; anemia.*
• CNS: *seizures.*
• GI: nausea, vomiting, diarrhea, cheilosis, glossitis.
• GU: amenorrhea, testicular atrophy, impotence.
• Metabolic: Addison-like wasting syndrome, profound hyperuricemia due to increased cell lysis.
• Skin: transient hyperpigmentation, rash, urticaria, anhidrosis.
• Other: gynecomastia, alopecia, *irreversible pulmonary fibrosis, commonly termed "busulfan lung."*

Interactions
None significant.

Incompatibility
None.

Administration guidelines
• The dosage regimen for adults is as follows: Give 4 to 12 mg P.O. daily until WBC

Common reactions are in *italics;* life-threatening reactions in **bold italics**.

count falls to 15,000/mm³; then stop the drug until WBC count rises to 50,000/mm³ and resume treatment as before. Or give 4 to 8 mg P.O. daily until WBC count falls to 10,000 to 20,000/mm³; then reduce daily dosage as needed to maintain WBC count at this level (usually 2 mg daily).
• The dosage regimen for children is as follows: Give 0.06 to 0.12 mg/kg or 1.8 to 4.6 mg/m² P.O. daily; adjust dosage to maintain WBC count at 20,000/mm³, but never less than 10,000/mm³.
• Do not give the drug to a patient with chronic myelogenous leukemia, which is known to be resistant to the drug.
• Because high-dose therapy has been associated with seizures, use the drug cautiously in patients with a history of head trauma or seizures or in patients receiving other drugs that lower the seizure threshold.

Carboplatin
Paraplatin

Pharmacologic classification
Carboplatin is an alkylating agent that is cell cycle–nonspecific.

Indications
Advanced ovarian carcinoma

Adverse reactions
• Blood: *bone marrow depression, thrombocytopenia, leukopenia, neutropenia, hemolytic anemia.*
• CNS: peripheral neuropathy.
• GI: *nausea, vomiting,* constipation, diarrhea, electrolyte loss, hepatotoxicity.
• GU: renal toxicity.
• Local: pain at injection site.
• Other: alopecia, hypersensitivity, ototoxicity, pain, asthenia.

Interactions
Nephrotoxic agents: produce additive nephrotoxicity of carboplatin.
Phenytoin: may decrease phenytoin serum levels.

Incompatibility
Sodium bicarbonate 200 mM solution causes a 13% loss of carboplatin activity in 24 hours. Fluorouracil and ifosfamide with etoposide cause some loss of carboplatin activity in 24 hours.

Administration guidelines
• Reconstitute with D₅W, 0.9% sodium chloride solution, or sterile water for injection to make a concentration of 10 mg/ml.
• Dilute carboplatin with 0.9% sodium chloride solution or D₅W.
• Store unopened vials at room temperature. Once reconstituted and diluted as directed, solution is stable at room temperature for 8 hours. Because the drug does not contain antibacterial preservatives, unused drug should be discarded after 8 hours.
• Do not use needles or I.V. administration sets containing aluminum because carboplatin may precipitate and lose potency.
• Although drug is promoted as causing less nausea and vomiting than cisplatin, it can cause severe emesis. Antiemetic therapy may be required.

Carmustine
(BCNU)
BiCNU

Pharmacologic classification
Carmustine is an alkylating agent (nitrosourea) that is cell cycle–nonspecific.

Indications
Palliative treatment of the following:
• brain tumors: glioblastoma, brain-stem glioma, medulloblastoma, astrocytoma, epenymoma, and metastatic brain tumors.
• multiple myeloma
• Hodgkin's disease
• malignant lymphomas

Adverse reactions
• Blood: *cumulative bone marrow depression* (dose-limiting, usually occurring 4 to 6 weeks after a dose); *leukopenia, thrombocytopenia,*

Common reactions are in *italics;* life-threatening reactions in ***bold italics.***

acute leukemia or bone marrow dysplasia may occur after long-term use.
• GI: *nausea, possibly severe, lasting 2 to 6 hours after dose; vomiting.*
• GU: nephrotoxicity.
• Hepatic: reversible hepatotoxicity.
• Metabolic: possible hyperuricemia in lymphoma patients when rapid cell lysis occurs.
• Skin: hyperpigmentation upon accidental contact of drug with skin; alopecia.
• Local: *intense pain at infusion site;* phlebitis (rare).
• Other: *pulmonary fibrosis.*

Interactions
Cimetidine: increases the bone marrow toxicity of carmustine. The mechanism of this interaction is unknown. Avoid concomitant use.

Incompatibility
Some data indicate that solutions of carmustine in 5% dextrose injection in PVC containers are rapidly degraded; avoid admixture of the drug in PVC containers. The manufacturer recommends that only glass containers be used for administration.

Carmustine is rapidly degraded in aqueous solutions at a pH greater than 6. Therefore, do not admix with solutions containing sodium bicarbonate or administer through a common tubing or site. As a precaution, don't mix carmustine with other drugs during administration.

Administration guidelines
• To reduce nausea, give an antiemetic before administering carmustine.
• Reconstitute the 100-mg vial with the 3 ml of absolute alcohol provided by the manufacturer; then dilute further with 27 ml of sterile water for injection. Resultant solution contains 3.3 mg carmustine/ml in 10% ethanol. Dilute in 0.9% sodium chloride solution or D_5W for I.V. infusion. Give at least 250 ml over 1 to 2 hours. Discard excess drug. To reduce pain on infusion, dilute further or slow infusion rate.
• Wear gloves to administer carmustine infusion and when changing I.V. tubing. Avoid contact with skin because carmustine will cause a brown stain. If drug comes into contact with skin, wash off thoroughly.

• Solution is unstable in plastic I.V. bags. Administer only in glass containers.
• At first sign of extravasation, discontinue infusion and infiltrate area with liberal injections of 0.5 mEq/ml sodium bicarbonate solution.
• Reconstituted solution may be refrigerated for 24 hours.
• Carmustine may decompose at temperatures above 80° F (26° C). Discard if powder liquefies or appears oily—a sign of decomposition.
• Avoid all I.M. injections when platelet count is below 100,000/mm³.
• Carmustine has been applied topically in concentrations of 0.5% to 2% to treat mycosis fungoides.

Chlorambucil
Leukeran

Pharmacologic classification
Chlorambucil is an alkylating agent of the nitrogen mustard type that is cell cycle–nonspecific.

Indications
Chronic lymphatic leukemia and malignant lymphomas including lymphosarcoma, giant follicular lymphoma, and Hodgkin's disease

Adverse reactions
• Blood: *neutropenia,* delayed up to 3 weeks, lasting up to 10 days after last dose; *thrombocytopenia; anemia;* myelosuppression (usually moderate, gradual, and rapidly reversible).
• CNS: seizures (with high doses).
• GI: *nausea, vomiting, stomatitis,* anorexia, diarrhea.
• GU: *azoospermia, infertility,* sterile cystitis (rare).
• Hepatic: hepatotoxicity
• Metabolic: hyperuricemia.
• Skin: rash, pruritus, *exfoliative dermatitis,* peripheral neuropathy (rare).
• Other: *pulmonary fibrosis,* drug fever, alopecia (rare), sterility.

Common reactions are in *italics;* life-threatening reactions in **bold italics.**

Interactions
None reported.

Incompatibility
None.

Administration guidelines
• Oral suspension can be prepared in the pharmacy by crushing tablets and mixing powder with a suspending agent and simple syrup.
• Store tablets in a tightly closed, light-resistant container.
• To prevent hyperuricemia with resulting uric acid nephropathy, allopurinol may be used with adequate hydration. Monitor uric acid level.

Cisplatin
(cis-platinum)
Platinol, Platinol AQ

Pharmacologic classification
Cisplatin is an alkylating agent that is cell cycle–nonspecific.

Indications
Metastatic testicular tumors, metastatic ovarian tumors, and advanced bladder cancer

Adverse reactions
• Blood: *mild myelosuppression in 25% to 30% of patients; **leukopenia; thrombocytopenia; anemia;** nadir in circulating platelet and leukocyte levels in 7 to 10 days, with 21-day recovery.
• CNS: peripheral neuropathy, loss of taste, **seizures,** headache.
• EENT: *tinnitus, high-frequency hearing loss may occur in both ears;* blurred vision, changes in ability to see colors.
• GI: *nausea and vomiting, beginning 1 to 4 hours after dose and lasting 24 hours;* diarrhea; metallic taste; stomatitis.
• GU: *renal toxicity (dose-limiting).*
• Other: **anaphylactoid reaction,** hyperuricemia, **hypomagnesemia, hypocalcemia,** hypokalemia.

Interactions
Aminoglycosides: potentiate cumulative nephrotoxicity caused by cisplatin through additive toxicity. Don't use aminoglycosides within 2 weeks of cisplatin therapy.
Loop diuretics, such as furosemide: increase the risk of ototoxicity. Closely monitor the patient's audiologic status.
Phenytoin: may decrease serum levels of phenytoin.

Incompatibility
D_5W (100 mg and 75 mg/liter concentration) causes some loss or decomposition of cisplatin; sodium bicarbonate 5% solution causes a bright gold precipitate to form within 8 to 24 hours at 77° F (25° C); and 0.1% NaCl or water causes some degree of cisplastin decomposition. Etoposide with mannitol and potassium chloride cause a precipitate to form within 24 hours; fluorouracil causes some degree of cisplatin loss; mesna causes cisplatin to be undetectable or only weakly so after 1 hour; and thiotepa causes a yellow precipitate.

Administration guidelines
• Reconstitute a 10-mg vial with 10 ml and a 50-mg vial with 50 ml of sterile water for injection to yield a concentration of 1 mg/ml. Drug may be diluted further in a saline-containing solution for I.V. infusion.
• Do not use aluminum needles for reconstitution or administration of cisplatin; a black precipitate may form. Use stainless steel needles.
• Drug is stable for 24 hours in 0.9% sodium chloride solution at room temperature. Do not refrigerate because precipitation may occur. Discard any solution containing precipitate.
• Infusions are most stable in chloride-containing solutions (such as 0.9% sodium chloride, 0.45% sodium chloride, and 0.22% sodium chloride).
• Avoid contact with skin. If contact occurs, wash drug off immediately with soap and water.
• Patient must be well-hydrated before administration to limit nephrotoxicity and ototoxicity.
• Hydration and forced diuresis (using manni-

Common reactions are in *italics;* life-threatening reactions in **bold italics.**

tol or furosemide) continue for 24 hours after administration to ensure adequate urine output (via indwelling catheter).
• Discontinue drug if signs of neurotoxicity appear.

Cladribine
(2-chlorodeoxyadenosine)
Leustatin

Pharmacologic classification
Cladribine is an antimetabolite agent that is a purine nucleoside analogue. It enters tumor cells and disrupts cellular metabolism.

Indications
Active hairy cell leukemia

Adverse reactions
Blood: *severe neutropenia, anemia, thrombocytopenia.*
• CNS: *headache, fatigue, dizziness, insomnia, asthenia.*
• CV: *tachycardia, edema.*
• EENT: *epistaxis.*
• GI: *nausea, decreased appetite, vomiting, diarrhea, constipation, abdominal pain.*
• Respiratory: *abnormal breath or chest sounds, cough, shortness of breath.*
• Skin: *rash, pruritus, erythema,* purpura, petechiae.
• Other: *fever, **infection,** local reactions at the injection site, chills, asthenia, diaphoresis, malaise, trunk pain, myalgia, arthralgia,* hyperuricemia.

Interactions
None reported.

Incompatibility
Don't use with solutions that contain dextrose because studies show increased degradation of cladribine.

Administration guidelines
• For a 24-hour infusion, add the calculated dose to a 500-ml infusion bag of 0.9% sodium chloride injection and infuse over 24 hours. Once diluted, administer promptly or begin within 8 hours. Because the drug con-

tains no bacteriostatic agents, use strict aseptic technique to prepare the admixture. Repeat daily for 7 consecutive days.
• Alternatively, prepare a 7-day infusion using bacteriostatic sodium chloride injection, which contains 0.9% benzyl alcohol. Studies show acceptable physical and chemical stability using Pharmacia Deltec medication cassettes. First, pass the calculated amount of drug through a disposable 0.22-micron hydrophilic syringe filter into a sterile infusion reservoir. Next, add sufficient bacteriostatic sodium chloride injection to bring the total volume to 100 ml. Clamp off the line, then disconnect and discard the filter. If necessary, aseptically aspirate air bubbles from the reservoir using a new filter or a sterile vent filter assembly.
• Because the calculated dose dilutes the benzyl alcohol preservative, 7-day infusion solutions prepared for patients weighing more than 187 lb (85 kg) may have reduced preservative effectiveness.
• Refrigerate unopened vials at 36° to 46° F (2° to 8° C) and protect from light. Although freezing doesn't adversely affect the drug, a precipitate may form; this will disappear if you warm the drug to room temperature gradually and shake the vial vigorously. Don't heat or microwave; don't refreeze.
• In addition to being administered for active hairy cell leukemia, cladribine has been used to treat advanced cutaneous T-cell lymphomas, chronic lymphocytic leukemia, malignant lymphomas, acute myeloid leukemias, mycosis fungoides, and Sézary syndrome.

Cyclophosphamide
Cytoxan, Neosar

Pharmacologic classification
Cyclophosphamide is chemically related to alkylating agents and is cell cycle–nonspecific.

Common reactions are in *italics;* life-threatening reactions in ***bold italics.***

Indications

Treatment of the following cancers:
• malignant lymphomas (stages II and IV of the Ann Arbor staging system), Hodgkin's disease, lymphocytic lymphoma (nodular or diffuse), mixed-cell type lymphoma, histiocytic lymphoma, Burkitt's lymphoma
• multiple myeloma
• leukemias: chronic lymphocytic leukemia, chronic granulocytic leukemia, acute myelogenous and monocytic leukemia, and acute lymphoblastic (stem-cell) leukemia in children
• mycosis fungoides (advanced disease)
• neuroblastoma (disseminated disease)
• adenocarcinoma of the ovary
• retinoblastoma
• carcinoma of the breast

Adverse reactions

• Blood: *leukopenia* (nadir between days 8 and 15, recovery in 17 to 28), *thrombocytopenia, anemia.*
• CV: *cardiotoxicity,* hemorrhagic cardial necrosis.
• GI: *nausea and vomiting beginning within 6 hours, lasting 4 hours;* anorexia; stomatitis; mucositis; diarrhea.
• GU: *hemorrhagic cystitis,* bladder fibrosis, nephrotoxicity; gonadal suppression.
• Metabolic: hyperuricemia, syndrome of inappropriate ADH secretion.
• Other: *reversible alopecia in 50% of patients* (especially with high doses), secondary malignancies, *pulmonary fibrosis,* fever, *anaphylaxis,* dermatitis.

Interactions

Allopurinol, chloramphenicol, chloroquine, imipramine, phenothiazines, potassium iodide, vitamin A: may inhibit cyclophosphamide metabolism.
Barbiturates, chloral hydrate, and *phenytoin:* all known inducers of hepatic microsomal enzymes that increase the rate of metabolism of cyclophosphamide.
Doxorubicin: may potentiate cardiotoxic effects of this drug.
Succinylcholine: may prolong respiratory distress and apnea when administered as an adjunct to anesthesia in patients undergoing cyclophosphamide therapy. This may occur

up to several days after the discontinuation of cyclophosphamide. Cyclophosphamide depresses the activity of pseudochlorphosphamide, the enzyme responsible for the inactivation of succinylcholine. Use cautiously.

Incompatibility

None reported.

Administration guidelines

• Reconstitute vials with appropriate volume of bacteriostatic or sterile water for injection to give a concentration of 20 mg/ml.
• Reconstituted solution is stable 6 days if refrigerated or 24 hours at room temperature.
• Give cyclophosphamide by direct I.V. push over 3 minutes into a free-flowing I.V. line or by infusion in 0.9% sodium chloride solution or D_5W.
• Oral doses should be taken with or after a meal. Higher oral doses (400 mg) may be tolerated better if divided into smaller doses.
• Give with cold foods such as ice cream to improve toleration of oral dose.
• Don't give drug P.O. at bedtime because voiding afterward is too infrequent to avoid cystitis.
• Push fluids (3 liters daily) to prevent hemorrhagic cystitis. Some clinicians use uroprotectant agents such as mesna. If hemorrhagic cystitis occurs, the drug will need to be discontinued. Cystitis can occur months after therapy has been discontinued.
• Reduce dosage of cyclophosphamide if patient is concomitantly receiving corticosteroid therapy and develops viral or bacterial infections. Also adjust dosage if patient has renal impairment.

Cytarabine
(ara-C, cytosine arabinoside)
Cytosar-U

Pharmacologic classification

Cytarabine is an antimetabolite agent that is cell cycle–specific in the S phase.

Common reactions are in *italics;* life-threatening reactions in ***bold italics.***

Indications
Remission induction in acute nonlymphocytic leukemia, treatment of acute lymphocytic leukemia and the blast phase of chronic myelocytic leukemia, and meningeal leukemia when administered by the intrathecal route

Adverse reactions
• Blood: *leukopenia* (nadir 7 to 9 days after drug stopped), anemia, **thrombocytopenia,** reticulocytopenia (platelet nadir occurring on day 10), *megaloblastosis.*
• CNS: neurotoxicity, neuritis and peripheral neuropathy (with high doses).
• EENT: *keratitis,* conjunctivitis.
• GI: *nausea;* diarrhea; dysphagia; reddened area at juncture of lips, followed by sore mouth, oral ulcers in 5 to 10 days; vomiting (high dose given via rapid I.V. may cause projectile vomiting).
• Hepatic: hepatotoxicity (usually mild and reversible).
• Metabolic: hyperuricemia.
• Skin: rash, alopecia.
• Other: flulike syndrome.

Interactions
Digoxin: oral absorption may be impaired due to temporary damage to GI mucosa caused by cytarabine.
Methotrexate: reduced effectiveness related to decreased cellular uptake caused by cytarabine.

Incompatibility
Additive drug incompatibilities with cytarabine include carbenicillin disodium (pH is outside of stability range for carbenicillin); cephalothin sodium, 2 g concentration (immediate precipitation); fluorouracil (altered UV spectra for cytarabine within 1 hour at room temperature); gentamicin sulfate, 240 mg concentration, hydrocortisone sodium succinate, or methylprednisolone sodium (physically incompatible); heparin sodium (haze formation); lincomycin HCL (fine precipitate forms); nafcillin sodium (heavy crystalline precipitate forms); oxacillin sodium (pH outside stability range for oxacillin); and penicillin G sodium (pH outside stability range for penicillin).

Administration guidelines
• To reduce nausea, give an antiemetic before administering cytarabine.
• To reconstitute the 100-mg vial for I.V. administration, use 5 ml bacteriostatic water for injection (20 mg/ml); for the 500-mg vial, use 10 ml bacteriostatic water for injection (50 mg/ml).
• Further dilute drug with D₅W or 0.9% sodium chloride solution for continuous I.V. infusion.
• For intrathecal injection, dilute drug in 5 to 15 ml lactated Ringer's solution, Elliot's B solution, or 0.9% sodium chloride solution with no preservative, and administer after withdrawing an equivalent volume of CSF.
• Do not reconstitute the drug with bacteriostatic diluent for intrathecal administration because the preservative, benzyl alcohol, has been associated with a higher incidence of neurologic toxicity.
• Reconstituted solutions are stable for 48 hours at room temperature. Infusion solutions up to a concentration of 5 mg/ml are stable for 7 days at room temperature. Discard cloudy reconstituted solution.
• Dose modification may be required in thrombocytopenia, leukopenia, renal or hepatic disease, and after other chemotherapy or radiation therapy.
• Maintain high fluid intake and give allopurinol, if ordered, to avoid urate nephropathy in leukemia induction therapy.
• Pyridoxine supplements may be administered to prevent neuropathies; reportedly, however, prophylactic use of pyridoxine does not prevent cytarabine neurotoxicity.
• Discontinue drug if polymorphonuclear granulocyte count falls below 1,000/mm³, or if platelet count falls below 50,000/mm³ during maintenance therapy (not during remission induction therapy).

Dacarbazine
(DTIC)
DTIC-Dome

Pharmacologic classification
Dacarbazine is an alkylating agent that is cell cycle–nonspecific.

Common reactions are in *italics;* life-threatening reactions in ***bold italics.***

Indications
Metastatic malignant melanoma; second-line therapy for Hodgkin's disease

Adverse reactions
• Blood: *leukopenia and thrombocytopenia* (nadir between 3 and 4 weeks), anemia.
• CNS: confusion, headache, paresthesia.
• EENT: blurred vision.
• GI: *severe nausea and vomiting beginning within 1 to 3 hours in 90% of patients, lasting 1 to 12 hours; anorexia;* diarrhea (rare).
• Hepatic: hepatotoxicity
• Skin: photoxicity, urticaria.
• Local: severe pain if I.V. solution infiltrates or if solution is too concentrated; tissue damage.
• Other: *anaphylaxis, flulike syndrome* (fever, malaise, myalgia beginning 7 days after treatment is stopped and possibly lasting 7 to 21 days), alopecia, facial flushing, renal impairment.

Interactions
None reported.

Incompatibility
Is incompatible with Y-site injection of heparin sodium (25 mg/ml concentration). A white, flocculent precipitate forms immediately.

Administration guidelines
• To minimize nausea and vomiting, administer dacarbazine by I.V. infusion and hydrate patient 4 to 6 hours before therapy.
• To reconstitute the drug for I.V. administration, use sterile water for injection with a concentration of 10 mg/ml (9.9 ml for 100-mg vial, 19.7 ml for 200-mg vial).
• Dilute drug further with D_5W to a volume of 100 to 200 ml for I.V. infusion over 30 minutes. Increase volume or slow the rate of infusion to decrease pain at infusion site.
• Administer drug by I.V. push over 1 to 2 minutes.
• A change in the solution's color from ivory to pink indicates some drug degradation. During infusion, protect the solution from light to avoid possible drug breakdown.
• Discard refrigerated solution after 72 hours; discard room temperature solution after 8 hours.
• Reduce dosage when giving repeated doses to a patient with severely impaired renal function.
• Use lower dose if renal function or bone marrow is impaired. Stop drug if WBC count falls to 3,000/mm³ or platelet count drops to 100,000/mm³.

Dactinomycin (actinomycin D)
Cosmegen

Pharmacologic classification
Dactinomycin is an antibiotic antineoplastic that is cell cycle–nonspecific.

Indications
Wilms' tumor, rhabdomyosarcoma, and testicular and uterine carcinomas; also used in the palliative treatment of Ewing's sarcoma and sarcoma botryoides as well as treatment for various types of sarcomas, carcinomas, and adenocarcinomas when given by the isolation-perfusion technique (either as palliative treatment or as an adjunct to resection of a tumor)

Adverse reactions
• Blood: *anemia, leukopenia, thrombocytopenia, pancytopenia,* agranulocytosis.
• GI: *anorexia, nausea, vomiting,* diarrhea, abdominal pain, *stomatitis,* esophagitis, pharyngitis.
• Hepatic: *hepatotoxicity.*
• Skin: *erythema;* desquamation; *hyperpigmentation of skin, especially in previously irradiated areas; acnelike eruptions (reversible).*
• Local: phlebitis, severe damage to soft tissue.
• Other: *anaphylaxis,* reversible alopecia, malaise, fever.

Interactions
None reported.

Common reactions are in *italics;* life-threatening reactions in ***bold italics.***

Incompatibility
Powder for injection must be reconstituted with sterile water that does not contain preservatives to prevent possible precipitation. Cellulose ester membrane filters, such as those used in I.V. fluid sterilization or administration, have been shown to partially remove dactinomycin.

Administration guidelines
• To reduce nausea, give an antiemetic before administering dactinomycin.
• To reconstitute for I.V. administration, add 1.1 ml of sterile water for injection to drug to give a concentration of 0.5 mg/ml. Do not use a diluent containing preservatives because a precipitate may form.
• Wear gloves when preparing and administering this drug.
• May dilute further with D_5W or 0.9% sodium chloride solution for administration by I.V. infusion.
• Discard any unused solution because it doesn't contain any preservatives.
• Administer by I.V. push into the tubing of a freely flowing I.V. infusion. Do not administer through an in-line I.V. filter.
• Discontinue drug if diarrhea and stomatitis develop. Resume therapy when these conditions subside.

Daunorubicin hydrochloride (DNR)
Cerubidine

Pharmacologic classification
Daunorubicin is an antibiotic antineoplastic agent that is cell cycle–nonspecific.

Indications
Remission induction in acute nonlymphocytic leukemia (myelogenous, monocytic, erythroid) in adults and for remission induction in acute lymphocytic leukemia in children and adults

Adverse reactions
• Blood: *bone marrow suppression* (dose-limiting), anemia, pancytopenia (nadir between 10 to 14 days), leukopenia, thrombocytopenia.

• CV: *irreversible cardiomyopathy* (dose-related), ECG changes, arrhythmias, pericarditis, myocarditis.
• GI: *nausea, vomiting, stomatitis, esophagitis,* anorexia, diarrhea.
• GU: nephrotoxicity, transient red urine.
• Hepatic: *hepatoxicity.*
• Metabolic: hyperuricemia.
• Skin: rash.
• Local: *severe cellulitis or tissue slough if drug extravasates.*
• Other: *generalized alopecia,* fever, chills.

Interactions
Hepatoxic drugs: may increase the risk of hepatoxicity.

Incompatibility
Is incompatible with fludarabine phosphate because it causes a slight haze (visible under high intensity light) to form in 4 hours at room temperature. Admixture with heparin sodium or dexamethasone phosphate results in the formation of a precipitate.

Administration guidelines
• Use antiemetics to prevent or treat nausea and vomiting.
• To reconstitute the drug for I.V. administration, add 4 ml of sterile water for injection to a 20-mg vial to give a concentration of 5 mg/ml.
• Drug may be diluted further into 100 ml of D_5W or 0.9% sodium chloride solution and infused over 40 to 45 minutes.
• For I.V. push administration, withdraw reconstituted drug into syringe containing 10 to 15 ml of 0.9% sodium chloride solution, and inject over 2 to 3 minutes into the tubing of a freely flowing I.V. infusion. Reconstituted solution is stable for 24 hours at room temperature.
• Reddish color of drug looks similar to that of doxorubicin. Do not confuse the two drugs.
• Erythematous streaking along the vein or facial flushing indicates too rapid drug administration.
• To prevent cardiomyopathy, limit cumulative dose to 550 mg/m² (450 mg/m² when patient has been receiving any other cardiotoxic

Common reactions are in *italics;* life-threatening reactions in **bold italics.**

agent, such as cyclophosphamide, or radiation therapy that encompasses the heart).
• Reduce dosage in patients with hepatic or renal impairment; in patients with serum bilirubin of 1.2 to 3 mg/dl, reduce dose by 25%; with serum bilirubin or creatinine levels over 3 mg/dl, reduce dose by 50%.
• Discontinue drug if patient develops signs of congestive heart failure or cardiomyopathy.

Dexamethasone (systemic)
Decadron, Dexone, Hexadrol, Sk-Dexamethasone

Dexamethasone acetate
Dalalone D.P., Decadron L.A., Decaject-L.A., Decameth L.A., Dexacen-LA, Dexasone-LA, Dexone-LA, Solurex-LA

Dexamethasone sodium phosphate
Ak-Dex, Dalalone, Decadrol, Decadron Phosphate, Decaject, Decameth, Dexacen LA-8, Dexasone, Dexon, Dexone, Hexadrol Phosphate, Solurex

---

Pharmacologic classification
Although not an antineoplastic agent, dexamethasone is a glucocorticoid used to treat neoplasms because of its immunosuppressant activity.

Indications
High doses may help prevent nausea and vomiting associated with emetogenic cancer chemotherapy, and may treat or prevent cerebral edema associated with brain tumors; also used in palliative treatment of leukemias and lymphomas in adults and acute leukemia in children

Adverse reactions
When administered in high doses or for prolonged periods, dexamethasone suppresses the release of corticotropin from the pituitary gland, stopping secretion of endogenous corticosteroids from the adrenal cortex. The degree and duration of related hypothalamic-pituitary-adrenal axis suppression varies, depending on the dose, frequency, and duration of glucocorticoid therapy.
• CNS: *euphoria, insomnia,* headache, psychotic behavior, pseudotumor cerebri, mental changes, nervousness, restlessness.
• CV: ***CHF,*** hypertension, edema.
• EENT: cataracts, glaucoma, thrush.
• GI: *peptic ulcer,* irritation, increased appetite.
• Immune: immunosuppression, increased susceptibility to infection.
• Metabolic: hypokalemia, sodium retention, fluid retention, weight gain, hyperglycemia, osteoporosis, growth suppression in children.
• Musculoskeletal: muscle atrophy, weakness.
• Skin: delayed healing, acne, skin eruptions, striae.
• Local: atrophy at I.M. injection sites.
• Other: pancreatitis, hirsutism, cushingoid symptoms, *withdrawal syndrome* (nausea, fatigue, anorexia, dyspnea, hypotension, hypoglycemia, myalgia, arthralgia, fever, dizziness, and fainting).
Sudden discontinuation may be fatal or may exacerbate the underlying disease. Acute adrenal insufficiency may follow increased stress (infection, surgery, trauma) or abrupt withdrawal after long-term therapy.

Interactions
Antacids, cholestyramine, colestipol: adsorb the corticosteroid (dexamethasone), thus decreasing the amount available for absorption by the body.
Barbiturates, phenytoin, and *rifampin:* may increase hepatic metabolism, decreasing corticosteroid effects.
Estrogens: may reduce the metabolism of dexamethasone by increasing the concentration of transcortin. The half-life of the corticosteroid is then prolonged because of increased protein-binding.
Isoniazid, salicylates: dexamethasone increases the metabolism of these drugs; causes hyperglycemia, requiring dosage adjustment of insulin or oral antidiabetic agents in diabetic patients; and may enhance hypokalemia associated with diuretic or amphotericin B therapy. The hypokalemia may in-

Common reactions are in *italics;* life-threatening reactions in ***bold italics.***

crease the risk of toxicity in patients receiving digitalis glycosides.
Oral anticoagulants: in rare cases, may be rendered less effective by unknown mechanisms.
Ulcerogenic drugs, such as the nonsteroidal anti-inflammatory agents: may increase the risk of GI ulceration.

Incompatibility
Is incompatible with the following additive drugs: amikacin sulfate at a 100 mg concentration (some dexamethasone decomposition); daunorubicin HCL or doxorubicin HCL (immediate milky precipitation); metaraminol bitartrate (altered UV spectra for dexamethasone within 1 hour at room temperature); and vancomycin HCL (physically incompatible). Don't mix with glycopyrrolate in same syringe because some glycopyrrolate decomposition will occur.

Administration guidelines
• Give oral form with food to avoid GI upset.
• Give I.M. injection deep into gluteal muscle. Rotate injection sites to prevent muscle atrophy. Avoid S.C. injection because atrophy and sterile abscesses may occur.
• When administering as direct I.V. injection, inject undiluted over at least 1 minute. When administering as an intermittent or continuous infusion, dilute solution according to manufacturer's instructions and give over the prescribed duration. If used for continuous infusion, change solution every 24 hours.
• During times of physiologic stress (trauma, surgery, infection), the patient may require additional steroids and may experience signs of steroid withdrawal; patients who were previously steroid-dependent may need systemic corticosteroids to prevent adrenal insufficency.
• After long-term therapy, reduce the drug gradually. Rapid reduction may cause withdrawal symptoms.
• Because adrenocorticoids increase susceptibility to and mask symptoms of infection, don't use dexamethasone (except in life-threatening situations) in viral or bacterial infections not controlled by anti-infective agents.

Doxorubicin hydrochloride
Adriamycin

Pharmacologic classification
Doxorubicin is an antibiotic antineoplastic agent that is cell cycle–nonspecific.

Indications
Disseminated neoplastic conditions such as acute lymphoblastic leukemia, acute myeloblastic leukemia, Wilms' tumor, neuroblastoma, soft-tissue and bone sarcomas, breast carcinoma, ovarian carcinoma, transitional cell bladder carcinoma, thyroid carcinoma, Hodgkin's disease and malignant lymphoma, bronchogenic carcinoma, and gastric carcinoma

Adverse reactions
• Blood: **leukopenia, especially agranulocytosis, during days 10 to 15, with recovery by day 21; thrombocytopenia.**
• CV: *cardiodepression, seen in such ECG changes as sinus tachycardia, T-wave flattening, ST-segment depression, and voltage reduction; arrhythmias;* **irreversible cardiomyopathy, sometimes with pulmonary edema.**
• GI: anorexia, *nausea, vomiting,* diarrhea, *stomatitis,* esophagitis.
• GU: transient red urine.
• Skin: *hyperpigmentation of nails, dermal creases, or skin, especially in previously irradiated areas;* severe tissue damage and necrosis on extravasation.
• Local: *severe cellulitis.*
• Other: hyperpigmentation of nails and dermal creases, *complete alopecia,* fever.

Interactions
May potentiate cyclophosphamide-induced cystitis and hepatotoxicity due to mercaptopurine.
Cyclophosphamide, daunorubicin: may potentiate the cardiotoxicity of doxorubicin through additive effects on the heart.
Digoxin: serum levels may be decreased.

Common reactions are in *italics;* life-threatening reactions in **bold italics.**

Incompatibility

Don't mix with furosemide, heparin sodium, fluorouracil, aminophylline, cephalosporins, dexamethasone sodium phosphate, or hydro-cortisone sodium phosphate because a pre-cipitate will form.

Administration guidelines

• To reconstitute, add 5 ml of 0.9% sodium chloride solution to the 10-mg vial, 10 ml to the 20-mg vial, and 25 ml to the 50-mg vial, to yield a concentration of 2 mg/ml.
• Drug may be further diluted with 0.9% so-dium chloride solution or D_5W and adminis-tered by I.V. infusion.
• Drug may be administered by I.V. push in-jection over 5 to 10 minutes into the tubing of a freely flowing I.V. infusion.
• The alternative dosage schedule (once-weekly dosing) has been found to cause a lower incidence of cardiomyopathy.
• If cumulative dose exceeds 550 mg/m² body surface area, 30% of patients develop cardiac adverse reactions, which begin 2 weeks to 6 months after stopping the drug.
• Too rapid administration may cause streak-ing along a vein or facial flushing.
• Discontinue the drug or slow the rate of in-fusion if tachycardia develops. Also discon-tinue the drug if hematopoietic toxicity becomes severe.
• Decrease dosage as follows if serum biliru-bin level increases: 50% of dose when biliru-bin level is 1.2 to 3 mg/dl; 25% of dose when bilirubin level exceeds 3 mg/dl.

Etoposide
(VP-16)
VePesid

Pharmacologic classification

Etoposide is a podophyllotoxin that is cell cycle–specific in the G_2 and late S phases.

Indications

Refractory testicular tumors and small-cell lung cancer

Adverse reactions

• Blood: *myelosuppression* (dose-limiting),

leukopenia, thrombocytopenia, anemia.
• CNS: headache, weakness, visual distur-bances, peripheral neuropathy (especially if administered with other neurotoxic medica-tions).
• CV: hypotension from rapid infusion, palpi-tation, tachycardia.
• GI: nausea and vomiting (in 30%), diarrhea, anorexia, *stomatitis.*
• Local: infrequent phlebitis; pain at I.V. site.
• Other: occasional fever, *reversible alopecia,* **anaphylaxis** (rare), generalized pain, chills, diaphoresis, fever, rash.

Interactions

Cisplatin: increased cytotoxicity against cer-tain tumors through an unknown mechanism.
Warfarin: possible increased effect.

Incompatibility

At a concentration of 1 mg/ml in 0.9% so-dium chloride or D_5W injection, crystalliza-tion may occur within 5 minutes after stirring the solution or within 30 minutes after allow-ing the solution to stand; therefore, this con-centration is not recommended for I.V. administration. If solutions of etoposide are prepared at concentrations above 0.4 mg/ml, a precipitate may form. The manufacturer recommends that the concentration not ex-ceed 0.4 mg/ml.

Plastic devices made of acrylic or ABS (a polymer composed of acrylonitrile, buta-diene, and styrene) have been reported to crack and leak when used with undiluted etoposide injection.

Administration guidelines

• Pretreatment with antiemetics may reduce frequency and duration of nausea and vomit-ing.
• To prepare solution, dilute prescribed dose to a concentration of 0.2 to 0.4 mg/ml with 0.9% sodium chloride solution or D_5W. Higher concentrations may crystallize. Discard solu-tion if cloudy.
• Solutions diluted to 0.2 mg/ml are stable for 96 hours at room temperature in plastic or glass unprotected from light; solutions di-luted to 0.4 mg/ml are stable for 48 hours under the same conditions.

Common reactions are in *italics;* life-threatening reactions in ***bold italics.***

• Administer infusion over 30 to 60 minutes to avoid hypotensive reactions.
• Intrapleural and intrathecal administration of this drug is contraindicated due to severe toxicity.
• Dosage reduction may be required for patients with impaired renal function.
• Refrigerate capsules.
• Have diphenhydramine, hydrocortisone, epinephrine, and airway available in case of anaphylaxis.
• Etoposide has produced complete remissions in small-cell lung cancer and testicular cancer.
• Discontinue drug if severe hematopoietic toxicity results.

Floxuridine
FUDR

Pharmacologic classification
Floxuridine is an antimetabolite agent that inhibits DNA synthesis.

Indications
Palliative management of GI adenocarcinoma metastatic to the liver; treatment of brain, breast, head, neck, gallbladder, and bile duct cancers

Adverse reactions
• Blood: *leukopenia, anemia, thrombocytopenia*
• CNS: cerebellar ataxia, vertigo, nystagmus, seizures, depression, hemiplegia, hiccups, lethargy
• EENT: blurred vision
• GI: *anorexia, stomatitis, cramps, nausea, vomiting, diarrhea, bleeding, enteritis*
• Hepatic: cholangitis, jaundice, elevated liver enzyme levels
• Skin: *erythema, dermatitis,* pruritus, rash

Interactions
None.

Incompatibility
Check with the pharmacist before administering with other drugs.

Administration guidelines
• Reconstitute with sterile water for injection. Dilute further in D_5W or 0.9% sodium chloride solution for actual infusion.
• Use an infusion pump with intra-arterial infusions.
• Refrigerated solution is stable for no more than 2 weeks.
• Discontinue the drug if the WBC count falls below 3,500/mm^3 or if platelet count falls below 100,000/mm^3.
• Severe skin and GI adverse reactions require stopping the drug. Use of antacid eases but probably won't prevent GI distress.
• Preparation of parenteral form is associated with carcinogenic, mutagenic, and teratogenic risks for personnel. Follow institutional policy to reduce risks.

Fludarabine phosphate
Fludara

Pharmacologic classification
Fludarabine is an antimetabolite agent that intereferes with DNA synthesis.

Indications
Palliative treatment of chronic lymphocytic leukemia and treatment of acute leukemias and lymphoid cancers

Adverse reactions
• Blood: *myelosuppression.*
• CNS: *fatigue, malaise, weakness,* paresthesia, headache, sleep disorder, depression, cerebellar syndrome, transient ischemic attack, agitation, *confusion; coma, death* (with high doses)
• CV: *edema,* angina, phlebitis, *arrhythmias, CHF,* supraventricular tachycardia, deep venous thrombosis, aneurysm, CVA, hemorrhage
• EENT: *visual disturbances,* hearing loss; delayed blindness (with high doses); sinusitis, pharyngitis, epistaxis
• GI: *nausea, vomiting,* diarrhea, constipation, *anorexia,* stomatitis, GI bleeding, esophagitis, mucositis
• GU: dysuria, urinary infection, urinary hesi-

Common reactions are in *italics;* life-threatening reactions in ***bold italics.***

tancy, proteinuria, hematuria, **renal failure**
• Respiratory: cough, *pneumonia,* dyspnea, upper respiratory infection, allergic pneumonitis, hemoptysis, hypoxia, bronchitis
• Skin: rash, pruritus, seborrhea
• Other: *fever, chills, infection,* pain, myalgia, tumor lysis syndrome, alopecia, **anaphylaxis,** diaphoresis, hyperglycemia, dehydration, liver failure, cholelithiasis.

Interactions
Other myelosuppressive agents: cause increased toxicity. Avoid concomitant use.

Incompatibility
Check with the pharmacist before administering with other drugs.

Administration guidelines
• Optimal duration of therapy has not been determined. Current recommendations suggest three additional cycles after achieving maximal response before discontinuing therapy.
• To prepare I.V. solution, add 2 ml of sterile water for injection to the solid cake of fludarabine. Dissolution should occur within 15 seconds; each ml will contain 25 mg of drug. Use within 8 hours of reconstitution. Fludarabine also can be diluted in 100 or 125 ml of D_5W or 0.9% sodium chloride solution.
• Follow institutional protocol regarding proper handling and disposal of chemotherapeutic agents.
• Refrigerate drug at 36° to 46° F (2° to 8° C).
• In addition to being used to treat B-cell chronic lymphocytic leukemia (CLL) in patients who have either not responded or responded inadequately to at least one standard alkylating agent regimen, the drug has been used investigationally to treat malignant lymphoma, macroglobulinemic lymphoma, prolymphocytic leukemia or prolymphocytoid variant of CLL, mycosis fungoides, hairy-cell leukemia, and Hodgkin's disease.

Fluorouracil
(5-FU)
Adrucil, Efudex, Fluoroplex

Pharmacologic classification
Fluorouracil is an antimetabolite agent that is cell cycle–specific in the S phase.

Indications
Palliative treatment of carcinoma of the colon, rectum, breast, stomach, and pancreas. The topical form may be used to treat superficial basal cell carcinomas.

Adverse reactions
• Blood: bone marrow depression (dose-limiting), **leukopenia** (nadir in 7 to 14 days), anemia, **thrombocytopenia.**
• CNS: acute cerebellar syndrome, drowsiness, *weakness, malaise,* euphoria.
• CV: mild angina, ECG changes.
• GI: *anorexia,* proctitis, paralytic ileus, *stomatitis,* mucositis, *diarrhea* (GI ulcer may precede leukopenia), *nausea, vomiting,* GI toxicity (dose-limiting).
• Skin: maculopapular rash, dryness, erythema, hyperpigmentation (especially in blacks), nail changes, pigmented palmar creases, *pruritus,* suppuration, *burning,* swelling, *scaling.*
• Other: photosensitivity (patient should avoid prolonged sun exposure), lacrimation, *reversible alopecia,* weakness, malaise, fever.

Interactions
Leucovorin calcium: given as a continuous infusion causes increased binding of fluorouracil to substrate, increased fluorouracil cell uptake, and increased inhibition of thymidine synthetase. Significance is unknown.

Incompatibility
Is incompatible with the following additive drugs: carboplatin (some loss of carboplatin); cisplatin (some loss of cisplatin); cytarabine (altered UV spectrum for cytarabine within 1 hour at room temperature); doxorubicin (solution color darkens from red to

Common reactions are in *italics;* life-threatening reactions in **bold italics.**

bluish-purple); and diazepam, droperidol, and ondansetron (immediate precipitation).

Administration guidelines
• Give an antiemetic before administering to decrease nausea and vomiting.
• To reconstitute, withdraw solution through a 5-micron filter and add to vial.
• Drug may be administered by I.V. push over 1 to 2 minutes.
• Drug may be further diluted in D_5W or 0.9% sodium chloride solution for infusions up to 24 hours in duration.
• Use plastic I.V. containers for administering continuous infusions. Solution is more stable in plastic I.V. bags than in glass bottles.
• Do not use cloudy solution. If crystals form, redissolve by warming at 140° F (60° C). Allow solution to cool to body temperature before using.
• Use new vein site for each dose.
• Do not refrigerate fluorouracil.
• Drug can be diluted in 120 ml of a 0.2% sodium bicarbonate solution and administered orally.
• Apply topical drug while using plastic gloves. Wash hands immediately after handling medication. Avoid topical use with occlusive dressings.
• Apply topical solution with caution near eyes, nose, and mouth.
• Topical application to larger ulcerated areas may cause systemic toxicity.
• For superficial basal cell carcinoma confirmed by biopsy, use 5% strength. Apply 1% concentration on the face. Reserve higher concentrations for thicker-skinned areas or resistant lesions. Occlusion may be required.
• Discontinue drug or reduce dose if intractable vomiting, stomatitis, diarrhea, GI ulceration, or GI bleeding occurs; if the leukocyte count falls below 3,000/mm³; or if the platelet count falls below 100,000/mm³.

Fluoxymesterone
Android F, Halotestin, Hysterone

Pharmacologic classification
Fluoxymesterone is an androgen agent.

Indications
Palliative treatment of androgen-responsive recurrent breast cancer in women who are more than 1 year but less than 5 years postmenopausal or who have been proven to have a hormone-dependent tumor

Adverse reactions
• Androgenic: in females; deepening of voice, clitoral enlargement, changes in libido; in males; *prepubertal premature epiphyseal closure,* priapism, phallic enlargement; postpubertal testicular atrophy, oligospermia, decreased ejaculatory volume, impotence, gynecomastia, epididymitis.
• Blood: polycythemia; suppression of clotting factors II, V, VII, and X.
• CNS: headache, anxiety, mental depression, generalized paresthesia.
• CV: edema.
• GI: gastroenteritis, nausea, vomiting, diarrhea, constipation, change in appetite, *weight gain.*
• GU: bladder irritability.
• Hepatic: cholestatic hepatitis, ***liver cell tumors,*** jaundice.
• Skin: acne, *oily skin, hirsutism,* flushing, sweating, male pattern baldness.
• Other: hypercalcemia, hepatocellular cancer (with long-term use).

Interactions
Anticoagulants: may be potentiated, resulting in increased prothrombin time.
Insulin, oral antidiabetic drug: in patients with diabetes, decreased blood glucose levels may require adjustment of dosage.
Oxyphenbutazone: serum concentrations may increase.

Incompatibility
None.

Administration guidelines
• Discontinue drug if hypocalcemia, edema, hypersensitivity reaction, priapism, or excessive sexual stimulation develops; or if virilization occurs in females.

Common reactions are in *italics;* life-threatening reactions in ***bold italics.***

• Administer with food or meals if GI upset occurs.
• When used in breast cancer, subjective effects may not be seen for about 1 month and objective effects on clinical symptoms not for 3 months.

Flutamide
Eulexin

Pharmacologic classification
Flutamide is a nonsteroidal antiandrogen.

Indications
Metastatic prostatic carcinoma

Adverse reactions
• CNS: *loss of libido, numbness or tingling of hands or feet, drowsiness, confusion,* nervousness.
• CV: edema, hypertension.
• GI: *diarrhea, nausea, vomiting.*
• GU: *impotence.*
• Metabolic: gynecomastia, elevation of hepatic enzymes, hepatitis.
• Skin: rash, photosensitivity.
• Other: *hot flashes.*

Interactions
None reported.

Incompatibility
None.

Administration guidelines
• Flutamide must be taken continuously with the agent used for medical castration (such as leuprolide acetate) to produce full benefit of therapy. Leuprolide suppresses testosterone production, whereas flutamide inhibits testosterone action at the cellular level. Together they can impair the growth of androgen-responsive tumors.
• Generally, the drug is taken in three divided doses daily.

Goserelin acetate
Zoladex

Pharmacologic classification
Goserelin is a synthetic decapeptide analogue of luteinizing hormone-releasing hormone.

Indications
Advanced carcinoma of the prostate

Adverse reactions
• Blood: anemia.
• CNS: lethargy, pain (worse in the first 30 days), dizziness, insomnia, anxiety, depression, headache, chills, fever.
• CV: edema, ***CHF, arrhythmias, cerebrovascular accident,*** hypertension, ***myocardial infarction,*** peripheral vascular disorder, chest pain.
• EENT: upper respiratory infection.
• GI: nausea, vomiting, diarrhea.
• GU: decreased erections, *impotence, lower urinary tract symptoms,* renal insufficiency, urinary obstruction.
• Skin: rash, sweating.
• Other: *hot flashes, sexual dysfunction,* gout, hyperglycemia, weight increase, breast swelling and tenderness.

Interactions
None reported.

Incompatibility
None.

Administration guidelines
• The implant comes in a preloaded syringe. If the package is damaged, do not use the syringe. Make sure that the drug is visible in the translucent chamber of the syringe.
• Give the drug every 28 days, always under direct supervision of a doctor. Local anesthesia may be used before injection.
• Administer the drug in the upper abdominal wall using aseptic technique. After cleaning the area with an alcohol swab (and injecting a local anesthetic, if prescribed), stretch the

Common reactions are in *italics;* life-threatening reactions in ***bold italics.***

patient's skin with one hand while grasping the barrel of the syringe with the other. Insert the needle into the subcutaneous fat; then change the needle direction to parallel the abdominal wall. Push the needle in until the hub touches the patient's skin; then withdraw it about 1 cm (this creates a gap for the drug to be injected) before depressing the plunger completely.
• After inserting the needle, don't aspirate because blood will be seen instantly in the chamber if a large vessel is penetrated (a new syringe and injection site then will be needed).
• Store the drug at room temperature, not to exceed 77° F (25° C).

Hydroxyurea
Hydrea

Pharmacologic classification
Hydroxyurea is an antimetabolite agent that is cell cycle-specific in the S phase.

Indications
Melanoma; resistant chronic myelocytic leukemia; recurrent, metastatic, or inoperable ovarian carcinoma; and primary squamous cell (epidermoid) carcinomas of the head and neck, excluding the lip

Adverse reactions
• Blood: *bone marrow depression* (dose-limiting), *leukopenia, thrombocytopenia,* anemia, *megaloblastosis.*
• CNS: drowsiness, hallucinations, seizures, headache.
• GI: *anorexia, nausea, vomiting, diarrhea,* stomatitis, constipation.
• GU: increased BUN and serum creatinine levels.
• Metabolic: hyperuricemia.
• Skin: rash, pruritus, facial erythema.
• Other: alopecia, fever, chills.

Interactions
None.

Incompatibility
None.

Administration guidelines
• If patient can't swallow capsule, he may empty contents into water and take immediately.
• Dose modification may be required following other chemotherapy or radiation therapy.
• Store capsules in tight container at room temperature. Avoid exposure to excessive heat.
• Discontinue drug if inflammation of the mucous membranes is severe, if leukocyte count is less than 2,500/mm³, or if platelet count is less than 100,000/mm³.

Ifosfamide
Ifex

Pharmacologic classification
Ifosfamide is an alkylating agent that is cell cycle–nonspecific.

Indications
Third-line chemotherapeutic agent for germ-cell testicular cancer

Adverse reactions
• Blood: *leukopenia, myelosuppression, thrombocytopenia.*
• CNS: *lethargy and confusion* (with high doses), *coma.*
• GI: *nausea, vomiting.*
• GU: *hemorrhagic cystitis* (dose-limiting), *hematuria,* nephrotoxicity, dysuria, urinary frequency.
• Hepatic: elevated liver enzymes.
• Other: *alopecia,* phlebitis.

Interactions
Allopurinol: may increase the activity and bone marrow toxicity of ifosfamide, prolonging its half-life by an unknown mechanism.
Chloral hydrate, phenobarbital, phenytoin: may increase the activity of ifosfamide by induction of hepatic microsomal enzymes, increasing the conversion of ifosfamide to its active form.
Corticosteroids: may decrease the effectiveness of ifosfamide by inhibiting the enzymes that convert the drug to its active form.

Common reactions are in *italics;* life-threatening reactions in ***bold italics.***

Incompatibility

Incompatible with mesna with epirubicin. Over 50% of epirubicin is lost in 7 days at room temperature.

Administration guidelines

• To reconstitute a 1-g vial of the drug, use 20 ml sterile water for injection to yield a solution of 50 mg/ml or 30 ml sterile water for injection to yield a solution of 100 mg/ml; 0.9% sodium chloride solution may also be used for reconstitution.
• Use reconstituted solution within 8 hours because it contains no preservatives.
• Drug can be further diluted with D_5W or 0.9% sodium chloride solution for I.V. infusion. This solution is stable for 7 days at room temperature.
• Drug may be given by I.V. push injection in a minimum of 75 ml 0.9% sodium chloride solution over at least 30 minutes.
• I.V. infusions for periods up to 5 days can be used to administer ifosfamide.
• Infusing each dose over 2 hours or longer will decrease possibility of cystitis.
• Push fluids (at least 2 liters daily) and administer with mesna to prevent hemorrhagic cystitis. Avoid giving the drug at bedtime because infrequent voiding during the night may increase the possibility of cystitis. Bladder irrigation with 0.9% sodium chloride solution may decrease the possibility of cystitis.
• Encourage patients to void every 2 hours during the day and twice during the night. Catheterization is required for patients unable to void.

Interferon gamma-1b
Actimmune

Pharmacologic classification

Interferon gamma-1b is an antibiotic antineoplastic agent used to treat neoplastic disease because of its potent phagocyte-activating properties as well as its ability for oxidative metabolism of tissue macrophages.

Indications

Reduction of the frequency and severity of serious infections associated with cancer chemotherapy

Adverse reactions

• Blood: **bone marrow suppression** (at high doses).
• CNS: *headache, chills (flulike syndrome),* fatigue, decreased mental status, gait disturbance.
• GI: nausea, vomiting, diarrhea.
• Metabolic: elevated hepatic enzymes (at high doses).
• Skin: rash.
• Local: erythema or tenderness at the injection site.
• Other: fever, myalgia, arthralgia.

Interactions

Myelosuppressive agents: may cause possible additive myelosuppression. Use together with caution.
Zidovudine: increases plasma levels of zidovudine. Dosage adjustments will be necessary.

Incompatibility

None.

Administration guidelines

• Ensure that patient who will self-administer the drug has a copy of the patient information leaflet, which will help him use the drug safely and effectively. Teach the patient the correct method of drug administration and of medical waste disposal.
• Discomfort from the flulike syndrome commonly associated with this drug may be minimized by taking the drug at bedtime.
• The preferred injection site is the deltoid or anterior thigh.
• Refrigerate drug immediately. Vials must be refrigerated (36° to 46° F [2° to 8° C]); do not freeze. Do not shake the vial; avoid excessive agitation. Discard vials that have been left at room temperature for more than 12 hours.
• Each vial is for single dose only. Because the drug does not contain a preservative, discard the unused contents.

Common reactions are in *italics;* life-threatening reactions in ***bold italics.***

• This drug is also used to treat chronic granulomatous disease.

Leucovorin calcium (citrovorum factor, folinic acid)
Wellcovorin

Pharmacologic classification
Leucovorin calcium is calcium salt of folinic acid (active reduced form of folic acid). Although not an antineoplastic agent, this drug is given with selected antineoplastic agents to prevent or decrease hematologic toxicity of the antineoplastic agent being given.

Indications
Prevention or reduction of hematological toxicity associated with selected antineoplastic agents

Adverse reactions
• Skin: hypersensitivity reactions (rash, pruritus, erythema).
• Other: *bronchospasm*.

Interactions
Fluorouracil: give at lower doses because of increased toxicity.
Phenytoin: may decrease serum phenytoin concentrations and possibly increase frequency of seizures. Although this interaction has occurred solely in patients receiving folic acid, it should be considered when leucovorin is administered. The mechanism by which this occurs appears to be an increased metabolic clearance of phenytoin or a redistribution of phenytoin in the CSF and brain.
Phenytoin, primidone: may decrease serum folate levels, producing symptoms of folate deficiency. After chemotherapy with folic acid antagonists, parenteral administration is preferable to oral dosing because vomiting may cause loss of the leucovorin. To treat an overdose of folic acid antagonists, administer leucovorin within 1 hour, if possible; it is usually ineffective after a 4-hour delay. Leucovorin has no effect on other methotrexate toxicities.

Incompatibility
Drug is incompatible with droperidol (immediate precipitation) and foscarnet sodium (cloudy yellow solution).

Administration guidelines
• Begin leucovorin administration 24 hours after the beginning of the methotrexate infusion and continue until plasma methotrexate levels are below 5×10^{-8}M.
• To prepare leucovorin for parenteral use, add 5 ml of bacteriostatic water for injection to vial containing 50 mg of base drug.
• When giving more than 25 mg, administer drug parenterally.
• Store at room temperature in a light-resistant container, away from high-moisture areas.

Leuprolide acetate
Lupron, Lupron Depot

Pharmacologic classification
Leuprolide acetate is a synthetic nonpeptide analogue of gonadotropic-releasing hormone or leutinizing hormone–releasing hormone.

Indications
Palliative treatment of advanced prostate cancer

Adverse reactions
• CNS: dizziness, numbness, headache, blurred vision, muscle pain.
• CV: angina, *MI*, arrhythmias, CHF.
• Endocrine: *hot flashes,* breast tenderness, gynecomastia.
• GI: nausea, vomiting, constipation, anorexia.
• GU: infertility, impaired spermatogenesis.
• Skin: pruritus, rash.
• Local: redness and induration at injection site.
• Other: peripheral edema, decreased libido, transient bone pain during first week of treatment.

Common reactions are in *italics;* life-threatening reactions in ***bold italics.***

Interactions
None reported.

Incompatibility
None reported.

Administration guidelines
• Administer the injection using only the syringe provided by the manufacturer. If another syringe must be substituted, a low-dose insulin syringe (U-100, 0.5 ml) may be appropriate. Use a 22G needle for injection. Never use a needle smaller than 22G for depot injection.
• Erythema or induration may develop at injection site.
• Never administer by I.V. injection.
• A depot injection should be given monthly under the supervision of a doctor. Use the supplied diluent to reconstitute drug. Draw 1 mg into syringe with a 22G needle; discard any extra diluent. Inject into vial and shake well. Suspension will appear milky.
• Discard solution if particulate matter is visible or if the solution is discolored.
• The depot injection will remain stable for 24 hours after reconstitution; however, use it immediately, because there is no preservative in the drug.
• Store at room temperature under 86° F (30° C), and protect from light and heat.

Levamisole hydrochloride
Ergamisol

Pharmacologic classification
Levamisole is an immunomodulator.

Indications
Adjuvant treatment in combination with fluorouracil after surgical resection in patients with Dukes' stage C colon cancer

Adverse reactions
• Blood: *leukopenia, thrombocytopenia,* anemia, granulocytopenia, *agranulocytosis,* neutropenia.
• CNS: *fatigue, dizziness, headache, paresthesia,* ataxia, *somnolence, depression, nervousness, insomnia, anxiety,* forgetfulness,

blurred vision, confusion, paranoia, seizures, tremor.
• CV: chest pain.
• EENT: abnormal tearing, blurred vision, conjunctivitis, epistaxis, *altered sense of smell.*
• GI: *nausea, vomiting, diarrhea, constipation, flatulence, stomatitis, anorexia, dysgeusia, abdominal pain, dyspepsia.*
• Skin: *dermatitis,* rash, *alopecia, pruritus,* **exfoliative dermatitis,** skin discoloration, *urticaria.*
• Other: *fever,* rigors, edema, *infection,* hyperbilirubinemia, flulike syndrome, *arthralgia, myalgia.*

Interactions
Alcohol: disulfiram-like reaction occurs.
Phenytoin: results in increased phenytoin levels. Monitor plasma phenytoin levels and decrease dosage as needed.
Warfarin: prolongs prothrombin time, which necessitates close monitoring.

Incompatibility
None.

Administration guidelines
• Don't use levamisole in higher than recommended dosage or administer more frequently than indicated.
• Begin levamisole therapy when patient is out of hospital, ambulatory, maintaining normal oral nutrition, has well-healed wounds, and is fully recovered from any postsurgical complications.
• If levamisole therapy begins 7 to 20 days after surgery, start fluorouracil with the second course of levamisole therapy. It should begin no sooner than 21 days and no later than 35 days after surgery. If levamisole is deferred until 21 to 30 days after surgery, begin fluorouracil therapy with the first course of levamisole.
• Dosage modifications are based on hematologic parameters. Don't begin or continue fluorouracil therapy until WBC count is above 3,500/mm³. When WBC count is above 3,500/mm³ and fluorouracil is restarted, reduce dosage by 20%. If WBC count stays below

Common reactions are in *italics;* life-threatening reactions in **bold italics.**

2,500/mm³ for over 10 days after fluorouracil is withdrawn, discontinue levamisole.
• Discontinue therapy with both levamisole and fuorouracil if platelet count drops below 100,000/mm³.

Lomustine
(CCNU)
CeeNU

Pharmacologic classification
Lomustine is an alkylating agent (nitrosourea) that is cell cycle–nonspecific.

Indications
Brain tumors and Hodgkin's disease

Adverse reactions
• Blood: *bone marrow depression* (dose-limiting); *leukopenia,* delayed up to 6 weeks, lasting 1 to 2 weeks; *thrombocytopenia,* delayed up to 4 weeks, lasting 1 to 2 weeks; *anemia.*
• CNS: lethargy, ataxia, dysarthria.
• GI: *nausea and vomiting, beginning within 4 to 5 hours and lasting 24 hours;* stomatitis.
• GU: nephrotoxicity, progressive azotemia.
• Other: hepatotoxicity, alopecia, pulmonary toxicity.

Interactions
None reported.

Incompatibility
None.

Administration guidelines
• To avoid nausea, give antiemetic before administering.
• Give 2 to 4 hours after meals. Lomustine will be more completely absorbed if taken when the stomach is empty.
• Dose modification may be required in patients with decreased platelets, leukocytes, or erythrocytes and in patients receiving other myelosuppressive drugs.
• Lomustine may be given alone or in combination with other drugs, and it is usually not administered more often than every 6 weeks because bone marrow toxicity is cumulative and delayed.
• Store drug below 104° F (40° C).

Mechlorethamine hydrochloride (nitrogen mustard)
Mustargen

Pharmacologic classification
Mechlorethamine is an alkylating agent that is cell cycle–nonspecific.

Indications
I.V. administration for palliative treatment of Hodgkin's disease (stages III and IV), lymphosarcoma, chronic myelocytic or chronic lymphocytic leukemia, polycythemia vera, mycosis fungoides, and bronchogenic carcinoma; administered intrapericardially, intraperitoneally, or intrapleurally for the palliative treatment of metastatic carcinoma resulting in effusion.

Adverse reactions
• Blood: *thrombocytopenia, granulocytopenia lymphocytopenia,* nadir of myelosuppression occurring by days 4 to 10 and lasting 10 to 21 days; mild anemia beginning in 2 to 3 weeks, possibly lasting 7 weeks.
• CNS: drowsiness, vertigo, paresthesia (especially with high doses), *seizures, cerebral degeneration, coma.*
• EENT: tinnitus, *metallic taste* (immediately after dose), deafness.
• GI: *nausea, vomiting, and anorexia* beginning within 1 hour and lasting 8 to 24 hours, diarrhea.
• GU: oligomenorrhea, amenorrhea, azoospermia, delayed spermatogenesis, sterility.
• Metabolic: hyperuricemia.
• Local: thrombophlebitis, sloughing, severe irritation if drug extravasates or touches skin, rash.
• Other: alopecia, herpes zoster, leukemia (rare).

Interactions
Anticoagulants, aspirin: increased risk of bleeding. Avoid concomitant use.
Cyclophosphamide, procarbazine: possible increased risk of hepatotoxicity.

Common reactions are in *italics;* life-threatening reactions in ***bold italics.***

Incompatibility
Check with pharmacist before administering with any other drug.

Administration guidelines
• To reconstitute powder, use 10 ml of sterile water for injection or 0.9% sodium chloride solution to yield 1 mg/ml.
• Solution is very unstable. Prepare it immediately before infusion and use within 20 minutes. Discard unused solution.
• Administer drug I.V. push over a few minutes into the tubing of a freely flowing I.V. infusion.
• Don't dilute mechlorethamine into a large volume of I.V. solution because the drug may react with the diluent and is not stable for a prolonged period.
• Treatment of extravasation includes local injections of a 0.125M sodium thiosulfate solution. Prepare solution by mixing 4 ml of sodium thiosulfate 10% with 6 ml of sterile water for injection. Also apply ice packs for 6 to 12 hours to minimize local reactions.
• During intracavitary administration, turn patient from side to side every 15 minutes for 1 hour to distribute drug.
• Avoid contact with skin or mucous membranes. Wear gloves when preparing solution and during administration to prevent accidental skin contact. If contact occurs, wash with copious amounts of water.

Melphalan
(L-phenylalanine mustard)
Alkeran

Pharmacologic classification
Melphalan is an alkylating agent that is cell cycle-nonspecific.

Indications
Palliative treatment for multiple myeloma

Adverse reactions
• Blood: bone marrow depression (dose-limiting); *leukopenia, thrombocytopenia, agranulocytosis;* acute nonlymphocytic leukemia may develop with chronic use.
• GI: mild nausea and vomiting, diarrhea, stomatitis.
• Skin: dermatitis.
• Other: hypersensitivity reaction, alopecia,

pneumonitis, pulmonary fibrosis, anaphylaxis.

Interactions
None reported.

Incompatibility
None.

Administration guidelines
• Give oral dose all at one time.
• Administer melphalan on an empty stomach because absorption is decreased by food.
• Frequent hematologic monitoring, including a CBC, is necessary for accurate dosage adjustments and prevention of toxicity.
• Discontinue therapy temporarily or reduce dosage if leukocyte count falls below 3,000/mm³ or platelet count falls below 100,000/mm³.

Mercaptopurine
(6-MP)
Purinethol

Pharmacologic classification
Mercaptopurine is an antimetabolite agent that is cell cycle–specific in the S phase.

Indications
Acute lymphatic (lymphocytic, lymphoblastic) leukemia and acute myelogenous (and acute myelomonocytic) leukemia

Adverse reactions
• Blood: bone marrow suppression (dose-limiting), decreased RBC count, *leukopenia, thrombocytopenia,* anemia (all may persist several days after drug is stopped).
• GI: *nausea, vomiting, and anorexia* (in 25% of patients); diarrhea, painful oral ulcers, GI ulceration.
• Hepatic: *jaundice, hepatic necrosis.*
• Metabolic: hyperuricemia.
• Skin: hyperpigmentation, rash.
• Other: fever, headache.

Interactions
Allopurinol: at doses of 300 to 600 mg/day, increases the toxic effects of mercaptopu-

Common reactions are in *italics;* life-threatening reactions in **bold italics.**

rine, especially myelosuppression; inhibits mercaptopurine metabolism. Reduce dosage of mercaptopurine to 25% to 30% of original amount.
Other hepatotoxic drugs: increased potential for hepatotoxicity. Use mercaptopurine cautiously.
Warfarin: decreased anticoagulant activity due to an unknown mechanism.

Incompatibility
None.

Administration guidelines
• Dosage modifications may be required following chemotherapy or radiation therapy, in depressed neutrophil or platelet count, and in impaired hepatic or renal function.
• Discontinue drug if hepatic tenderness or signs of bone marrow toxicity or toxic hepatitis occur.
• Store tablets at room temperature and protect from light.
• This drug is sometimes ordered as 6-mercaptopurine. The numeral 6 is part of the drug name and does not signify the number of dosage units.

Mesna
Mesnex

Pharmacologic classification
Mesna is a thiol derivative. Although it is not an antineoplastic agent, it is given with ifosfamide to prevent ifosfamide-induced hemorrhagic cystitis.

Indications
Ifosfamide-induced hemorrhagic cystitis

Adverse reactions
• CNS: headache, fatigue.
• CV: hypotension.
• GI: bad taste, soft stools, diarrhea, nausea, vomiting.
• Other: allergy.
Note: Because mesna is given with ifosfamide, adverse reactions attributable to mesna alone are difficult to identify.

Interactions
None reported.

Incompatibility
Because drug is physically incompatible with cisplatin, don't add to cisplatin infusions. Drug is also incompatible with carboplatin (more than 10% carboplatin loss within 24 hours at room temperature) and ifosfamide with epirubicin (more than 50% epirubicin is lost in 7 days at room temperature).

Administration guidelines
• Discard any unused mesna from open ampules. It will form an inactive oxidation product (dimesna) when exposed to oxygen.
• Dilute the appropriate dose in D_5W injection, 0.9% sodium chloride injection, or lactated Ringer's injection to a concentration of 20 mg/ml.
• Once diluted, the solution is stable for 24 hours at room temperature.
• Administer by bolus or as a 24-hour infusion.

Methotrexate, methotrexate sodium
Folex, Mexate

Pharmacologic classification
Methotrexate is an antimetabolite agent that is cell cycle-specific in the S phase.

Indications
Gestational choriocarcinoma, chorioadenoma destruens, hydatidiform mole, acute lymphocytic leukemia, meningeal leukemia, breast cancer, epidermoid cancers of the head and neck, advanced mycosis fungoides, lung cancer, advanced malignant lymphoma, and nonmetastatic osteosarcoma

Adverse reactions
• Blood: bone marrow depression (dose-limiting), *leukopenia and thrombocytopenia* (nadir occurring in 7 to 14 days), *anemia.*
• CNS: *arachnoiditis* within hours of intrathecal use; subacute neurotoxicity may begin a few weeks later, *necrotizing demyelinating leukoencephalopathy* a few years later.
• GI: *nausea, vomiting, stomatitis, diarrhea* leading to *hemorrhagic enteritis and interstinal perforation,* gingivitis, pharyngitis.
• GU: *tubular necrosis.*

Common reactions are in *italics;* life-threatening reactions in **bold italics.**

• Hepatic: *hepatic dysfunction leading to cirrhosis* or **hepatic fibrosis.**
• Metabolic: hyperuricemia.
• Respiratory: **pulmonary fibrosis,** pneumonitis.
• Skin: photosensitivity, *urticaria,* pruritus, hyperpigmentation, rash; exposure to sun may aggravate psoriatic lesions.
• Other: alopecia, **pulmonary interstitial infiltrates.** Long-term use in children may cause osteoporosis.

Interactions
Immunizations: may be ineffective; risk of disseminated infection with live virus vaccines.
NSAIDs, salicylates, sulfonamides, sulfonylureas: may increase the therapeutic and toxic effects of methotrexate by displacing methotrexate from plasma proteins, increasing the concentrations of free methotrexate. Avoid using these agents with methotrexate if possible.
Phenytoin: serum levels may be decreased, resulting in an increased risk of seizures.
Probenecid, salicylates: increase the therapeutic and toxic effects of methotrexate by inhibiting the renal tubular secretion of methotrexate. Lower methotrexate dosage.

Incompatibility
Drug is incompatible with the following additive drugs: bleomycin sulfate (a substantial loss of bleomycin activity); prednisolone sodium phosphate (altered UV spectra for both drugs within 1 hour at room temperature); droperidol (immediate precipitation); heparin sodium 2500 units/1 ml concentration (turbidity or precipitate forms within 5 minutes); metoclopramide (physically incompatible); and ranitidine (immediate white turbidity).

Administration guidelines
• Before oral administration, administer an antacid.
• Methotrexate may be given undiluted by I.V. push injection at a rate of 10 mg/minute.
• Dilute powdered form to 5 mg/2 ml of sterile water.
• Drug can be diluted to a higher volume with 0.9% sodium chloride solution for I.V. infusion.

• Use reconstituted solutions of preservative-free drug within 24 hours after mixing.
• For intrathecal administration, use preservative-free formulations only. Dilute with unpreserved 0.9% sodium chloride solution, and further dilute with either lactated Ringer's or Elliot's B solution, to a final concentration of 1 mg/ml.
• Discontinue drug if diarrhea or ulcerative stomatitis occurs.
• Leucovorin rescue is necessary with high-dose protocols (doses greater than 100 mg).
• Dose modification may be required in impaired hepatic or renal function, bone marrow depression, aplasia, leukopenia, thrombocytopenia, or anemia. Use cautiously in infection, peptic ulcer, ulcerative colitis, and in very young, old, or debilitated patients.
• Don't use methotrexate when the potential for "third spacing" exists.

Methylprednisolone
Medrol, Meprolone

Methylprednisolone acetate
depMedalone, Depoject, Depo-Medrol, Depopred, Depo-Predate, Duralone, Durameth, Medralone, Medrone, M-Prednisol, Rep-Pred

Methylprednisolone sodium succinate
A-metha-Pred, Solu-Medrol

Pharmacologic classification
Although not an antineoplastic agent, methylprednisolone is a glucocorticoid used to treat neoplasms because of its immunosuppressant effect.

Indications
Palliative treatment of leukemias and lymphomas in adults and acute leukemia of childhood

Adverse reactions
When administered in high doses or for prolonged therapy, methylprednisolone suppresses release of corticotropin from the pituitary gland; in turn, the adrenal cortex

Common reactions are in *italics;* life-threatening reactions in **bold italics.**

stops secreting endogenous corticosteroids. The degree and duration of hypothalamic-pituitary-adrenal axis suppression varies, depending on the dose, frequency, and duration of glucocorticoid therapy.
• CNS: *euphoria, insomnia,* headache, psychotic behavior, mood swings, pseudotumor cerebri, mental changes, nervousness, restlessness.
• CV: CHF, hypertension, edema.
• EENT: cataracts, glaucoma, thrush.
• GI: *peptic ulcer,* increased appetite.
• Immune: immunosuppression, increased susceptibility to infection.
• Metabolic: hypokalemia, sodium retention, fluid retention, weight gain, hyperglycemia, osteoporosis, growth suppression in children.
• Musculoskeletal: muscle atrophy, weakness.
• Skin: delayed healing, acne, skin eruptions, striae.
• Other: pancreatitis, hirsutism, cushingoid symptoms, withdrawal syndrome (nausea, fatigue, anorexia, dyspnea, hypotension, hypoglycemia, myalgia, arthralgia, fever, dizziness, and fainting). Sudden withdrawal may be fatal or may exacerbate the underlying disease. ***Acute adrenal insufficency may occur with increased stress (infection, surgery, trauma) or abrupt withdrawal after long-term therapy.***

Interactions
Adrenocorticoids: may decrease the effects of oral anticoagulants by unknown mechanisms.
Antacids, cholestyramine, colestipol: adsorb the corticosteroid (methylprednisolone), thus decreasing the amount absorbed and its effectiveness.
Barbiturates, phenytoin, rifampin: may cause decreased corticosteroid effects because of increased hepatic metabolism.
Estrogens: may reduce the metabolism of corticosteroids by increasing the concentration of transcortin. The half-life of the corticosteroid is then prolonged because of increased protein binding.
Glucocorticoids: increase the metabolism of isoniazid and salicylates; cause hyperglycemia, requiring dosage adjustment of insulin or oral antidiabetic agents in diabetic

patients. Also, may enhance hypokalemia associated with diuretic or amphotericin B therapy. The hypokalemia may increase the risk of toxicity in patients receiving digitalis glycosides.
Ulcerogenic drugs such as NSAIDs: may increase the risk of GI ulceration.

Incompatibility
Injections of methylprednisolone acetate and methylprednisolone sodium succinate have been reported to be incompatible with various drugs, but the compatibility depends on several factors (such as concentrations of the drugs, resulting pH, temperatures). Consult specialized references for specific compatibility information. Do not dilute methylprednisolone acetate sterile suspension or mix it with any other solution.

Administration guidelines
• Give oral form with food when possible to avoid GI upset.
• Give I.M. injection deep into gluteal muscle. Rotate injection sites to prevent muscle atrophy. Avoid S.C. injection, because atrophy and sterile abscesses may occur. Dermal atrophy may occur with large doses of acetate salt. Use multiple small injections rather than a single large dose.
• When administering as direct I.V. injection, inject diluted drug into a vein or free-flowing compatible I.V. solution over at least 1 minute.
• When administering as an intermittent or continuous infusion, dilute solution according to manufacturer's instructions and give over the prescribed duration. If used for continuous infusion, change solution every 24 hours. Don't use acetate form for I.V. use.
• Discard reconstituted solutions after 48 hours.
• During times of physiologic stress (trauma, surgery, infection), the patient may require additional steroids and may experience signs of steroid withdrawal; patients who were previously steroid-dependent may need systemic corticosteroids to prevent adrenal insufficency.
• After long-term therapy, the drug dosage should be reduced gradually. Rapid reduction may cause withdrawal symptoms.

Common reactions are in *italics;* life-threatening reactions in ***bold italics.***

Mitomycin
Mutamycin

Pharmacologic classification
Mitomycin is an antineoplastic antibiotic agent that is cell cycle–nonspecific.

Indications
Disseminated adenocarcinoma of the stomach and pancreas

Adverse reactions
• Blood: ***bone marrow suppression, thrombocytopenia, leukopenia*** (may be delayed up to 8 weeks and may be cumulative with successive doses).
• CNS: paresthesia.
• GI: nausea, vomiting, anorexia, stomatitis, hepatotoxicity.
• Respiratory: ***interstitial pneumonitis.***
• Local: ***desquamation, induration, pruritus, pain at injection site,*** tissue necrosis with extravasation, cellulitis, ulceration, sloughing.
• Other: reversible alopecia; purple coloration of nail beds; fever; ***microangiopathic hemolytic anemia syndrome characterized by thrombocytopenia, renal toxicity, and hypertension.***

Interactions
Dextran, urokinase: enhance the cytotoxic activity of mitomycin. Through a series of enzymatic processes, these agents increase autolysis of cells, adding to the cell death caused by mitomycin.
Vinca alkaloids: may cause severe bronchospasms and respiratory distress.

Incompatibility
Drug is incompatible with a number of solutions. Consult specialized references for specific information. Also incompatible with bleomycin sulfate (some loss of bleomycin activity) and sargramostim (slight haze, visible with high intensity light, forms in 30 minutes).

Administration guidelines
• Reconstitute 5-mg vial with 10 ml of sterile water for injection; and 20-mg vial with 40 ml of sterile water to yield 0.5 mg/ml.
• Drug may be administered by I.V. push injection slowly over 5 to 10 minutes into the tubing of a freely flowing I.V. infusion.
• Drug can be further diluted to 100 to 150 ml with 0.9% sodium chloride solution or D_5W for I.V. infusion (over 30 to 60 minutes or longer).
• Reconstituted solution remains stable for 1 week at room temperature and for 2 weeks if refrigerated.
• Mitomycin has been used intra-arterially to treat certain tumors—for example, into hepatic artery for colon cancer. It has also been given as a continuous daily infusion.
• An unlabeled use of this drug is to treat small bladder papillomas. It is instilled directly into the bladder in a concentration of 20 mg/20 ml sterile water.

Mitotane
Lysodren

Pharmacologic classification
Mitotane is an antineoplastic agent that alters hormone balance.

Indications
Inoperable adrenal cortical carcinoma

Adverse reactions
• CNS: *depression, somnolence, lethargy, vertigo,* brain damage and dysfunction (with long-term, high-dose therapy).
• GI: *severe nausea, vomiting,* diarrhea, anorexia.
• Metabolic: adrenal insufficiency.
• Skin: dermatitis, maculopapular rash.

Interactions
None significant.

Incompatibility
None.

Administration guidelines
• Give an antiemetic before administering drug to reduce nausea and vomiting.

Common reactions are in *italics;* life-threatening reactions in ***bold italics.***

• Reduce dosage if GI or skin adverse reactions are severe.
• Obese patients may need higher dosage and may have longer lasting adverse reactions because drug distributes mostly to body fat.
• Adequate trial is at least 3 months, but therapy can continue if clinical benefits are observed.

Mitoxantrone hydrochloride
Novantrone

Pharmacologic classification
Mitoxantrone is an antibiotic antineoplastic agent.

Indications
Acute nonlymphocytic leukemia in adults

Adverse reactions
• CNS: *seizures,* headache.
• Blood: bone marrow suppression, thrombocytopenia, leukopenia.
• CV: *CHF, arrhythmias,* ECG changes, chest pain, tachycardia, hypotension, asymptomatic decreases in left ventricular ejection fraction.
• EENT: conjunctivitis.
• GI: *nausea, vomiting, diarrhea, abdominal pain, mucositis, stomatitis, bleeding.*
• GU: urinary tract infection, renal failure.
• Respiratory: cough, dyspnea, pneumonia.
• Skin: alopecia, petechiae, ecchymosis, urticaria, rashes.
• Other: jaundice, sepsis, fungal infections, fever, phlebitis at injection site (rare), tissue necrosis after extravasation (rare).

Interactions
None reported.

Incompatibility
Drug is incompatible with heparin; a precipitate may form. Specific compatibility data on other drugs are not available.

Administration guidelines
• Do not use intrathecally. Safety of administration by routes other than I.V. has not been established.

• To prepare, dilute solutions to at least 50 ml with either 0.9% sodium chloride solution or D_5W. Inject slowly into tubing of a freely running I.V. solution of 0.9% sodium chloride or D_5W over at least 3 minutes. Discard unused infusion solutions appropriately.
• Discontinue drug or reduce dose if WBC count drops below 3,000/mm^3 or platelet count falls below 75,000/mm^3.

Paclitaxel
Taxol

Pharmacologic classification
Paclitaxel is a miscellaneous antineoplastic agent that prevents depolymerization of cellular microtubules, thus inhibiting the normal reorganization of the microtubule network necessary for mitosis and other vital cellular functions.

Indications
Metastatic ovarian carcinoma after failure of first-line or subsequent chemotherapy

Adverse reactions
• Blood: *bone marrow suppression, neutropenia, leukopenia, thrombocytopenia,* anemia, infections, *bleeding.*
• CV: *bradycardia, hypotension, abnormal ECG.*
• GI: *nausea, vomiting, diarrhea, mucositis.*
• Skin: alopecia.
• Other: hypersensitivity reactions *(anaphylaxis),* peripheral neuropathy, *myalgia, arthralgia.*

Interactions
Cisplatin: may cause additive myelosuppressive effects. Use together cautiously.
Ketoconazole: inhibits paclitaxel metabolism. Use together cautiously.

Incompatibility
Check with pharmacist before administering with any other drug.

Administration guidelines
• Severe hypersensitivity reactions have occurred in up to 2% of patients treated in

---

Common reactions are in *italics;* life-threatening reactions in ***bold italics.***

early clinical trials. To reduce the incidence or severity of these reactions, pretreat patients with corticosteroids, such as dexamethasone and antihistamines. Both H_1-receptor antagonists, such as diphenhydramine, and H_2-receptor antagonists, such as cimetidine or ranitidine, may be used.
• Dilute the concentrate before infusion. Compatible solutions include 0.9% sodium chloride injection, D_5W, dextrose 5% in 0.9% sodium chloride injection, and dextrose 5% in lactated Ringer's injection. Dilute to a final concentration of 0.3 to 1.2 mg/ml. Prepare and store infusion solutions in glass containers. Administer drug using an in-line 0.22-micron filter.
• The undiluted concentrate shouldn't come in contact with polyvinylchloride I.V. bags or tubing. Store diluted solution in glass or polypropylene plastic bottles, or use polypropylene or polyolefin bags. Administer through polyethylene-lined administration sets.
• Follow institutional protocol for the safe handling, preparation, and administration of chemotherapeutic drugs. Dispose of all waste materials properly.

Pentostatin
(2′-deoxycoformycin, DCF)

Pharmacologic classification
Pentostatin is a miscellaneous antineoplastic agent that inhibits the enzyme adenosine deaminase, causing an increase in intracellular levels of deoxyadenosine triphosphate. This leads to cell damage and death.

Indications
Hairy cell leukemia that is refractory to alpha interferon in adults

Adverse reactions
• Blood: **bone marrow suppression, leukopenia, anemia, thrombocytopenia, lymphadenopathy**
• CNS: *headache, neurologic symptoms, anxiety, confusion, depression, dizziness, insomnia, nervousness, paresthesia, somnolence, abnormal thinking,* **seizures**
• CV: **arrhythmias,** *abnormal ECG, thrombophlebitis,* **hemorrhage**

• EENT: abnormal vision, conjunctivitis, ear pain, eye pain, epistaxis, pharyngitis, rhinitis, sinusitis
• GI: *nausea, vomiting, anorexia, diarrhea, constipation, flatulence, stomatitis*
• GU: *hematuria, dysuria, increased BUN and creatinine levels*
• Hepatic: *elevated liver function tests*
• Metabolic: weight loss, peripheral edema, increased lactate dehydrogenase
• Respiratory: *cough, bronchitis, dyspnea,* lung edema, *pneumonia*
• *Skin: ecchymosis, petechiae, rash,* skin disorder, *eczema, dry skin, herpes simplex or zoster, maculopapular rash, vesiculobullous rash, pruritus, seborrhoa, discoloration, sweating,* **exfoliative dermatitis**
• Other: fever, infection, *fatigue,* pain, **allergic reactions,** chills, sepsis, chest pain, abdominal pain, back pain, flulike syndrome, asthenia, malaise, myalgia, arthralgia

Interactions
Fludarabine: severe or fatal pulmonary toxicity. Avoid concomitant use.
Vidarabine: increases the incidence or severity of adverse reactions associated with either drug. Avoid concomitant use.

Incompatibility
Check with pharmacist before administering with any other drug.

Administration guidelines
• Make sure patient is adequately hydrated before therapy. Administer 500 to 1,000 ml of D_5W in 0.45% sodium chloride injection as ordered. Give 500 ml of D_5W after drug is given.
• Follow institutional guidelines for proper handling, administration, and disposal of chemotherapeutic agents. Treat all spills and waste products with 5% solution sodium hypochlorite. Wear protective clothing and polyethylene gloves.
• Add 5 ml sterile water for injection to the vial containing pentostatin powder for injection. Mix thoroughly to make a solution of 5 mg/ml. Administer drug by I.V. bolus injection or dilute further in 25 or 50 ml of D_5W or 0.9% sodium chloride injection and infuse over 20 to 30 minutes.

Common reactions are in *italics;* life-threatening reactions in **bold italics**.

• Withhold drug or discontinue in CNS toxicity, a severe rash, or an active infection. Resume drug when the infection clears. Also avoid drug in patients with renal damage (creatinine clearance of 60 ml/minute or less).
• Temporarily withhold the drug if the absolute neutrophil count falls below 200/mm³ and the pretreatment level was over 500/mm³. No recommendations exist regarding dosage adjustments in patients with anemia, neutropenia, or thrombocytopenia.
• Drug should only be used in patients who have hairy cell leukemia refractory to alpha interferon. This is defined as disease that progresses after a minimum of 3 months of treatment with alpha interferon or disease that does not respond after 6 months of therapy.
• The optimal duration of therapy is unknown. Current recommendations suggest two additional courses of therapy after a complete response. If the patient has not had a partial response after 6 months of therapy, discontinue the drug. If the patient has had only a partial response, continue the drug for another 6 months or for two courses of therapy after a complete response.

Pipobroman
Vercyte

Pharmacologic classification
Pipobroman is an alkylating agent. Its mechanism of action is unknown.

Indications
Chronic granulocytic leukemia in patients refractory to busulfan

Adverse reactions
• Blood: *bone marrow suppression, leukopenia, thrombocytopenia, anemia*
• GI: *nausea, vomiting, diarrhea*
• Skin: rash

Interactions
None known.

Incompatibility
None.

Administration guidelines
• Administer drug in divided doses daily and continue as long as needed to maintain satisfactory clinical response.
• If leukocyte count falls too rapidly, discontinue the drug until rate of decrease levels off.
• Initiate maintenance therapy when leukocyte count approaches 10,000/mm³. If relapse is rapid (doubling of leukocyte count in 70 days), continuous treatment is indicated. Intermittent therapy is adequate if more than 70 days are required to double leukocyte count.
• If leukocyte count falls to less than 3,000/mm³, or if platelet count is reduced to less than 150,000/mm³, temporarily discontinue the drug, cautiously reinstating it when the leukocyte or platelet count has risen.

Plicamycin (mithramycin)
Mithracin

Pharmacologic classification
Plicamycin is an antibiotic antineoplastic agent that forms a complex with DNA, thus inhibiting RNA synthesis. It also inhibits osteocytic activity, blocking calcium and phosphorus resorption from bone.

Indications
Malignant testicular tumors and hypercalcemia and hypercalciuria associated with a variety of advanced neoplasms

Adverse reactions
• Blood: *bone marrow suppression, thrombocytopenia, leukopenia, bleeding syndrome* (may range from epistaxis to generalized hemorrhage)
• GI: *nausea, vomiting,* anorexia, diarrhea, stomatitis, metallic taste
• GU: proteinuria; increased BUN and serum creatinine levels
• Metabolic: *decreased serum calcium,* potassium, and phosphorus levels; *elevated liver enzyme levels*
• Skin: *facial flushing;* periorbital pallor, usually the day before toxic symptoms occur
• Local: extravasation causes irritation, cellulitis

Common reactions are in *italics;* life-threatening reactions in ***bold italics.***

Interactions
None significant.

Incompatibility
Check with pharmacist before administering with another drug.

Administration guidelines
• Before administering drug, give an antiemetic as ordered to reduce nausea and vomiting.
• To prepare I.V. solution, add 4.9 ml sterile water for injection to vial and shake to dissolve. Then dilute for I.V. infusion in 1,000 ml D_5W or 0.9% sodium chloride solution.
• Store lyophilized powder in refrigerator. It remains stable after reconstitution for 24 hours and 48 hours when refrigerated. Diluted solutions are stable for 4 to 6 hours. Discard unused drug properly.
• Preparation of parenteral form is associated with carcinogenic, mutagenic, and teratogenic risks for personnel. Follow institutional policy to reduce risks.
• Slow infusion reduces nausea that develops with I.V. push.
• Avoid extravasation. Plicamycin is a vesicant. If I.V. solution infiltrates, stop immediately; use ice packs. Restart I.V. infusion.
• Avoid contact with skin or mucous membranes.
• Therapeutic effect in hypercalcemia may not be seen for 24 to 48 hours and may last 3 to 15 days.

Prednisone
Meticorten, Orasone, Panasol, Prednicen-M, Sk-Prednisone

Pharmacologic classification
Although not an antineoplastic agent, prednisone is an adrenocorticoid used to treat neoplasms because of its immunosuppressant effects.

Indications
Palliative treatment of leukemias and lymphomas in adults and acute leukemia in children

Adverse reactions
When administered in high doses or for prolonged periods, prednisone suppresses re-

lease of corticotropin from the pituitary gland; in turn, the adrenal cortex stops secreting endogenous corticosteroids. The degree and duration of hypothalamic-pituitary-adrenal axis suppression varies, depending on the dose, frequency, and duration of glucocorticoid therapy.
• CNS: *euphoria, insomnia,* headache, psychotic behavior, mood swings, pseudotumor cerebri, mental changes, nervousness, restlessness.
• CV: ***CHF,*** hypertension, edema.
• EENT: cataracts, glaucoma, thrush.
• GI: *peptic ulcer,* increased appetite.
• Immune: immunosuppression, increased susceptibility to infection.
• Metabolic: hypokalemia, sodium retention, fluid retention, weight gain, hyperglycemia, osteoporosis, growth suppression in children.
• Musculoskeletal: muscle atrophy, weakness.
• Skin: delayed healing, acne, skin eruptions, striae.
• Other: pancreatitis, hirsutism, cushingoid symptoms, withdrawal syndome (nausea, fatigue, anorexia, dyspnea, hypotension, hypoglycemia, myalgia, arthralgia, fever, dizziness, and fainting). Sudden withdrawal may be fatal or may exacerbate the underlying disease. ***Acute adrenal insufficency may occur with increased stress (infection, surgery, trauma) or abrupt withdrawal after long-term therapy.***

Interactions
Antacids, cholestyramine, colestipol: adsorb the corticosteroid (prednisone), thus decreasing the amount of the drug absorbed by the body and decreasing its effectiveness.
Barbiturates, phenytoin, rifampin: may decrease corticosteroid effects because of increased hepatic metabolism.
Estrogens: may reduce the metabolism of corticosteroids by increasing the concentration of transcortin. The half-life of the corticosteroid is then prolonged because of increased protein binding.
Glucocorticoids: increase the metabolism of isoniazid and salicylates; cause hyperglycemia, requiring dosage adjustment of insulin or oral antidiabetic agents in diabetic patients; and may enhance hypokalemia asso-

ciated with diuretic or amphotericin B therapy. The hypokalemia may increase the risk of toxicity in patients receiving digitalis glycosides.
Oral anticoagulants: in rare cases, effects decreased by unknown mechanisms.
Ulcerogenic drugs such as NSAIDs: may increase the risk of GI ulceration.

Incompatibility
None.

Administration guidelines
• Give with food when possible to avoid GI upset.
• During times of physiologic stress (trauma, surgery, infection), the patient may require additional steroids and may experience signs of steroid withdrawal; patients who were previously steroid-dependent may need systemic corticosteroids to prevent adrenal insufficiency.
• After long-term therapy, the drug should be reduced gradually. Rapid reduction may cause withdrawal symptoms.
• Because adrenocorticoids increase susceptibility to and mask symptoms of infection, prednisone should not be used (except in life-threatening situations) in viral or bacterial infections not controlled by anti-infective agents.

Procarbazine hydrochloride
Matulane

Pharmacologic classification
Procarbazine is an antibiotic antineoplastic agent that is cell cycle–specific in the S phase.

Indications
Stage III and IV Hodgkin's disease

Adverse reactions
• Blood: ***bone marrow suppression*** (dose-limiting), pancytopenia, hemolysis, ***bleeding tendency, thrombocytopenia, leukopenia, anemia.***
• CNS: paresthesia and neuropathy, myalgia, arthralgia, fatigue, lethargy, headache, nervousness, depression, insomnia, nightmares, *hallucinations,* confusion, ***seizures.***

• CV: hypotension, tachycardia, syncope.
• EENT: retinal hemorrhage, nystagmus, photophobia, diplopia, papilledema, altered hearing abilities.
• GI: *nausea, vomiting, anorexia,* stomatitis, dry mouth, dysphagia, diarrhea, constipation.
• GU: decreased spermatogenesis, infertility, hematuria.
• Skin: dermatitis, pruritus, flushing, hyperpigmentation, photosensitivity.
• Other: chills, fever, pneumonitis, reversible alopecia, ***pleural effusion.***

Interactions
Alcohol: can cause a disulfiram-like reaction through a poorly defined mechanism.
CNS depressants: enhances CNS depression through an additive mechanism.
Digoxin: serum levels may be decreased.
Levodopa, MAO inhibitors or tyramine-rich foods, sympathomimetics, tricyclic antidepressants: can cause a hypertensive crisis, tremors, excitation, and cardiac palpitations through inhibition of MAO by procarbazine.
Meperidine: may result in severe hypotension and death.

Incompatibility
None.

Administration guidelines
• Nausea and vomiting may be decreased if taken at bedtime and in divided doses.
• Store capsules in a dry environment.
• Stop the drug if the following occur: bleeding or bleeding tendencies, stomatitis, diarrhea, paresthesia, neuropathy, confusion, or hypersensitivity.

Semustine
(methyl CCNU)

Pharmacologic classification
Semustine is a nitrosourea compound that probably acts as an alkylating agent.

Indications
Advanced GI tumors, brain tumors, Hodgkin's disease, and malignant lymphoma

Common reactions are in *italics;* life-threatening reactions in ***bold italics.***

Adverse reactions
• Blood: *delayed thrombocytopenia* (about 4 weeks) and *leukopenia* (about 6 weeks). *Myelosuppression* may be cumulative.
• GI: *acute nausea and vomiting 2 to 6 hours after administration, anorexia.*
• GU: *renal toxicity.*
• Hepatic: *elevated liver enzymes.*
• Other: **pulmonary fibrosis** with prolonged use.

Interactions
Not known.

Incompatibility
None.

Administration guidelines
• Drug should be taken on an empty stomach to ensure absorption.
• Capsules are usually refrigerated but are stable for 1 year at room temperature. Avoid high temperatures and excessive moisture.
• Administer drug every 6 to 8 weeks.

Streptozocin
Zanosar

Pharmacologic classification
Streptozocin is an antineoplastic antibiotic agent with alkylating activity and is cell cycle–nonspecific.

Indications
Metastatic islet cell carcinoma of the pancreas

Adverse reactions
• Blood: **bone marrow suppression, leukopenia, thrombocytopenia, anemia.**
• CNS: lethargy, confusion.
• GI: *nausea and vomiting* (dose-limiting), diarrhea.
• GU: *renal toxicity* (evidenced by azotemia, glucosuria, and renal tubular acidosis), mild proteinuria, nephrogenic diabetes insipidus.
• Hepatic: elevated liver enzymes, liver dysfunction.
• Metabolic: hyperglycemia, hypoglycemia.
• Local: *sloughing, severe irritation if extravasation occurs.*

Interactions
Doxorubicin: prolonged elimination and half-life, requiring reduced dosage of doxorubicin.
Nitrosurea compounds such as *carmustine:* may increase hematological toxicity.
Other nephrotoxic drugs: may potentiate the nephrotoxicity caused by streptozocin.
Phenytoin: may decrease the effects of streptozocin on the pancreas.

Incompatibility
None reported.

Administration guidelines
• Reconstitute drug with 9.5 ml of 0.9% sodium chloride solution to yield 100 mg/ml.
• Use streptozocin within 12 hours of reconstitution. The reconstituted solution is a golden color that changes to dark brown upon decomposition.
• The product contains no preservatives and is not intended as a multiple-dose vial.
• Drug may be administered by rapid I.V. push injection.
• Drug may be further diluted in 10 to 200 ml of D_5W in water to infuse over 10 to 15 minutes. It can also be infused over 6 hours.
• Wear gloves during preparation or administration. If skin contact occurs, wash off solution immediately with soap and water. Follow recommended procedures for the safe preparation, administration, and disposal of chemotherapeutic agents.
• Administer phenytoin concomitantly to protect pancreatic beta cells from cytotoxicity.
• Keep dextrose 50% at bedside because of risk of hypoglycemia from sudden release of insulin.

Tamoxifen citrate
Nolvadex

Pharmacologic classification
Tamoxifen is a nonsteroidal antiestrogen.

Indications
Treatment of metastatic breast cancer or prevention of its recurrence

Common reactions are in *italics;* life-threatening reactions in **bold italics.**

Adverse reactions
• Blood: transient fall in WBC or platelet count.
• CNS: headache, dizziness, depression, confusion.
• CV: thrombosis, peripheral edema.
• EENT: blurred vision, decreased visual acuity, corneal changes.
• GI: *nausea,* vomiting, anorexia.
• GU: vaginal discharge and bleeding.
• Metabolic: hypercalcemia.
• Skin: rash, photosensitivity.
• Other: hot flashes, temporary bone or tumor pain, brief exacerbation of pain from osseous metastases.

Interactions
None reported.

Incompatibility
None.

Administration guidelines
• Administer medication on time despite nausea, if vomiting becomes a problem, premedicate patient with an antiemetic.
• Reassure the patient that bone pain during therapy usually indicates the drug will produce a good response; tell the patient to request an analgesic from doctor.

Teniposide (VM-26)
Vumon

Pharmacologic classification
Teniposide is a semisynthetic derivative of podophyllotoxin that arrests cell mitosis and causes breaks in DNA.

Indications
Induction therapy in patients with refractory childhood acute lymphoblastic leukemia and treatment of neuroblastoma and malignant lymphomas

Adverse reactions
• Blood: **bone marrow suppression** (dose-limiting), **leukopenia, neutropenia, thrombocytopenia, anemia.**
• CV: hypotension from rapid infusion.
• GI: nausea and vomiting.

• Local: *phlebitis at injection site with extravasation.*
• Other: alopecia (rare), **anaphylaxis** (rare), sensitivity reactions (chills, fever, urticaria, tachycardia, **bronchospasm,** dyspnea, hypotension, flushing), mucositis.

Interactions
None significant.

Incompatibility
Check with pharmacist before administering with another drug.

Administration guidelines
• Some clinicians may decide to use this drug in spite of the patient's history of hypersensitivity reactions because the drug's benefits may outweigh its risks. Pretreat such a patient with antihistamines and corticosteroids before the infusion begins and observe him closely during drug administration.
• Dilute drug in either D_5W or 0.9% sodium chloride injection to a final concentration of 0.1, 0.2, 0.4, or 1 mg/ml. Discard cloudy solution. Prepare and store the drug in glass containers. Infuse over 45 to 90 minutes to prevent hypotension.
• Solutions containing 0.5 to 1 mg/ml are stable for 4 hours; those containing 0.1 to 0.2 mg/ml are stable for 6 hours.
• Avoid extravasation. Because extravasation of drug can result in local tissue necrosis or sloughing, be certain to ensure careful placement of the I.V. catheter.
• Monitor blood pressure before infusion and at 30-minute intervals during infusion. If systolic blood pressure falls below 90 mm Hg, stop infusion.
• Don't administer through a membrane-type in-line filter because the diluent may dissolve the filter.
• Have on hand diphenhydramine, hydrocortisone, epinephrine, and appropriate emergency equipment to establish an airway in case of anaphylaxis.
• Drug may be given by local bladder instillation for bladder cancer.
• Preparation of parenteral form is associated with carcinogenic, mutagenic, and teratogenic risks for personnel. Follow institutional policy to reduce risks.

Common reactions are in *italics;* life-threatening reactions in ***bold italics.***

Testolactone
Teslac

Pharmacologic classification
Testolactone is an antineoplastic agent that alters hormone balance, which in turn alters the neoplastic process.

Indications
Palliative treatment of advanced or disseminated breast cancer in pre- or postmenopausal women in whom ovarian function has been terminated. Testolactone is contraindicated in male breast cancer and is not recommended for premenopausal women.

Adverse reactions
• CNS: paresthesia, peripheral neuropathy.
• CV: increased blood pressure, edema.
• GI: nausea, vomiting, diarrhea.
• Metabolic: hypercalcemia.
• Other: alopecia.

Interactions
Oral anticoagulants: cause increased pharmacologic effects. Monitor carefully.

Incompatibility
None.

Administration guidelines
• Administer drug daily in four equal doses.
• Adequate trial period is 3 months. Inform patient that therapeutic response isn't immediate.

Thioguanine
(6-thioguanine, 6-TG)
Lanvis

Pharmacologic classification
Thioguanine is an antimetabolite agent that is cell cycle–specific in the S phase.

Indications
Nonlymphocytic leukemias

Adverse reactions
• Blood: ***bone marrow suppression*** (dose-limiting), ***leukopenia, anemia, thrombocytopenia*** (occurs slowly over 2 to 4 weeks).
• GI: nausea, vomiting, stomatitis, diarrhea, anorexia.
• Hepatic: ***hepatotoxicity,*** jaundice.
• Metabolic: hyperuricemia.

Interactions
None reported.

Incompatibility
None.

Administration guidelines
• Total daily dosage can be given at one time.
• Give dose between meals to facilitate complete absorption.
• Dose modification may be required in renal or hepatic dysfunction.
• Stop drug if hepatotoxicity or hepatic tenderness occurs. Watch for jaundice; may reverse if drug stopped promptly.
• Keep in mind that this drug is sometimes ordered as 6-thioguanine. The numeral 6 is part of the drug name and does not signify dosage units.

Thiotepa
(TESPA, TSPA)

Pharmacologic classification
Thiotepa is an alkylating agent that is cell cycle–nonspecific.

Indications
Palliative treatment of adenocarcinoma of the breast or ovary, superficial papillary carcinoma of the urinary bladder, and for controlling intracavitary effusions secondary to diffuse or localized neoplastic diseases of various serosal cavities

Adverse reactions
• Blood: ***bone marrow suppression*** (dose-limiting), ***leukopenia*** (beginning within 5 to 30 days), ***thrombocytopenia, neutropenia, anemia.***
• CNS: dizziness, headache.
• GI: *nausea, vomiting,* anorexia.

Common reactions are in *italics;* life-threatening reactions in ***bold italics.***

- GU: amenorrhea, decreased spermatogenesis.
- Metabolic: hyperuricemia.
- Skin: hives, rash.
- Local: intense pain at administration site.
- Other: headache, fever, tightness of throat.

Interactions
Succinylcholine: may cause prolonged apnea.
Pseudocholinesterase (the enzyme that deactivates succinylcholine): may be inactivated by thiotepa. Use with extreme caution.

Incompatibility
Drug is incompatible with cisplatin, causing a yellow precipitate.

Administration guidelines
- Reconstitute drug with 1.5 ml of sterile water for injection to yield 10 mg/ml. The solution is clear to slightly opaque.
- A 1 mg/ml solution is considered isotonic.
- Use sterile water for injection to reconstitute. Refrigerated solution is stable for 5 days.
- Refrigerate dry powder; protect from light.
- Drug can be given by all parenteral routes, including direct injection into the tumor.
- Drug may be mixed with procaine 2%, epinephrine 1:1,000, or both for local use.
- Drug may be further diluted to larger volumes with 0.9% sodium chloride solution, D_5W, or lactated Ringer's solution for administration by I.V. infusion, intracavitary injection, or perfusion therapy.
- Withhold fluids for 8 to 10 hours before bladder instillation. Instill 60 ml of drug into bladder by catheter; ask patient to retain for 2 hours. Reduce to 30 ml if discomfort is great. Reposition patient every 15 minutes for maximum area contact.
- Stop drug or decrease dosage if WBC count falls below 4,000/mm³ or if platelet count falls below 150,000/mm³.

Vinblastine sulfate (VLB)
Velban

Pharmacologic classification
Vinblastine is a Vinca alkaloid agent that is cell cycle–specific in the M phase.

Indications
Palliative treatment of generalized Hodgkin's disease (stages III and IV, Ann Arbor modification of the Rye staging system), lymphocytic lymphoma, histiocytic lymphoma, advanced mycosis fungoides, advanced testicular cancer, Kaposi's sarcoma, Letterer-Siwe disease, choriocarcinoma resistant to other chemotherapeutic agents, and carcinoma of the breast unresponsive to appropriate endocrine surgery and hormonal therapy

Adverse reactions
- Blood: **bone marrow suppression** (dose-limiting), **leukopenia** (nadir occurs on days 4 to 10 and lasts another 7 to 14 days), **thrombocytopenia, anemia.**
- CNS: depression, *paresthesia, peripheral neuropathy and neuritis, numbness, loss of deep tendon reflexes, muscle pain, weakness*, malaise, **seizures**.
- CV: hypertension, myocardial infarction, cerebrovascular accident.
- EENT: pharyngitis.
- GI: *nausea, vomiting, stomatitis*, ulcer, bleeding, *constipation, ileus, anorexia, weight loss*, abdominal pain.
- GU: oligospermia, aspermia, urine retention.
- Skin: dermatitis, vesiculation.
- Local: *irritation, phlebitis*, cellulitis, necrosis or tissue damage if I.V. solution extravasates.
- Other: **acute bronchospasm,** reversible alopecia in 5% to 10% of patients, *pain in tumor site,* low fever.

Interactions
Methotrexate: increased cellular uptake of methotrexate. Lower the dosage of methotrexate to reduce the potential for toxicity.
Mitomycin-C: may cause severe bronchospasm and respiratory distress.
Phenytoin: causes decreased serum phenytoin levels.

Incompatibility
Drug is incompatible with furosemide (immediate precipitation) and heparin sodium at 200 units at 1 ml concentration (turbidity appears in 2 to 3 minutes).

Administration guidelines
- Give an antiemetic before administering drug to reduce nausea.

Common reactions are in *italics;* life-threatening reactions in **bold italics.**

• Reconstitute with 10 ml of preserved 0.9% sodium chloride solution injection for 1 mg/ml.

• Drug may be administered by I.V. push injection over 1 minute into the tubing of a freely flowing I.V. infusion.

• Dilution into larger volume is not recommended for infusion into peripheral veins. This method increases risk of extravasation. Drug may be administered as an I.V. infusion through a central venous catheter.

• Do not give more often than every 7 days to allow review of effect on leukocytes before next dose. Leukopenia may develop.

• Reduced dosage may be required in patients with liver disease.

• After giving, monitor for life-threatening acute bronchospasm reaction (most likely in a patient also receiving mitomycin).

• Do not confuse vinblastine with vincristine or vindesine.

• Treat extravasation with liberal injection of hyaluronidase into the site, followed by warm compresses. (Some clinicians use cold compresses.) Prepare hyaluronidase by adding 3 ml of 0.9% sodium chloride solution to the 150-unit vial.

Vincristine sulfate
Oncovin

Pharmacologic classification
Vincristine is a Vinca alkaloid that is cell cycle–specific in the M phase.

Indications
Acute leukemia, Hodgkin's disease, malignant lymphoma, rhabdomyosarcoma, neuroblastoma, and Wilms' tumor

Adverse reactions
• Blood: rapidly reversible mild anemia and leukopenia.

• CNS: neurotoxicity, *peripheral neuropathy,* sensory loss, *deep tendon reflex loss, paresthesia, wristdrop and footdrop,* ataxia, cranial nerve palsies (headache, *jaw pain,* hoarseness, vocal cord paralysis, visual disturbances), *muscle weakness and cramps,* depression, agitation, insomnia. Some neurotoxicities may be permanent.

• EENT: diplopia, optic and extraocular neuropathy, ptosis.

• GI: *constipation, cramps,* ileus that mimics acute abdomen, *nausea, vomiting,* anorexia, stomatitis, weight loss, dysphagia, ***intestinal necrosis.***

• GU: urine retention.

• Local: severe local reaction when extravasation occurs, *phlebitis,* cellulitis.

• Other: ***acute bronchospasm,*** *reversible alopecia,* syndrome of inappropriate antidiuretic hormone, blood pressure alterations.

Interactions
Asparaginase: decreases the hepatic clearance of vincristine.

Calcium channel blockers: enhance vincristine accumulation in cells.

Digoxin: decreases serum digoxin levels, which should be monitored.

Methotrexate: therapeutic effect of methotrexate increased, allowing lower dose and reducing potential for methotrexate toxicity.

Mitomycin: may increase the frequency of bronchospasm and acute pulmonary reactions.

Other neurotoxic drugs: increase neurotoxicity through an additive effect.

Incompatibility
Drug is incompatible with furosemide (immediate precipitation occurs).

Administration guidelines
• Drug may be administered by I.V. push injection over 1 minute into the tubing of a freely flowing I.V. infusion.

• Dilution into larger volumes is not recommended for infusion into peripheral veins: This method increases risk of extravasation. Drug may be administered as an I.V. infusion through a central venous catheter.

• Treat extravasation with cold compresses and prompt administration of 150 units of intradermal hyaluronidase, sodium bicarbonate, a local injection of hydrocortisone, or a combination of these treatments. However, some clinicians prefer to treat extravasation only with warm compresses.

• Because of the potential for neurotoxicity, don't give the drug more than once a week.

• Vials of 5 mg are for multiple dose use only. Don't give entire vial as a single dose.

Common reactions are in *italics;* life-threatening reactions in ***bold italics.***

Chemotherapy Acronyms and Protocols

ACRONYM & INDICATION	DRUG		DOSAGE
	Generic name	Trade name	
ABVD Hodgkin's disease	doxorubicin	Adriamycin	25 mg/m² I.V., days 1 and 15
	bleomycin	Blenoxane	10 units/m² I.V., days 1 and 15
	vinblastine	Velban	6 mg/m² I.V., days 1 and 15
	dacarbazine	DTIC-Dome	375 mg/m² I.V., days 1 and 15
			Repeat cycle every 28 days.
AC Bony sarcoma	doxorubicin	Adriamycin	75 to 90 mg/m² by 96-hour continuous I.V. infusion
	cisplatin	Platinol	90 to 120 mg/m² intra-arterially or I.V., day 6
			Repeat cycle every 28 days.
ACE (CAE) Small-cell lung cancer	doxorubicin	Adriamycin	45 mg/m² I.V., days 1 to 3
	cyclophosphamide	Cytoxan	1 g/m² I.V., days 1 to 5
	etoposide (VP-16)	VePesid	50 mg/m² I.V., days 1 to 5
			Repeat cycle every 21 days.
AP Ovarian cancer, epithelial	doxorubicin	Adriamycin	50 to 60 mg/m² I.V., day 1
	cisplatin	Platinol	50 to 60 mg/m² I.V., day 1
			Repeat cycle every 21 days.
ASHAP Malignant lymphoma	doxorubicin	Adriamycin	10 mg/m² daily by continuous I.V. infusion, days 1 to 4
	cisplatin	Platinol	25 mg/m² daily by continuous I.V. infusion, days 1 to 4
	(cytarabine ara-C)	Cytosar-U	1,500 mg/m² I.V. immediately after completion of doxorubicin and cisplatin therapy
	methylprednisolone	Solu-Medrol	500 mg I.V. daily, days 1 to 5
			Repeat cycle every 21 to 25 days.

(continued)

ACRONYM & INDICATION	DRUG		DOSAGE
	Generic name	Trade name	
BACON Non–small cell lung cancer	bleomycin	Blenoxane	30 units I.V. q 6 weeks, day 2
	doxorubicin	Adriamycin	40 mg/m² I.V. q 4 weeks, day 1
	lomustine (CCNU)	CeeNU	65 mg/m² P.O. q 8 weeks, day 1
	vincristine	Oncovin	0.75 to 1 mg/m² I.V. q 6 weeks, day 2
	mechlorethamine (nitrogen mustard)	Mustargen	8 mg/m² I.V. q 4 weeks, day 1
			Repeat cycle as indicated in protocol.
BACOP Malignant lymphoma	bleomycin	Blenoxane	5 units/m² I.V., days 15 and 22
	doxorubicin	Adriamycin	25 mg/m² I.V., days 1 and 8
	cyclophosphamide	Cytoxan	650 mg/m² I.V., days 1 and 8
	vincristine	Oncovin	1.4 mg/m² (2 mg maximum) I.V., days 1 and 8
	prednisone	Deltasone	60 mg/m² P.O., days 15 to 28
			Repeat cycle every 28 days.
BCP Multiple myeloma	carmustine	BiCNU	75 mg/m² I.V., day 1
	cyclophosphamide	Cytoxan	400 mg/m² I.V., day 1
	prednisone	Deltasone	75 mg P.O., days 1 to 7
			Repeat cycle every 28 days.
BEP Genitourinary cancer	bleomycin	Blenoxane	30 units I.V., days 2, 9, and 16
	etoposide (VP-16)	VePesid	100 mg/m², days 1 to 5
	cisplatin	Platinol	20 mg/m² I.V. over 30 minutes, days 1 to 5
			Repeat cycle every 21 days.
BHD Malignant melanoma	carmustine	BiCNU	100 to 150 mg/m² I.V. q 6 weeks
	hydroxyurea	Hydrea	1,480 mg/m² P.O. q 3 weeks, days 1 to 5
	dacarbazine	DTIC-Dome	100 to 150 mg/m² I.V. q 3 weeks, days 1 to 5
			Repeat cycle as indicated in protocol.

ACRONYM & INDICATION	DRUG		DOSAGE
	Generic name	Trade name	
CAF (FAC) Breast cancer	cyclophosphamide	Cytoxan	100 mg/m² P.O., days 1 to 14
	doxorubicin	Adriamycin	30 mg/m² I.V., days 1 and 8
	fluorouracil (5-FU)	Adrucil	400 to 500 mg/m² I.V., days 1 and 8
			Repeat cycle every 28 days for 6 cycles.
or	cyclophosphamide	Cytoxan	500 mg/m² I.V., day 1
	doxorubicin	Adriamycin	50 mg/m² I.V., day 1
	fluorouracil (5-FU)	Adrucil	500 mg/m² I.V., day 1
			Repeat cycle every 21 days for 8 to 10 cycles.
CAMP Non–small cell lung cancer	cyclophosphamide	Cytoxan	300 mg/m² I.V., days 1 and 8
	doxorubicin	Adriamycin	20 mg/m² I.V., days 1 and 8
	methotrexate sodium	Folex	15 mg/m² I.V., days 1 and 8
	procarbazine	Matulane	100 mg/m² P.O., days 1 to 10
			Repeat cycle every 28 days.
CAP Genitourinary cancer	cisplatin	Platinol	60 mg/m² I.V., day 1
	doxorubicin	Adriamycin	40 mg/m² I.V., day 1
	cyclophosphamide	Cytoxan	400 mg/m² I.V., day 1
			Repeat cycle every 21 days.
CAP Non–small cell lung cancer	cyclophosphamide	Cytoxan	400 mg/m² I.V., day 1
	doxorubicin	Adriamycin	40 mg/m² I.V., day 1
	cisplatin	Platinol	60 mg/m² I.V., day 1
			Repeat cycle every 28 days.
CAP (PAC) Ovarian cancer, epithelial	cisplatin	Platinol	50 mg/m² I.V., day 1
	doxorubicin	Adriamycin	50 mg/m² I.V., day 1
	cyclophosphamide	Cytoxan	500 mg/m² I.V., day 1
			Repeat cycle every 21 days for 8 cycles.
CAV (VAC) Small-cell lung cancer	cyclophosphamide	Cytoxan	750 mg/m² I.V., day 1
	doxorubicin	Adriamycin	50 mg/m² I.V., day 1
	vincristine	Oncovin	2 mg/m² I.V., day 1
			Repeat cycle every 21 days for 4 to 6 cycles.

(continued)

ACRONYM & INDICATION	DRUG		DOSAGE
	Generic name	Trade name	
CAVe Hodgkin's disease	lomustine (CCNU)	CeeNU	100 mg/m² I.V., day 1
	doxorubicin	Adriamycin	60 mg/m² I.V., day 1
	vinblastine	Velban	5 mg/m² I.V., day 1
			Repeat cycle every 6 weeks.
CC Ovarian cancer, epithelial	carboplatin	Paraplatin	300 mg/m² I.V., day 1
	cyclophosphamide	Cytoxan	600 mg/m² I.V., day 1
			Repeat cycle every 20 days.
CD (DC) Leukemia— ANLL, consolidation	cytarabine (ara-C)	Cytosar-U	3,000 mg/m² I.V. q 12 hours for 6 days
	daunorubicin	Cerubidine	30 mg/m² I.V. daily for 3 days, after cytarabine therapy (days 7 to 9)
			Cycle is not repeated.
CDC Ovarian cancer, epithelial	carboplatin	Paraplatin	300 mg/m² I.V., day 1
	doxorubicin	Adriamycin	40 mg/m² I.V., day 1
	cyclophosphamide	Cytoxan	500 mg/m² I.V., day 1
			Repeat cycle every 28 days.
CF Head and neck cancer	cisplatin	Platinol AO	100 mg/m² I.V., day 1
	(fluorouracil 5-FU)	Adrucil	1,000 mg/m² daily by continuous I.V. infusion, days 1 to 5
			Repeat cycle every 21 to 28 days.
or	carboplatin	Paraplatin	400 mg/m² I.V., day 1
	fluorouracil (5-FU)	Adrucil	1,000 mg/m² daily by continuous I.V. infusion, days 1 to 5
			Repeat cycle every 21 to 28 days.
CFL Head and neck cancer	cisplatin	Platinol	100 mg/m² I.V., day 1
	fluorouracil (5-FU)	Adrucil	600 to 800 mg/m² daily by continuous I.V. infusion, days 1 to 5
	leucovorin calcium	Wellcovorin	200 to 300 mg/m² I.V. daily, days 1 to 5
			Repeat cycle every 21 days.
CFM Breast cancer	cyclophosphamide	Cytoxan	500 mg/m² I.V., day 1
	fluorouracil (5-FU)	Adrucil	500 mg/m² I.V., day 1
	mitoxantrone	Novantrone	10 mg/m² I.V., day 1
			Repeat cycle every 21 days.

ACRONYM & INDICATION	DRUG		DOSAGE
	Generic name	Trade name	
CFPT Breast cancer	cyclophosphamide	Cytoxan	150 mg/m^2 I.V., days 1 to 5
	fluorouracil (5-FU)	Adrucil	300 mg/m^2 I.V., days 1 to 5
	prednisone	Deltasone	10 mg P.O. t.i.d. for first 7 days of each course
	tamoxifen	Nolvadex	10 mg P.O. b.i.d. (daily through each course)
			Repeat cycle every 6 weeks.
CHAP Ovarian cancer, epithelial	cyclophosphamide	Cytoxan	300 to 500 mg/m^2 I.V., days 1 and 8
	altretamine	Hexalen	150 mg/m^2 P.O., days 1 to 7
	doxorubicin	Adriamycin	30 to 50 mg/m^2 I.V., day 1
	cisplatin	Platinol	50 mg/m^2 I.V., day 1
			Repeat cycle every 28 days.
ChIVPP Hodgkin's disease	chlorambucil	Leukeran	6 mg/m^2 P.O., days 1 to 14 (10 mg/day maximum)
	vinblastine	Velban	6 mg/m^2 I.V., days 1 to 8 (10 mg/day maximum)
	procarbazine	Matulane	50 mg P.O., days 1 to 14 (150 mg/day maximum)
	prednisone	Deltasone	40 mg/m^2 P.O., days 1 to 14 (25 mg/m^2 for child)
CHOP Malignant lymphoma	cyclophosphamide	Cytoxan	750 mg/m^2 I.V., day 1
	doxorubicin	Adriamycin	50 mg/m^2 I.V., day 1
	vincristine	Oncovin	1.4 mg/m^2 (2 mg maximum) I.V., day 1
	prednisone	Deltasone	100 mg/m^2 P.O., days 1 to 5
			Repeat cycle every 21 to 28 days for minimum of 6 cycles or until 2 cycles after disappearance of lymphoma.
CHOP-Bleo Malignant lymphoma	cyclophosphamide	Cytoxan	750 mg/m^2 I.V., day 1
	doxorubicin	Adriamycin	50 mg/m^2 I.V., day 1
	vincristine	Oncovin	2 mg I.V., days 1 and 5
	prednisone	Deltasone	100 mg P.O., days 1 to 5
	bleomycin	Blenoxane	15 units I.V., days 1 and 5
			Repeat cycle every 21 days.

(continued)

ACRONYM & INDICATION	DRUG		DOSAGE
	Generic name	Trade name	
CISCA Genitourinary cancer	cyclophosphamide	Cytoxan	650 mg/m² I.V., day 1
	doxorubicin	Adriamycin	50 mg/m² I.V., day 1
	cisplatin	Platinol	70 to 100 mg/m² I.V., day 2
			Repeat cycle every 21 to 28 days.
CMF Breast cancer	cyclophosphamide	Cytoxan	100 mg/m² P.O., days 1 to 14, or 400 to 600 mg/m² I.V., day 1
	methotrexate	Folex	40 to 60 mg/m² I.V., days 1 and 8
	fluorouracil (5-FU)	Adrucil	400 to 600 mg/m² I.V., days 1 and 8
			Repeat cycle every 28 days.
CMFVP (Cooper's) Breast cancer	cyclophosphamide	Cytoxan	2 to 2.5 mg/kg P.O. daily for 9 months
	methotrexate	Folex	0.7 mg/kg/week I.V. for 8 weeks, then every other week for 7 months
	fluorouracil (5-FU)	Adrucil	12 mg/kg/week I.V. for 8 weeks, then weekly for 7 months
	vincristine	Oncovin	0.035 mg/kg (2 mg/week maximum) I.V. for 5 weeks, then once monthly
	prednisone	Deltasone	0.75 mg/kg P.O. daily, days 1 to 10, then taper over next 40 days and discontinue
			Repeat cycle as indicated in protocol.
CMFVP (SWOG) Breast cancer	cyclophosphamide	Cytoxan	60 mg/m² P.O. daily for 1 year
	methotrexate	Folex	15 mg/m² I.V. weekly for 1 year
	fluorouracil (5-FU)	Adrucil	300 mg/m² I.V. weekly for 1 year
	vincristine	Oncovin	0.625 mg/m² I.V. weekly for 1 year
	prednisone	Deltasone	30 mg/m² P.O., days 1 to 14; 20 mg/m², days 15 to 28; 10 mg/m², days 29 to 42
			Repeat cycle every 6 weeks.
COAP Leukemia— AML, induction	cyclophosphamide	Cytoxan	100 mg/m² I.V. or P.O., days 1 to 5
	vincristine	Oncovin	2 mg/m² I.V., day 1
	cytarabine (ara-C)	Cytosar-U	100 mg/m² I.V., days 1 to 5
	prednisone	Deltasone	100 mg P.O., days 1 to 5
			Repeat cycle only if leukemia persists.

ACRONYM & INDICATION	DRUG		DOSAGE
	Generic name	Trade name	
COB Head and neck cancer	cisplatin	Platinol	100 mg/m^2 I.V., day 1
	vincristine	Oncovin	1 mg I.V., days 2 and 5
	bleomycin	Blenoxane	30 units by continuous I.V. infusion, days 2 to 5
			Repeat cycle every 21 days.
COMLA Malignant lymphoma	cyclophosphamide	Cytoxan	1,500 mg/m^2 I.V., day 1
	vincristine	Oncovin	1.4 mg/m^2 (2.5 mg maximum) I.V., days 1, 8, and 15
	methotrexate	Folex	120 mg/m^2 I.V., days 22, 29, 36, 43, 50, 57, 64, and 71
	leucovorin calcium	Wellcovorin	25 mg/m^2 P.O. q 6 hours for four doses, beginning 24 hours after methotrexate dose
	cytarabine (ara-C)	Cytosar-U	300 mg/m^2 I.V., days 22, 29, 36, 43, 50, 57, 64, and 71
			Repeat cycle every 21 days.
COP Malignant lymphoma	cyclophosphamide	Cytoxan	800 to 1,000 mg/m^2 I.V., day 1
	vincristine	Oncovin	1.4 mg/m^2 (2 mg maximum) I.V., day 1
	prednisone	Deltasone	60 mg/m^2 P.O., days 1 to 5
			Repeat cycle every 21 days.
COP-BLAM Malignant lymphoma	cyclophosphamide	Cytoxan	400 mg/m^2 I.V., day 1
	vincristine	Oncovin	1 mg/m^2 I.V., day 1
	prednisone	Deltasone	40 mg/m^2 P.O., days 1 to 10
	bleomycin	Blenoxane	15 mg I.V., day 14
	doxorubicin	Adriamycin	40 mg/m^2, day 1
	procarbazine	Matulane	100 mg/m^2, days 1 to 10
COPE Small-cell lung cancer	cyclophosphamide	Cytoxan	750 mg/m^2 I.V., day 1
	cisplatin	Platinol	20 mg/m^2 I.V., days 1 to 3
	etoposide (VP-16)	VePesid	100 mg/m^2 I.V., days 1 to 3
	vincristine	Oncovin	2 mg/m^2 I.V., day 3
			Repeat cycle every 21 days.

(continued)

ACRONYM & INDICATION	DRUG		DOSAGE
	Generic name	**Trade name**	
COPP Malignant lymphoma	cyclophosphamide	Cytoxan	400 to 650 mg/m² I.V., days 1 and 8
	vincristine	Oncovin	1.4 to 1.5 mg/m² (2 mg maximum) I.V., days 1 and 8
	procarbazine	Matulane	100 mg/m² P.O., days 1 to 10 or 1 to 14
	prednisone	Deltasone	40 mg/m² P.O., days 1 to 14
			Repeat cycle every 28 days.
CP Ovarian cancer, epithelial	cyclophosphamide	Cytoxan	1,000 mg/m² I.V., day 1
	cisplatin	Platinol	50 to 60 mg/m² I.V., day 1
			Repeat cycle every 21 days.
CV Small-cell lung cancer	cisplatin	Platinol	50 mg/m² I.V., day 1
	etoposide (VP-16)	VePesid	60 mg/m² I.V., days 1 to 5
			Repeat cycle every 21 to 28 days.
or	cisplatin	Platinol	75 mg/m² I.V., day 2
	etoposide (VP-16)	VePesid	125 mg/m² I.V., days 1, 3, and 5
			Repeat cycle every 28 days.
CV Non–small cell lung cancer	cisplatin	Platinol	60 to 80 mg/m² I.V., day 1
	etoposide (VP-16)	VePesid	120 mg/m² I.V., days 4, 6, and 8
			Repeat cycle every 21 to 28 days.
CVEB Genitourinary cancer	cisplatin	Platinol	40 mg/m² I.V., days 1 to 5
	vinblastine	Velban	7.5 mg/m² I.V., day 1
	etoposide (VP-16)	VePesid	100 mg/m² I.V., days 1 to 5
	bleomycin	Blenoxane	30 units I.V. weekly
			Repeat cycle every 21 days.
CVI (VIC) Non–small cell lung cancer	carboplatin	Paraplatin	300 mg/m² I.V., day 1
	etoposide (VP-16)	VePesid	60 to 100 mg/m² I.V., day 1
	ifosfamide	Ifex	1.5 g/m² I.V., days 1, 3, and 5
	mesna	Mesnex	Dosage is 20% of ifosfamide dose, given immediately before and at 4 and 8 hours after ifosfamide infusion
			Repeat cycle every 28 days.

ACRONYM & INDICATION	DRUG		DOSAGE
	Generic name	Trade name	
CVP Leukemia— CLL, blast crisis	cyclophosphamide	Cytoxan	300 mg/m^2 P.O., days 1 to 5
	vincristine	Oncovin	1.4 mg/m^2 (2 mg maximum) I.V., day 1
	prednisone	Deltasone	100 mg/m^2 P.O., days 1 to 5
			Repeat cycle every 21 days.
CVP Malignant lymphoma	cyclophosphamide	Cytoxan	400 mg/m^2 P.O., days 1 to 5
	vincristine	Oncovin	1.4 mg/m^2 (2 mg maximum) I.V., day 1
	prednisone	Deltasone	100 mg/m^2 P.O., days 1 to 5
			Repeat cycle every 21 days.
CVPP Hodgkin's disease	lomustine (CCNU)	CeeNU	75 mg/m^2 P.O., day 1
	vinblastine	Velban	4 mg/m^2 I.V., days 1 and 8
	procarbazine	Matulane	100 mg/m^2 P.O., days 1 to 14
	prednisone	Deltasone	30 mg/m^2 P.O., days 1 to 14 (cycles 1 and 4 only)
			Repeat cycle every 28 days.
CYADIC Soft-tissue sarcoma	cyclophosphamide	Cytoxan	600 mg/m^2 I.V., day 1
	doxorubicin	Adriamycin	15 mg/m^2 by continuous I.V. infusion, days 1 to 4
	dacarbazine	DTIC-Dome	250 mg/m^2 by continuous I.V. infusion, days 1 to 4
			Repeat cycle every 21 to 28 days.
CYVADIC Bony sarcoma	cyclophosphamide	Cytoxan	600 mg/m^2 I.V., day 1
	vincristine	Oncovin	1.4 mg/m^2 (2 mg maximum) I.V. weekly for 6 weeks, then on day 1 of future cycles
	doxorubicin	Adriamycin	15 mg/m^2 by continuous I.V. infusion, days 1 to 4
	dacarbazine	DTIC-Dome	250 mg/m^2 by continuous I.V. infusion, days 1 to 4
			Repeat cycle every 21 to 28 days.
CYVADIC Soft-tissue sarcoma	cyclophosphamide	Cytoxan	500 mg/m^2 I.V., day 1
	vincristine	Oncovin	1.4 mg/m^2 (2 mg maximum) I.V., days 1 and 5
	doxorubicin	Adriamycin	50 mg/m^2 I.V., day 1
	dacarbazine	DTIC-Dome	250 mg/m^2 I.V., days 1 to 5
			Repeat cycle every 21 days.

(continued)

ACRONYM & INDICATION	DRUG		DOSAGE
	Generic name	**Trade name**	
DC Leukemia— pediatric AML, induction	daunorubicin	Cerubidine	45 to 60 mg/m² I.V., days 1 to 3
	cytarabine (ara-C)	Cytosar-U	100 mg/m² I.V. or S.C. q 12 hours for 5 to 7 days
			Repeat cycle if remission does not occur.
DCPM Leukemia— pediatric AML, induction	daunorubicin	Cerubidine	25 mg/m² I.V., day 1
	cytarabine (ara-C)	Cytosar-U	80 mg/m² I.V., days 1 to 3
	prednisone	Deltasone	40 mg/m² P.O. daily
	mercaptopurine (6-MP)	Purinethol	100 mg/m² P.O. daily
			Repeat cycle weekly until remission occurs.
DCT Leukemia— ANLL, induction	daunorubicin	Cerubidine	60 mg/m² I.V., days 1 to 3
	cytarabine (ara-C)	Cytosar-U	200 mg/m² daily by continuous I.V. infusion, days 1 to 5
	thioguanine (6-TG)	Lanvis	100 mg/m² P.O. q 12 hours, days 1 to 5
			Repeat cycle on day 14 if remission does not occur.
DHAP Hodgkin's disease	dexamethasone	Decadron	40 mg P.O. or I.V., days 1 to 4
	cisplatin	Platinol	100 mg/m² by continuous I.V. infusion, day 1
	cytarabine (ara-C)	Cytosar-U	2 g/m² I.V. q 12 hours for two doses, day 2
			Repeat cycle every 3 to 4 weeks.
DTIC-ACTD Malignant melanoma	dacarbazine	DTIC-Dome	750 mg/m² I.V., day 1
	dactinomycin (actinomycin D)	Cosmegen	1 mg/m² I.V., day 1
			Repeat cycle every 28 days.
DVP Leukemia— ALL, induction	daunorubicin	Cerubidine	45 mg/m² I.V., days 1 to 4
	vincristine	Oncovin	2 mg/m² (2 mg maximum) I.V. weekly for 4 weeks
	prednisone	Deltasone	45 mg/m² P.O. for 28 to 35 days
EP Small-cell or non–small cell lung cancer	cisplatin	Platinol	75 to 100 mg/m² I.V., day 1
	etoposide (VP-16)	VePesid	75 to 100 mg/m² I.V., days 1 to 3
			Repeat cycle every 21 to 28 days.

ACRONYM & INDICATION	DRUG		DOSAGE
	Generic name	Trade name	
ESHAP Malignant lymphoma	etoposide (VP-16)	VePesid	40 mg/m^2 by I.V. infusion, days 1 to 4
	cisplatin	Platinol	25 mg/m^2 daily by continuous I.V. infusion, days 1 to 4
	cytarabine (ara-C)	Cytosar-U	2 g/m^2 I.V. immediately after completion of etoposide and cisplatin therapy
	methylpred-nisolone	Solu-Medrol	500 mg I.V. daily, days 1 to 4
			Repeat cycle every 21 to 28 days.
EVA Hodgkin's disease	etoposide (VP-16)	VePesid	100 mg/m^2 I.V., days 1 to 3
	vinblastine	Velban	6 mg/m^2 I.V., day 1
	doxorubicin	Adriamycin	50 mg/m^2 I.V., day 1
			Repeat cycle every 28 days.
FAC (CAF) Breast cancer	fluorouracil (5-FU)	Adrucil	500 mg/m^2 I.V., days 1 and 8
	doxorubicin	Adriamycin	50 mg/m^2 I.V., day 1
	cyclophosphamide	Cytoxan	500 mg/m^2 I.V., day 1
			Repeat cycle every 21 days.
FAM Colon cancer, gastric cancer	fluorouracil (5-FU)	Adrucil	600 mg/m^2 I.V., days 1, 8, 29, and 36
	doxorubicin	Adriamycin	30 mg/m^2 I.V., days 1 and 29
	mitomycin	Mutamycin	10 mg/m^2 I.V., day 1
			Repeat cycle every 8 weeks.
FAM Non–small cell lung cancer	fluorouracil (5-FU)	Adrucil	600 mg/m^2 I.V., days 1, 8, 29, and 36
	doxorubicin	Adriamycin	30 mg/m^2 I.V., days 1 and 29
	mitomycin	Mutamycin	10 mg/m^2 I.V., day 1
			Repeat cycle every 8 weeks.
FAM Pancreatic cancer	fluorouracil (5-FU)	Adrucil	600 mg/m^2 I.V., days 1, 8, 29, and 36
	doxorubicin	Adriamycin	30 mg/m^2 I.V., days 1 and 29
	mitomycin	Mutamycin	10 mg/m^2 I.V., day 1
			Repeat cycle every 8 weeks.

(continued)

ACRONYM & INDICATION	DRUG		DOSAGE
	Generic name	**Trade name**	
FAME Gastric cancer	fluorouracil (5-FU)	Adrucil	350 mg/m² I.V., days 1 to 5 and 36 to 40
	doxorubicin	Adriamycin	40 mg/m² I.V., days 1 and 36
	semustine (methyl CCNU)		150 mg/m² P.O., day 1
			Repeat cycle every 10 weeks.
FCE Gastric cancer	fluorouracil (5-FU)	Adrucil	900 mg/m² by continuous I.V. infusion, days 1 to 5
	cisplatin	Platinol	20 mg/m² I.V., days 1 to 5
	etoposide (VP-16)	VePesid	90 mg/m² I.V., days 1, 3, and 5
			Repeat cycle every 21 days.
F-CL Colon cancer	fluorouracil (5-FU)	Adrucil	370 to 400 mg/m² I.V., days 1 to 5
	leucovorin calcium	Wellcovorin	200 mg/m² daily I.V., days 1 to 5, begun 15 minutes before fluorouracil infusion
			Repeat cycle every 21 days.
or	fluorouracil (5-FU)	Adrucil	100 mg/m² daily by continuous I.V. infusion, days 1 to 4
	leucovorin calcium	Wellcovorin	200 mg/m² daily I.V., days 1 to 4
			Repeat cycle every 28 days.
5 + 2 Leukemia— ANLL, consolidation	cytarabine (ara-C)	Cytosar-U	100 mg/m² I.V. q 12 hours for 6 days
	daunorubicin	Cerubidine	45 mg/m² I.V., days 1 and 2
FL Genitourinary cancer	flutamide	Eulexin	250 mg P.O. t.i.d.
	leuprolide acetate	Lupron	1 mg S.C. daily
or	flutamide	Eulexin	250 mg P.O. t.i.d.
	leuprolide acetate	Lupron Depot	7.5 mg I.M. q 28 days
			Repeat cycle every 28 days.

ACRONYM & INDICATION	DRUG		DOSAGE
	Generic name	Trade name	
FLe Colon cancer	levamisole	Ergamisol	50 mg P.O. t.i.d. for 3 days, repeated q 2 weeks for 1 year
	fluorouracil (5-FU)	Adrucil	450 mg/m² I.V. for 5 days; then, after a pause of 4 weeks, 450 mg/m² I.V. weekly for 48 weeks
FMS Pancreatic cancer	fluorouracil (5-FU)	Adrucil	600 mg/m² I.V., days 1, 8, 29, and 36
	mitomycin	Mutamycin	10 mg/m² I.V., day 1
	streptozocin	Zanosar	1 g/m² I.V., days 1, 8, 29, and 36 *Repeat cycle every 8 weeks.*
FMV Colon cancer	fluorouracil (5-FU)	Adrucil	10 mg/kg I.V., days 1 to 5
	semustine (methyl CCNU)		175 mg/m² P.O., day 1
	vincristine	Oncovin	1 mg/m² (2 mg maximum) I.V., day 1 *Repeat cycle every 35 days.*
FZ Genitourinary cancer	flutamide	Eulexin	250 P.O. t.i.d.
	goserelin acetate	Zoladex	3.6 mg implant S.C. q 4 weeks
HDAC Leukemia— ANLL, consolidation	cytarabine (ara-C)	Cytosar-U	3,000 mg/m² I.V. over 1 hour q 12 hours, days 1 to 6 *Cycle not repeated.*
HDMTX (high-dose methotrexate) Bony sarcoma	methotrexate	Folex	12 g/m² I.V. (20 g maximum)
	leucovorin calcium	Wellcovorin	15 to 25 mg I.V. or P.O. q 6 hours for 10 doses, beginning 24 hours after methotrexate dose (serum methotrexate levels must be monitored) *Repeat cycle every 4 to 16 weeks.*
Hexa-CAF Ovarian cancer, epithelial	altretamine	Hexalen	150 mg/m² P.O., days 1 to 14
	cyclophosphamide	Cytoxan	150 mg/m² P.O., days 1 to 14
	methotrexate	Folex	40 mg/m², days 1 and 8
	fluorouracil (5 FU)	Adrucil	600 mg/m² I.V., days 1 and 8 *Repeat cycle every 28 days.*

(continued)

ACRONYM & INDICATION	DRUG		DOSAGE
	Generic name	Trade name	
IMF Breast cancer	ifosfamide	Ifex	1.5 g/m² I.V., days 1 and 8
	mesna	Mesnex	Dosage is 20% of ifosfamide dose, given immediately before and at 4 and 8 hours after ifosfamide infusion
	methotrexate	Folex	40 mg/m² I.V., days 1 and 8
	fluorouracil (5-FU)	Adrucil	600 mg/m² I.V., days 1 and 8
			Repeat cycle every 28 days.
L-VAM Genitourinary cancer	leuprolide acetate	Lupron	1 mg S.C. daily
	vinblastine	Velban	1.5 mg/m² by continuous I.V. infusion, days 2 to 7
	doxorubicin	Adriamycin	50 mg/m² by 24-hour continuous I.V. infusion, day 1
	mitomycin	Mutamycin	10 mg/m² I.V., day 2
			Repeat VAM cycle every 28 days.
MACC Non-small cell lung cancer	methotrexate	Folex	30 to 40 mg/m² I.V., day 1
	doxorubicin	Adriamycin	30 to 40 mg/m² I.V., day 1
	cyclophospamide	Cytoxan	400 to 600 mg/m² I.V., day 1
	lomustine (CCNU)	CeeNU	30 to 40 mg/m² P.O., day 1
			Repeat cycle every 21 to 28 days.
MACOP-B Malignant lymphoma	methotrexate	Folex	100 mg/m² I.V., weeks 2, 6, and 10; then 300 mg/m² I.V. for 4 hours, weeks 2, 6, and 10
	leucovorin calcium	Wellcovorin	15 mg P.O. q 6 hours for 6 doses, beginning 24 hours after methotrexate
	doxorubicin	Adriamycin	50 mg/m² I.V., weeks 1, 3, 5, 7, 9, and 11
	cyclophospamide	Cytoxan	350 mg/m² I.V., weeks 1, 3, 5, 7, 9, and 11
	vincristine	Oncovin	1.4 mg/m² I.V. (2 mg maximum), weeks 2, 4, 8, 10, and 12
	bleomycin	Blenoxane	10 mg/m² I.V., weeks 4, 8, and 12
	prednisone	Deltasone	75 mg P.O. daily
			Repeat cycle as indicated in protocol.

ACRONYM & INDICATION	DRUG		DOSAGE
	Generic name	Trade name	
MAID Bony sarcoma	mesna	Mesnex	Uroprotection 1.5 g/m² by continuous I.V. infusion, days 1 to 4
	doxorubicin	Adriamycin	15 mg/m² by continuous I.V. infusion, days 1 to 3
	ifosfamide	Ifex	1.5 g/m² by continuous I.V. infusion, days 1 to 3
	dacarbazine	DTIC-Dome	250 mg/m² by continuous I.V. infusion, days 1 to 3
			Repeat cycle every 21 to 28 days.
MAP Head and neck cancer	mitomycin	Mutamycin	8 mg/m² I.V., day 1
	doxorubicin	Adriamycin	40 mg/m² I.V., day 1
	cisplatin	Platinol	60 mg/m² I.V., day 1
			Repeat cycle every 28 days.
m-BACOD Malignant lymphoma	bleomycin	Blenoxane	4 units/m² I.V., day 1
	doxorubicin	Adriamycin	45 mg/m² I.V., day 1
	cyclophosphamide	Cytoxan	600 mg/m² I.V., day 1
	vincristine	Oncovin	1 mg/m² I.V., day 1
	dexamethasone	Decadron	6 mg/m² I.V., days 1 to 5
	methotrexate	Folex	200 mg/m² I.V., days 8 and 15
	leucovorin calcium	Wellcovorin	10 mg/m² P.O. q 6 hours for 8 doses, beginning 24 hours after methotrexate dose
			Repeat cycle every 21 days.
MBC Head and neck cancer	methotrexate	Folex	40 mg/m² I.M. or I.V., days 1 and 15
	bleomycin	Blenoxane	10 units/m² I.M. or I.V., weekly
	cisplatin	Platinol	50 mg/m² I.V., day 1
			Repeat cycle every 21 days.
MC Leukemia— ANLL, consolidation	mitoxantrone	Novantrone	12 mg/m² I.V. daily, days 1 and 2
	cytarabine (ara-C)	Cytosar-U	100 mg/m² daily by continuous I.V. infusion, days 1 to 5
			Repeat cycle in 28 days.
MC Leukemia— ANLL, induction	mitoxantrone	Novantrone	12 mg/m² I.V., days 1 to 3 and 17 to 18
	cytarabine (ara-C)	Cytosar-U	100 mg/m² daily by continuous I.V. infusion, days 1 to 7 and 17 to 21

(continued)

ACRONYM & INDICATION	DRUG		DOSAGE
	Generic name	Trade name	
MF Head and neck cancer	methotrexate	Folex	125 to 150 mg/m² I.V., day 1
	fluorouracil (5-FU)	Adrucil	600 mg/m² I.V., beginning 1 hour after methotrexate dose
	leucovorin calcium	Wellcovorin	10 mg/m² I.V. or P.O. q 6 hours for 5 doses, beginning 24 hours after methotrexate dose
			Repeat cycle weekly.
MICE (ICE) Small-cell and non–small cell lung cancer	mesna	Mesnex	Dosage is 20% of ifosfamide doses given I.V. immediately before and at 4 and 8 hours after ifosfamide infusion
	ifosfamide	Ifex	2,000 mg/m² I.V., days 1 to 3
	carboplatin	Paraplatin	300 to 350 mg/m² I.V., day 1
	etoposide (VP-16)	VePesid	60 to 100 mg/m² I.V., days 1 to 3
MINE Malignant lymphoma	mesna	Mesnex	1.3 to 1.5 g/m² I.V., days 1 to 3 with ifosfamide; then 500 mg P.O. 4 hours after each ifosfamide dose
	ifosfamide	Ifex	1.3 to 1.5 g/m² I.V., days 1 to 3
	mitoxantrone	Novantrone	8 to 10 mg/m² I.V., day 1
	etoposide (VP-16)	VePesid	65 mg/m² I.V., days 1 to 3
			Repeat cycle every 28 days.
MM Leukemia — ALL, maintenance	mercaptopurine (6-MP)	Purinethol	50 mg/m² P.O. daily
	methotrexate	Folex	20 mg/m² P.O. or I.V. weekly
			Repeat cycle weekly.
MOF Colon cancer	fluorouracil (5-FU)	Adrucil	10 mg/kg/day I.V., days 1 to 5
	semustine (methyl CCNU)		175 mg/m² P.O., day 1
	vincristine	Oncovin	1 mg/m² (2 mg maximum) I.V., day 1
			Repeat cycle every 35 days.

ACRONYM & INDICATION	DRUG		DOSAGE
	Generic name	**Trade name**	
MOP Pediatric brain tumors	mechlorethamine (nitrogen mustard)	Mustargen	6 mg/m² I.V., days 1 and 8
	vincristine	Oncovin	1.4 mg/m² (2 mg maximum) I.V., days 1 and 8
	procarbazine	Matulane	100 mg/m² P.O., days 1 to 14 *Repeat cycle every 28 days.*
MOPP Hodgkin's disease	mechlorethamine (nitrogen mustard)	Mustargen	6 mg/m² I.V., days 1 and 8
	vincristine	Oncovin	1.4 mg/m² (2 mg maximum) I.V., days 1 and 8
	procarbazine	Matulane	100 mg/m² P.O., days 1 to 14
	prednisone	Deltasone	40 mg/m² P.O., days 1 to 14 *Repeat cycle every 28 days.*
MP Multiple myeloma	melphalan (L-phenylalanine mustard)	Alkeran	8 mg/m² P.O., days 1 to 4
	prednisone	Deltasone	40 mg/m² P.O., days 1 to 7 *Repeat cycle every 28 days.*
m-PFL Genitourinary cancer	methotrexate	Folex	60 mg/m², day 1
	cisplatin	Platinol	25 mg/m² by continuous I.V. infusion, days 2 to 6
	fluorouracil (5-FU)	Adrucil	800 mg/m² by continuous I.V. infusion, days 2 to 6
	leucovorin calcium	Wellcovorin	500 mg/m² by continuous I.V. infusion, days 2 to 6 *Repeat cycle every 28 days for 4 cycles.*
M-2 Multiple myeloma	vincristine	Oncovin	0.03 mg/kg (2 mg maximum) I.V., day 1
	carmustine	BiCNU	0.5 mg/kg I.V., day 1
	cyclophosphamide	Cytoxan	10 mg/kg I.V, day 1
	melphalan (L-phenylalanine mustard)	Alkeran	0.25 mg/kg P.O., days 1 to 4
	prednisone	Deltasone	1 mg/kg, days 1 to 7, then taper over next 14 days *Repeat cycle every 35 days.*

(continued)

ACRONYM & INDICATION	DRUG		DOSAGE
	Generic name	Trade name	
MV Leukemia— AML, induction	mitoxantrone	Novantrone	10 mg/m² I.V., days 1 to 5
	etoposide (VP-16)	VePesid	100 mg/m² I.V., days 1 to 3
			Repeat cycle if remission does not occur.
MVAC Genitourinary cancer	methotrexate	Folex	30 mg/m² I.V., days 1, 15, and 22
	vinblastine	Velban	3 mg/m² I.V., days 2, 15, and 22
	doxorubicin	Adriamycin	30 mg/m² I.V., day 2
	cisplatin	Platinol	70 mg/m² I.V., day 2
			Repeat cycle every 28 days.
MVP Non–small cell lung cancer	mitomycin	Mutamycin	8 mg/m² I.V., days 1 and 29, and 71
	vinblastine	Velban	4.5 mg/m² I.V., days 1, 5, 22, 29, and then q 2 weeks
	cisplatin	Platinol	120 mg/m² I.V., days 1 and 29, then q 6 weeks
MVPP Hodgkin's disease	mechlorethamine (nitrogen mustard)	Mustargen	6 mg/m² I.V., days 1 and 8
	vinblastine	Velban	6 mg/m² I.V., days 1 and 8
	procarbazine	Matulane	100 mg/m² P.O., days 1 to 14
	prednisone	Deltasone	40 mg/m² P.O., days 1 to 14
			Repeat cycle every 42 days for 6 cycles.
OPEN Malignant lymphoma	vincristine	Oncovin	2 mg I.V., day 1
	prednisone	Deltasone	100 mg P.O. daily for 5 days
	etoposide (VP-16)	VePesid	100 mg/m² I.V. daily for 3 days
	mitoxantrone	Novantrone	10 mg/m² I.V., day 1
PCV Pediatric brain tumors	procarbazine	Matulane	60 mg/m² P.O., days 18 to 21
	lomustine (CCNU)	CeeNU	110 mg/m² P.O., day 1
	vincristine	Oncovin	1.4 mg/m² (2 mg maximum), days 8 and 29
			Repeat cycle every 6 to 8 weeks.

ACRONYM & INDICATION	DRUG		DOSAGE
	Generic name	Trade name	
PFL Head and neck cancer	cisplatin	Platinol	25 mg/m² by continuous I.V. infusion, days 1 to 5
	5-fluorouracil (5-FU)	Adrucil	800 mg/m² by continuous I.V. infusion, days 2 to 5 or 6
	leucovorin calcium	Wellcovorin	500 mg/m² by continuous I.V. infusion, days 1 to 5 or 6
			Repeat cycle every 28 days for 2 to 3 cycles.
PFL Non-small cell lung cancer	cisplatin	Platinol	25 mg/m² by continuous I.V. infusion, days 1 to 5
	fluorouracil (5-FU)	Adrucil	800 mg/m² by continuous I.V. infusion, days 2 to 6
	leucovorin calcium	Wellcovorin	500 mg/m² by continuous I.V. infusion, days 1 to 6
			Repeat cycle every 28 days.
ProMACE Malignant lymphoma	prednisone	Deltasone	60 mg/m² P.O., days 1 to 14
	methotrexate	Folex	1.5 g/m² I.V., day 14
	leucovorin calcium	Wellcovorin	50 mg/m² I.V. q 6 hours for 5 doses, beginning 24 hours after methotrexate dose
	doxorubicin	Adriamycin	25 mg/m² I.V., days 1 and 8
	cyclophosphamide	Cytoxan	650 mg/m² I.V., days 1 and 8
	etoposide (VP-16)	VePesid	120 mg/m² I.V., days 1 and 8
			Repeat cycle every 28 days; MOPP therapy to begin after the required number of ProMACE cycles (based on tumor response) are completed.

(continued)

ACRONYM & INDICATION	DRUG		DOSAGE
	Generic name	**Trade name**	
ProMACE/ cytaBOM Malignant lymphoma	cyclophosphamide	Cytoxan	650 mg/m^2 I.V., day 1
	doxorubicin	Adriamycin	25 mg/m^2 I.V., day 1
	etoposide (VP-16)	VePesid	120 mg/m^2 I.V., day 1
	prednisone	Deltasone	60 mg/m^2 P.O., days 1 to 14
	cytarabine (ara-C)	Cytosar-U	300 mg/m^2 I.V., day 8
	bleomycin	Blenoxane	5 mg/m^2 I.V., day 8
	vincristine	Oncovin	1.4 mg/m^2 I.V., day 8
	methotrexate	Folex	120 mg/m^2 I.V., day 8
	leucovorin calcium	Wellcovorin	25 mg/m^2 P.O. q 6 hours for 4 doses
			Repeat cycle every 28 days.
(pulse) VAC Soft-tissue sarcoma	vincristine	Oncovin	1.5 g/m^2 (2 mg maximum) I.V., day 1 or weekly, starting on day 1
	dactinomycin (actinomycin D)	Cosmegen	0.4 mg/m^2 I.V., day 1
	cyclophosphamide	Cytoxan	1,000 mg/kg I.V. or P.O., day 1
			Repeat cycle every 3 to 4 weeks.
7 + 3 (A + D) Leukemia— AML, induction	cytarabine (ara-C)	Cytosar-U	100 or 200 mg/m^2 by continuous I.V. infusion, days 1 to 7
	daunorubicin	Cerubidine	45 mg/m^2 I.V., days 1 to 3
TC Leukemia— ANLL, maintenance	thioguanine (6-TG)	Lanvis	40 mg/m^2 P.O. q 12 hours for 8 doses, days 1 to 4
	cytarabine (ara-C)	Cytosar-U	60 mg/m^2 S.C., day 5
			Repeat cycle weekly.

ACRONYM & INDICATION	DRUG		DOSAGE
	Generic name	**Trade name**	
T-2 Ewing's sarcoma	*Cycle #1* *Month 1* dactinomycin	Cosmegen	0.45mg/m² daily I.V., days 1 through 5
	doxorubicin	Adriamycin	20 mg/m² daily I.V., days 20 through 22 Radiation days 1 through 21, then 2 weeks' rest period
	Month 2 doxorubicin	Adriamycin	20 mg/m² daily I.V., days 8 through 10
	vincristine	Oncovin	1.5 to 2 mg/m² I.V., day 24 (maximum dose 2 mg)
	cyclophosphamide	Cytoxan	1,200 mg/m² I.V., day 24 Radiation days 8 through 28
	Month 3 vincristine	Oncovin	1.5 to 2 mg/m² I.V. daily, days 3, 9, and 15
	cyclophosphamide	Cytoxan	1,200 mg/m² I.V., day 9
	Cycle #2 Repeat cycle #1 without radiation		
	Cycle #3 *Month 1* dactinomycin	Cosmegen	0.45 mg/m² daily I.V., days 1 through 5
	doxorubicin	Adriamycin	20 mg/m² daily I.V., days 20 through 22
	Month 2 vincristine	Oncovin	1.5 to 2 mg/m² I.V., days 8, 15, 22, and 28
	cyclophosphamide	Cytoxan	1,200 mg/m² I.V., days 8 and 22
	Month 3 No drugs for 28 days		
	Cycle #4 Repeat cycle #3		
VA Wilms' tumor	vincristine	Oncovin	1.5 mg/m² (2 mg maximum) weekly
	dactinomycin (actinomycin D)	Cosmegen	0.4 mg/m² q 2 weeks
			Repeat cycle as indicated in protocol.

(continued)

ACRONYM & INDICATION	DRUG		DOSAGE
	Generic name	Trade name	
VAB Genitourinary cancer	vinblastine	Velban	4 mg/m² I.V., day 1
	dactinomycin (actinomycin D)	Cosmegen	1 mg/m² I.V., day 1
	bleomycin	Blenoxane	30 units I.V. push, then 20 units/m² by continuous I.V. infusion, days 1 to 3
	cisplatin	Platinol	120 mg/m² I.V., day 4
	cyclophosphamide	Cytoxan	600 mg/m² I.V., day 1 *Repeat cycle every 21 days.*
VAC Small-cell lung cancer	vincristine	Oncovin	2 mg I.V., day 1
	doxorubicin	Adriamycin	50 mg/m² I.V., day 1
	cyclophosphamide	Cytoxan	750 mg/m² I.V., day 1 *Repeat cycle every 21 days for 4 cycles.*
VAC Ovarian cancer, germ-cell	vincristine	Oncovin	1.2 to 1.5 mg/m² (2 mg maximum) I.V. weekly for 10 to 12 weeks, or q 2 weeks for 12 doses
	dactinomycin (actinomycin D)	Cosmegen	0.3 to 0.4 mg/m² I.V., days 1 to 5
	cyclophosphamide	Cytoxan	150 mg/m² I.V., days 1 to 5 *Repeat cycle every 28 days.*
VAC Wilms' tumor	vincristine	Oncovin	2 mg/m² (2 mg maximum) weekly for 10 to 12 weeks
	dactinomycin (actinomycin D)	Cosmegen	0.015 g/m² (0.5 mg maximum), days 1 to 5 q 3 months for 5 to 6 courses
	cyclophosphamide	Cytoxan	2.5 mg/kg daily P.O. for 2 years
VAD Multiple myeloma	vincristine	Oncovin	0.4 mg by continuous I.V. infusion, days 1 to 4
	doxorubicin	Adriamycin	9 to 10 mg/m² daily by continuous I.V. infusion, days 1 to 4
	dexamethasone	Decadron	40 mg P.O. on days 1 to 4, 9 to 12, and 17 to 20 *Repeat cycle every 25 to 35 days.*
VAP (VP + A) Leukemia—pediatric ALL, induction	vincristine	Oncovin	1.5 to 2 mg/m² (2 mg maximum) I.V. weekly for 4 weeks
	asparaginase	Elspar	10,000 units I.V., days 1 and 8 (other doses include 6,000 units/m² I.M. for 3 days/week or 25,000 units/m²)
	prednisone	Deltasone	40 mg/m² P.O., days 1 to 28, then taper over 7 days

ACRONYM & INDICATION	DRUG		DOSAGE
	Generic name	Trade name	
VATH Breast cancer	vinblastine	Velban	4.5 mg/m² I.V., day 1
	doxorubicin	Adriamycin	45 mg/m² I.V., day 1
	thiotepa	Thiotepa	12 mg/m² I.V., day 1
	fluoxymesterone	Halotestin	30 mg P.O. daily (through each course) *Repeat cycle every 21 days.*
VB Genitourinary cancer	vinblastine	Velban	3 to 4 mg/m² I.V., day 1
	methotrexate	Folex	30 to 40 mg/m² I.V., day 1 *Repeat cycle weekly.*
VBAP Multiple myeloma	vincristine	Oncovin	1 mg I.V., day 1
	carmustine	BiCNU	30 mg/m² I.V., day 1
	doxorubicin	Adriamycin	30 mg/m² I.V., day 1
	prednisone	Deltasone	100 mg P.O., days 1 to 4 *Repeat cycle every 21 days.*
VBC Malignant melanoma	vinblastine	Velban	6 mg/m² I.V., days 1 and 2
	bleomycin	Blenoxane	15 units/m² daily by continuous I.V. infusion, days 1 to 5
	cisplatin	Platinol	50 mg/m² I.V., day 5 *Repeat cycle every 28 days.*
VBP Genitourinary cancer	vinblastine	Velban	6 mg/m² I.V., days 1 and 2
	bleomycin	Blenoxane	30 units I.V. weekly
	cisplatin	Platinol	20 mg/m² I.V., days 1 to 5 *Repeat cycle every 21 to 28 days.*
VC Small-cell lung cancer	etoposide (VP-16)	VePesid	100 to 200 mg/m² I.V., days 1 to 3
	carboplatin	Paraplatin	50 to 125 mg/m² I.V., days 1 to 3 *Repeat cycle every 28 days.*
VCAP Multiple myeloma	vincristine	Oncovin	1 mg I.V., day 1
	cyclophosphamide	Cytoxan	100 mg/m² P.O., days 1 to 4
	doxorubicin	Adriamycin	25 mg/m² I.V., day 2
	prednisone	Deltasone	60 mg/m² P.O., days 1 to 4 *Repeat cycle every 28 days.*

(continued)

ACRONYM & INDICATION	DRUG		DOSAGE
	Generic name	**Trade name**	
VDP Malignant melanoma	vinblastine	Velban	5 mg/m² I.V., days 1 and 2
	dacarbazine	DTIC-Dome	150 mg/m² I.V., days 1 to 5
	cisplatin	Platinol	75 mg/m² I.V., day 5
			Repeat cycle every 21 to 28 days.
VIP Genitourinary cancer	vinblastine	Velban	0.11 mg/kg I.V., days 1 and 2
	ifosfamide	Ifex	1.2 g/m² I.V. over 30 minutes, days 1 to 5
	cisplatin	Platinol	20 mg/m² over 1 hour, days 1 to 5
	mesna	Mesnex	400 mg I.V., 15 minutes before ifosfamide, then 1.2 g by continuous I.V. infusion, days 1 to 5
			Repeat cycle every 21 days for 4 cycles.
or	etoposide (VP-16)	VePesid	75 mg/m² I.V., days 1 to 5
	ifosfamide	Ifex	1.2 g/m² I.V., days 1 to 5
	cisplatin	Platinol	20 mg/m², days 1 to 5
	mesna	Mesnex	400 mg I.V., 15 minutes before ifosfamide, then 1.2 g by continuous I.V. infusion, days 1 to 5
			Repeat cycle every 21 days for 4 cycles.

ICD-9-CM Classification of Neoplastic Disorders

The *International Classification of Diseases* 9th revision, *Clinical Modification (ICD-9-CM)* standardizes the classification of neoplastic diseases. Broadly speaking, this coding system is divided into these numeric groups:
• **140 to 195:** malignant neoplasms, stated or presumed to be primary, at specified sites, except for lymphatic and hematopoietic tissue
• **196 to 198:** malignant neoplasms, stated or presumed to be secondary, at specified sites
• **199:** malignant neoplasms, without specified site
• **200 to 208:** malignant neoplasms, stated or presumed to be primary, of lymphatic and hematopoietic tissue
• **210 to 229:** benign neoplasms
• **230 to 234:** carcinoma in situ
• **235 to 238:** neoplasms of uncertain behavior
• **239:** unspecified neoplasms.

In this classification system, you'll see these abbreviations:
NEC = not elsewhere classified
NOS = not otherwise specified.

MALIGNANT NEOPLASM OF LIP, ORAL CAVITY, AND PHARYNX (140 to 149)
Excludes carcinoma in situ (230.0)

140 Malignant neoplasm of lip
Excludes skin of lip (173.0)
  140.0 Upper lip, vermilion border
  NOS
  external
  lipstick area
  140.1 Lower lip, vermilion border
  NOS
  external
  lipstick area
  140.3 Upper lip, inner aspect
  buccal aspect
  frenulum
  mucosa
  oral aspect
  140.4 Lower lip, inner aspect
  buccal aspect
  frenulum

mucosa
oral aspect
  140.5 Lip, unspecified, inner aspect (not specified as upper or lower)
  buccal aspect
  frenulum
  mucosa
  oral aspect
  140.6 Commissure of lip
  Labial commissure
  140.8 Other sites of lip
  Malignant neoplasm of contiguous or overlapping sites of lip whose point of origin cannot be determined
  140.9 Lip, unspecified, vermilion border (not specified as upper or lower)
  NOS
  external
  lipstick area

141 Malignant neoplasm of tongue
  141.0 Base of tongue
  Dorsal surface of base of tongue
  Fixed part of tongue NOS
  141.1 Dorsal surface of tongue
  Anterior two-thirds of tongue, dorsal surface
  Dorsal tongue NOS
  Midline of tongue
  Excludes dorsal surface of base of tongue (141.0)
  141.2 Tip and lateral border of tongue
  141.3 Ventral surface of tongue
  Anterior two-thirds of tongue, ventral surface
  Frenulum linguae
  141.4 Anterior two-thirds of tongue, part unspecified
  Mobile part of tongue NOS
  141.5 Junctional zone
  Border of tongue at junction of fixed and mobile parts at insertion of anterior tonsillar pillar
  141.6 Lingual tonsil
  141.8 Other sites of tongue
  Malignant neoplasm of contiguous or overlapping sites of tongue whose point of origin cannot be determined

141.9 Tongue, unspecified
Tongue NOS

142 Malignant neoplasm of major salivary glands

Includes salivary ducts
Excludes malignant neoplasm of minor salivary glands:
NOS (145.9)
buccal mucosa (145.0)
soft palate (145.3)
tongue (141.0 to 141.9)
tonsil, palatine (146.0)
142.0 Parotid gland
142.1 Submandibular gland
Submaxillary gland
142.2 Sublingual gland
142.8 Other major salivary glands
Malignant neoplasm of contiguous or overlapping sites of salivary glands and ducts whose point of origin cannot be determined
142.9 Salivary gland, unspecified
Salivary gland (major) NOS

143 Malignant neoplasm of gum

Includes:
alveolar (ridge) mucosa
gingiva (alveolar, marginal)
interdental papillae
Excludes malignant odontogenic neoplasms (170.0 to 170.1)
143.0 Upper gum
143.1 Lower gum
143.8 Other sites of gum
Malignant neoplasm of contiguous or overlapping sites of gum whose point of origin cannot be determined
143.9 Gum, unspecified

144 Malignant neoplasm of floor of mouth

144.0 Anterior portion
Anterior to the premolar-canine junction
144.1 Lateral portion
144.8 Other sites of floor of mouth
Malignant neoplasm of contiguous or overlapping sites of floor of mouth whose point of origin cannot be determined
144.9 Floor of mouth, part unspecified

145 Malignant neoplasm of other and unspecified parts of mouth

Excludes mucosa of lips (140.0 to 140.9)
145.0 Cheek mucosa
Buccal mucosa
Cheek, inner aspect
145.1 Vestibule of mouth
Buccal sulcus (upper, lower)
Labial sulcus (upper, lower)
145.2 Hard palate
145.3 Soft palate
Excludes nasopharyngeal (posterior, superior) surface of soft palate (147.3)
145.4 Uvula
145.5 Palate, unspecified
Junction of hard and soft palate
Roof of mouth
145.6 Retromolar area
145.8 Other specified parts of mouth
Malignant neoplasm of contiguous or overlapping sites of mouth whose point of origin cannot be determined
145.9 Mouth, unspecified
Buccal cavity NOS
Minor salivary gland, unspecified site
Oral cavity NOS

146 Malignant neoplasm of oropharynx

146.0 Tonsil
NOS
faucial
palatine
Excludes lingual tonsil (141.6), pharyngeal tonsil (147.1)
146.1 Tonsillar fossa
146.2 Tonsillar pillars (anterior, posterior)
Faucial pillar
Glossopalatine fold
Palatoglossal arch
Palatopharyngeal arch
146.3 Vallecula
Anterior and medial surface of the pharyngoepiglottic fold
146.4 Anterior aspect of epiglottis
Epiglottis, free border (margin)
Glossoepiglottic fold(s)
Excludes epiglottis NOS (161.1), suprahyoid portion (161.1)
146.5 Junctional region
Junction of the free margin of the epiglottis, the aryepiglottic fold, and the pharyngoepiglottic fold
146.6 Lateral wall of oropharynx
146.7 Posterior wall of oropharynx
146.8 Other specified sites of oropharynx
Branchial cleft

Malignant neoplasm of contiguous or overlapping sites of oropharynx whose point of origin cannot be determined
146.9 Oropharynx, unspecified

147 Malignant neoplasm of nasopharynx
147.0 Superior wall
Roof of nasopharynx
147.1 Posterior wall
Adenoid
Pharyngeal tonsil
147.2 Lateral wall
Fossa of Rosenmüller
Opening of auditory tube
Pharyngeal recess
147.3 Anterior wall
Floor of nasopharynx
Nasopharyngeal (posterior, superior) surface of soft palate
Posterior margin of nasal septum and choanae
147.8 Other specified sites of nasopharynx
Malignant neoplasm of contiguous or overlapping sites of nasopharynx whose point of origin cannot be determined
147.9 Nasopharynx, unspecified
Nasopharyngeal wall NOS

148 Malignant neoplasm of hypopharynx
148.0 Postcricoid region
148.1 Pyriform sinus
Pyriform fossa
148.2 Aryepiglottic fold, hypopharyngeal aspect
Aryepiglottic fold or interarytenoid fold:
NOS
marginal zone
Excludes aryepiglottic fold or interarytenoid fold, laryngeal aspect (161.1)
148.3 Posterior hypopharyngeal wall
148.8 Other specified sites of hypopharynx
Malignant neoplasm of contiguous or overlapping sites of hypopharynx whose point of origin cannot be determined
148.9 Hypopharynx, unspecified
Hypopharyngeal wall NOS
Hypopharynx NOS

149 Malignant neoplasm of other and ill-defined sites with the lip, oral cavity, and pharynx
149.0 Pharynx, unspecified

149.1 Waldeyer's ring
149.8 Other
Malignant neoplasms of lip, oral cavity, and pharynx whose point of origin cannot be assigned to any one of the categories 140 to 148
Excludes "book leaf" neoplasm on ventral surface of tongue and floor of mouth (145.8)
149.9 Ill-defined

MALIGNANT NEOPLASM OF DIGESTIVE ORGANS AND PERITONEUM (150 to 159)
Excludes carcinoma in situ (230.1 to 230.9)

150 Malignant neoplasm of esophagus
150.0 Cervical esophagus
150.1 Thoracic esophagus
150.2 Abdominal esophagus
Excludes:
adenocarcinoma (151.0)
cardioesophageal junction (151.0)
150.3 Upper third of esophagus
Proximal third of esophagus
150.4 Middle third of esophagus
150.5 Lower third of esophagus
Distal third of esophagus
Excludes:
adenocarcinoma (151.0)
cardioesophageal junction (151.0)
150.8 Other specified part
Malignant neoplasm of contiguous or overlapping sites of esophagus whose point of origin cannot be determined
150.9 Esophagus, unspecified

151 Malignant neoplasm of stomach
151.0 Cardia
Cardiac orifice
Cardioesophageal junction
Excludes squamous cell carcinoma (150.2, 150.5)
151.1 Pylorus
Prepylorus
Pyloric canal
151.2 Pyloric antrum
Antrum of stomach NOS
151.3 Fundus of stomach
151.4 Body of stomach
151.5 Lesser curvature, unspecified
Lesser curvature, not classifiable to 151.1 to 151.4

151.6 Greater curvature, unspecified
Greater curvature, not classifiable to
151.0 to 151.4
151.8 Other specified sites of stomach
Anterior wall, not classifiable to 151.0 to
151.4
Posterior wall, not classifiable to 151.0 to
151.4
Malignant neoplasm of contiguous or
overlapping sites of stomach whose
point of origin cannot be determined
151.9 Stomach, unspecified
Carcinoma ventriculi
Gastric cancer

**152 Malignant neoplasm of small intestine,
including duodenum**
152.0 Duodenum
152.1 Jejunum
152.2 Ileum
Excludes ileocecal valve (153.4)
152.3 Meckel's diverticulum
152.8 Other specified sites of small intestine
Duodenojejunal junction
Malignant neoplasm of contiguous or
overlapping sites of small intestine
whose point of origin cannot be determined
152.9 Small intestine, unspecified

153 Malignant neoplasm of colon
153.0 Hepatic flexure
153.1 Transverse colon
153.2 Descending colon
153.3 Sigmoid colon
Left colon
Sigmoid (flexure)
Excludes rectosigmoid junction (154.0)
153.4 Cecum
Ileocecal valve
153.5 Appendix
153.6 Ascending colon
153.7 Splenic flexure
153.8 Other specified sites of large intestine
Malignant neoplasm of contiguous or
overlapping sites of colon whose
point of origin cannot be determined
Excludes:
ileocecal valve (153.4)
rectosigmoid junction (154.0)
153.9 Colon, unspecified
Large intestine NOS

**154 Malignant neoplasm of rectum, rectosig-
moid junction, and anus**
154.0 Rectosigmoid junction
Colon with rectum
Rectosigmoid (colon)
154.1 Rectum
Rectal ampulla
154.2 Anal canal
Anal sphincter
Excludes skin of anus (172.5, 173.5)
154.3 Anus, unspecified
Excludes anus:
margin (172.5, 173.5)
skin (172.5, 173.5)
perianal skin (172.5, 173.5)
154.8 Other
Anorectum
Cloacogenic zone
Malignant neoplasm of contiguous or
overlapping sites of rectum, rectosigmoid junction, and anus whose
point of origin cannot be determined

**155 Malignant neoplasm of liver and intra-
hepatic bile ducts**
155.0 Liver, primary
Carcinoma:
liver, specified as primary
hepatocellular
liver cell
Hepatoblastoma
155.1 Intrahepatic bile ducts
Canaliculi biliferi
Interlobular:
bile ducts
biliary canals
Intrahepatic:
biliary passages
canaliculi
gall duct
Excludes hepatic duct (156.1)
155.2 Liver not specified as primary or
secondary

**156 Malignant neoplasm of gallbladder and
extrahepatic bile ducts**
156.0 Gallbladder
156.1 Extrahepatic bile ducts
Biliary duct or passage NOS
Common bile duct
Cystic duct
Hepatic duct
Sphincter of Oddi

156.2 Ampulla of Vater
156.8 Other specified sites of gallbladder and extrahepatic bile ducts
Malignant neoplasm of contiguous or overlapping sites of gallbladder and extrahepatic bile ducts whose point of origin cannot be determined
156.9 Biliary tract, part unspecified
Malignant neoplasm involving both intrahepatic and extrahepatic bile ducts

157 Malignant neoplasm of pancreas
157.0 Head of pancreas
157.1 Body of pancreas
157.2 Tail of pancreas
157.3 Pancreatic duct
Duct of:
Santorini
Wirsung
157.4 Islets of Langerhans
Islets of Langerhans, any part of pancreas
157.8 Other specified sites of pancreas
Ectopic pancreatic tissue
Malignant neoplasm of contiguous or overlapping sites of pancreas whose point of origin cannot be determined
157.9 Pancreas, part unspecified

158 Malignant neoplasm of retroperitoneum and peritoneum
158.0 Retroperitoneum
Periadrenal tissue
Perinephric tissue
Perirenal tissue
Retrocecal tissue
158.8 Specified parts of peritoneum
Cul-de-sac (of Douglas)
Mesentery
Mesocolon
Omentum
Malignant neoplasm of contiguous or overlapping sites of retroperitoneum and peritoneum whose point of origin cannot be determined
Peritoneum:
parietal
pelvic
Rectouterine pouch
158.9 Peritoneum, unspecified

159 Malignant neoplasm of other and ill-defined sites within the digestive organs and peritoneum

159.0 Intestinal tract, part unspecified
Intestinal NOS
159.1 Spleen, not elsewhere classified
Angiosarcoma of spleen
Fibrosarcoma of spleen
Excludes:
Hodgkin's disease (201.0 to 201.9)
lymphosarcoma (200.1)
reticulosarcoma (200.0)
159.8 Other sites of digestive system and intra-abdominal organs
Malignant neoplasm of digestive organs and peritoneum whose point of origin cannot be assigned to any one of the categories 150 to 158
Excludes:
anus and rectum (154.8)
cardioesophageal junction (151.0)
colon and rectum (154.0)
159.9 Ill-defined
Alimentary canal or tract NOS
GI tract NOS
Excludes:
abdominal NOS (195.2)
intra-abdominal NOS (195.2)

MALIGNANT NEOPLASM OF RESPIRATORY AND INTRATHORACIC ORGANS (160 to 165)
Excludes carcinoma in situ (213.0 to 231.9)

160 Malignant neoplasm of nasal cavities, middle ear, and accessory sinuses
160.0 Nasal cavities
Cartilage of nose
Conchae, nasal
Internal nose
Septum of nose
Vestibule of nose
Excludes:
nasal bone (170.0)
nose NOS (195.0)
olfactory bulb (192.0)
posterior margin of septum and choanae (147.3)
skin of nose (172.3, 173.3)
turbinates (170.0)
160.1 Auditory tube, middle ear, and mastoid air cells
Antrum tympanicum
Eustachian tube
Tympanic cavity

Excludes:
  auditory canal (external) (172.2, 173.2)
  bone of ear (meatus) (170.0)
  cartilage of ear (171.0)
  ear (external, skin) (172.2, 173.2)
160.2 Maxillary sinus
  Antrum (of Highmore, maxillary)
160.3 Ethmoidal sinus
160.4 Frontal sinus
160.5 Sphenoidal sinus
160.8 Other
  Malignant neoplasm of contiguous or
    overlapping sites of nasal cavities,
    middle ear, and accessory sinuses
    whose point of origin cannot be de-
    termined
160.9 Accessory sinus, unspecified

161 Malignant neoplasm of larynx
161.0 Glottis
  Intrinsic larynx
  Laryngeal
  Commissure (anterior, posterior)
  True vocal cord
  Vocal cord NOS
161.1 Supraglottis
  Aryepiglottic fold or interarytenoid fold,
    laryngeal aspect
  Epiglottis (suprahyoid portion) NOS
  Extrinsic larynx
  False vocal cords
  Posterior (laryngeal) surface of epiglot-
    tis
  Ventricular bands
  Excludes:
    anterior aspect of epiglottis (146.4)
    aryepiglottic fold or interarytenoid
      fold:
      NOS (148.2)
      hypopharyngeal aspect (148.2)
      marginal zone (148.2)
161.2 Subglottis
161.3 Laryngeal cartilages
  Cartilage:
    arytenoid
    cricoid
    cuneiform
    thyroid
161.8 Other specified sites of larynx
  Malignant neoplasm of contiguous or
    overlapping sites of larynx whose
    point of origin cannot be determined
161.9 Larynx, unspecified

**162 Malignant neoplasm of trachea, bron-
chus, and lung**
162.0 Trachea
  Cartilage of trachea
  Mucosa of trachea
162.2 Main bronchus
  Carina
  Hilus of lung
162.3 Upper lobe, bronchus or lung
162.4 Middle lobe, bronchus or lung
162.5 Lower lobe, bronchus or lung
162.8 Other parts of bronchus or lung
  Malignant neoplasm of contiguous or
    overlapping sites of bronchus or
    lung whose point of origin cannot be
    determined
162.9 Bronchus and lung, unspecified

163 Malignant neoplasm of pleura
163.0 Parietal pleura
163.1 Visceral pleura
163.8 Other specified sites of pleura
  Malignant neoplasm of contiguous or
    overlapping sites of pleura whose
    point of origin cannot be determined
163.9 Pleura, unspecified

**164 Malignant neoplasm of thymus, heart,
and mediastinum**
164.0 Thymus
164.1 Heart
  Endocardium
  Epicardium
  Myocardium
  Pericardium
  Excludes great vessels (171.4)
164.2 Anterior mediastinum
164.3 Posterior mediastinum
164.8 Other
  Malignant neoplasm of contiguous or
    overlapping sites of thymus, heart,
    and mediastinum whose point of ori-
    gin cannot be determined
164.9 Mediastinum, part unspecified

**165 Malignant neoplasm of other and ill-
defined sites within the respiratory system and intrathoracic organs**
165.0 Upper respiratory tract, part unspecified
165.8 Other
  Malignant neoplasm of respiratory and

intrathoracic organs whose point of origin cannot be assigned to any one of the categories 160 to 164

165.9 Ill-defined sites within the respiratory system
Respiratory tract NOS
Excludes:
  intrathoracic NOS (195.1)
  thoracic NOS (195.1)

MALIGNANT NEOPLASM OF BONE, CONNECTIVE TISSUE, SKIN, AND BREAST (170 to 175)

Excludes carcinoma in situ:
  breast (233.0)
  skin (232.0 to 232.9)

170 Malignant neoplasm of bone and articular cartilage
Includes:
  cartilage (articular, joint)
  periosteum
Excludes:
  bone marrow NOS (202.9)
  cartilage:
    ear (171.0)
    eyelid (171.0)
    larynx (161.3)
    nose (160.0)
  synovia (171.0 to 171.9)

170.0 Bones of skull and face, except mandible
Bone:
  ethmoid
  frontal
  malar
  nasal
  occipital
  orbital
  parietal
  sphenoid
  temporal
  zygomatic
Maxilla (superior)
Turbinate
Upper jaw bone
Vomer
Excludes:
  carcinoma, any type except intraosseous or odontogenic:
    maxilla, maxillary (sinus) (160.2)
    upper jaw bone (143.0)
  jaw bone (lower) (170.1)

170.1 Mandible
Inferior maxilla
Jaw bone NOS
Lower jaw bone
Excludes carcinoma, any type except intraosseous or odontogenic:
  jaw bone NOS (143.9)
    lower (143.1)
  upper jaw bone (170.0)

170.2 Vertebral column, excluding sacrum and coccyx
Spinal column
Spine
Vertebra
Excludes sacrum and coccyx (170.6)

170.3 Ribs, sternum, and clavicle
Costal cartilage
Costovertebral joint
Xiphoid process

170.4 Scapula and long bones of upper limb
Acromion
Bones of upper limb NOS
Humerus
Radius
Ulna

170.5 Short bones of upper limb
Carpal
Cuneiform, wrist
Metacarpal
Navicular, of hand
Phalanges of hand
Pisiform
Scaphoid (of hand)
Semilunar or lunate
Trapezium
Trapezoid
Unciform

170.6 Pelvic bones, sacrum, and coccyx
Coccygeal vertebra
Ilium
Ischium
Pubic bone
Sacral vertebra

170.7 Long bones of lower limb
Bones of lower limb NOS
Femur
Fibula
Tibia

170.8 Short bones of lower limb
Astragalus (talus)
Calcaneus
Cuboid
Cuneiform, ankle

Metatarsal
Navicular (of ankle)
Patella
Phalanges of foot
Tarsal
170.9 Bone and articular cartilage, site
   unspecified

**171 Malignant neoplasm of connective and
   other soft tissue**
Includes:
   blood vessel
   bursa
   fascia
   fat
   ligament, except uterine
   muscle
   peripheral, sympathetic, and parasympa-
      thetic nerves and ganglia
   synovia
   tendon (sheath)
Excludes:
   cartilage of:
      articular (170.0 to 170.9)
      larynx (161.3)
      nose (160.0)
   connective tissue:
      breast (174.0 to 175.9)
      internal organs — code to malignant neo-
         plasm of the site (for example,
         leiomyosarcoma of stomach, 151.9)
   heart (164.1)
   uterine ligament (183.4)
171.0 Head, face, and neck
   Cartilage of:
      ear
      eyelid
171.2 Upper limb, including shoulder
   Arm
   Finger
   Forearm
   Hand
171.3 Lower limb, including hip
   Foot
   Leg
   Popliteal space
   Thigh
   Toe
171.4 Thorax
   Axilla
   Diaphragm
   Great vessels
   Excludes:
      heart (164.1)

   mediastinum (164.2 to 164.9)
   thymus (164.0)
171.5 Abdomen
   Abdominal wall
   Hypochondrium
   Excludes:
      peritoneum (158.8)
      retroperitoneum (158.0)
171.6 Pelvis
   Buttock
   Groin
   Inguinal region
   Perineum
   Excludes:
      pelvic peritoneum (158.8)
      retroperitoneum (158.0)
      uterine ligament, any (183.3 to 183.5)
171.7 Trunk, unspecified
   Back NOS
   Flank NOS
171.8 Other specified sites of connective
   and other soft tissue
   Malignant neoplasm of contiguous or
      overlapping sites of connective tis-
      sue whose point of origin cannot be
      determined
171.9 Connective and other soft tissue,
   site unspecified

172 Malignant melanoma of skin
Includes:
   melanocarcinoma
   melanoma (skin) NOS
Excludes:
   skin of genital organs (184.0 to 184.9,
      187.1 to 187.9)
   sites other than skin — code to malignant
      neoplasm of the site
172.0 Lip
   Excludes vermilion border of lip (140.0 to
      140.1, 140.9)
172.1 Eyelid, including canthus
172.2 Ear and external auditory canal
   Auricle (ear)
   Auricular canal, external
   External (acoustic) meatus
   Pinna
172.3 Other and unspecified parts of face
   Cheek (external)
   Chin
   Eyebrow
   Forehead
   Nose, external
   Temple
172.4 Scalp and neck

172.5 Trunk, except scrotum
Axilla
Breast
Buttock
Groin
Perianal skin
Perineum
Umbilicus
Excludes:
anal canal (154.2)
anus NOS (154.3)
scrotum (187.7)
172.6 Upper limb, including shoulder
Arm
Finger
Forearm
Hand
172.7 Lower limb, including hip
Ankle
Foot
Heel
Knee
Leg
Popliteal area
Thigh
Toe
172.8 Other specified sites of skin
Malignant melanoma of contiguous or
overlapping sites of skin whose
point of origin cannot be determined
172.9 Melanoma of skin, site unspecified

173 Other malignant neoplasm of skin
Includes malignant neoplasm of:
sebaceous glands
sudoriferous, sudoriparous glands
sweat glands
Excludes:
Kaposi's sarcoma (176.0 to 176.9)
malignant melanoma of skin (172.0 to
172.9)
skin of genital organs (184.0 to 184.9,
187.1 to 187.9)
173.0 Skin of lip
Excludes vermilion border of lip (140.0 to
140.1, 140.9)
173.1 Eyelid, including canthus
Excludes cartilage of eyelid (171.0)
173.2 Skin of ear and external auditory
canal
Auricle (ear)
Auricular canal, external
External meatus

Pinna
Excludes cartilage of ear (171.0)
173.3 Skin of other and unspecified parts
of face
Cheek, external
Chin
Eyebrow
Forehead
Nose, external
Temple
173.4 Scalp and skin of neck
173.5 Skin of trunk, except scrotum
Axillary fold
Perianal skin
Skin of:
abdominal wall
anus
back
breast
buttock
chest wall
groin
perineum
Umbilicus
Excludes:
anal canal (154.2)
anus NOS (154.3)
skin of scrotum (187.7)
173.6 Skin of upper limb, including shoul-
der
Arm
Finger
Forearm
Hand
173.7 Skin of lower limb, including hip
Ankle
Foot
Heel
Knee
Leg
Popliteal area
Thigh
Toe
173.8 Other specified sites of skin
Malignant neoplasm of contiguous or
overlapping sites of skin whose
point of origin cannot be determined
173.9 Skin, site unspecified

174 Malignant neoplasm of female breast
Includes:
breast (female):
connective tissue
soft parts

Paget's disease of:
  breast
  nipple
Excludes skin of breast (172.5, 173.5)
  174.0 Nipple and areola
  174.1 Central portion
  174.2 Upper-inner quadrant
  174.3 Lower-inner quadrant
  174.4 Upper-outer quadrant
  174.5 Lower-outer quadrant
  174.6 Axillary tail
  174.8 Other specified sites of female
    breast
    Ectopic sites
    Inner breast
    Lower breast
    Malignant neoplasm of contiguous or
      overlapping sites of breast whose
      point of origin cannot be determined
    Midline of breast
    Outer breast
    Upper breast
  174.9 Breast (female), unspecified

175 Malignant neoplasm of male breast
Excludes skin of breast (172.5, 173.5)
  175.0 Nipple and areola
  175.9 Other and unspecified sites of male
    breast
    Ectopic breast tissue, male

176 Kaposi's sarcoma
  176.0 Skin
  176.1 Soft tissue
    Includes:
      blood vessel
      connective tissue
      fascia
      ligament
      lymphatic(s) NEC
      muscle
    Excludes lymph glands and nodes
      (176.5)
  176.2 Palate
  176.3 GI sites
  176.4 Lung
  176.5 Lymph nodes
  176.8 Other specified sites
    Includes oral cavity NEC
  176.9 Unspecified
    Viscera NOS

**MALIGNANT NEOPLASM OF GENITOURI-
NARY ORGANS (179 to 189)**
Excludes carcinoma in situ (233.1 to 233.9)

**179 Malignant neoplasm of uterus, part
  unspecified**

180 Malignant neoplasm of cervix uteri
Includes invasive malignancy (carcinoma)
Excludes carcinoma in situ (233.1)
  180.0 Endocervix
    Cervical canal NOS
    Endocervical canal
    Endocervical gland
  180.1 Exocervix
  180.8 Other specified sites of cervix
    Cervical stump
    Squamocolumnar junction of cervix
    Malignant neoplasm of contiguous or
      overlapping sites of cervix uteri
      whose point of origin cannot be de-
      termined
  180.9 Cervix uteri, unspecified

181 Malignant neoplasm of placenta
  Choriocarcinoma NOS
  Chorioepithelioma NOS
  Excludes:
    chorioadenoma (destruens) (236.1)
    hydatidiform mole (630)
      malignant (236.1)
    invasive mole (236.1)
    male choriocarcinoma NOS (186.0 to
    186.9)

182 Malignant neoplasm of body of uterus
Excludes carcinoma in situ (233.2)
  182.0 Corpus uteri, except isthmus
    Cornu
    Endometrium
    Fundus
    Myometrium
  182.1 Isthmus
    Lower uterine segment
  182.8 Other specified sites of body of
    uterus
    Malignant neoplasm of contiguous or
      overlapping sites of body of uterus
      whose point of origin cannot be de-
      termined
    Excludes uterus NOS (179)

183 Malignant neoplasm of ovary and other uterine adnexa
Excludes Douglas' cul-de-sac (158.8)
  183.0 Ovary
    Use additional code, if desired, to identify any functional activity
  183.2 Fallopian tube
    Oviduct
    Uterine tube
  183.3 Broad ligament
    Mesovarium
    Parovarian region
  183.4 Parametrium
    Uterine ligament NOS
    Uterosacral ligament
  183.5 Round ligament
  183.8 Other specified sites of uterine adnexa
    Tubo-ovarian
    Utero-ovarian
    Malignant neoplasm of contiguous or overlapping sites of ovary and other uterine adnexa whose point of origin cannot be determined
  183.9 Uterine adnexa, unspecified

184 Malignant neoplasm of other and unspecified female genital organs
Excludes carcinoma in situ (233.3)
  184.0 Vagina
    Gartner's duct
    Vaginal vault
  184.1 Labia majora
    Greater vestibular (Bartholin's) gland
  184.2 Labia minora
  184.3 Clitoris
  184.4 Vulva, unspecified
    External female genitalia NOS
    Pudendum
  184.8 Other specified sites of female genital organs
    Malignant neoplasm of contiguous or overlapping sites of female genital organs whose point of origin cannot be determined
  184.9 Female genital organ, site unspecified
    Female genitourinary tract NOS

185 Malignant neoplasm of prostate
Excludes seminal vesicles (187.8)

186 Malignant neoplasm of testis
  Use additional code, if desired, to identify any functional activity.

186.0 Undescended testis
  Ectopic testis
  Retained testis
186.9 Other and unspecified testis
  Testis:
    NOS
    descended
    scrotal

187 Malignant neoplasm of penis and other male genital organs
  187.1 Prepuce
    Foreskin
  187.2 Glans penis
  187.3 Body of penis
    Corpus cavernosum
  187.4 Penis, part unspecified
    Skin of penis NOS
  187.5 Epididymis
  187.6 Spermatic cord
    Vas deferens
  187.7 Scrotum
    Skin of scrotum
  187.8 Other specified sites of male genital organs
    Seminal vesicle
    Tunica vaginalis
    Malignant neoplasm of contiguous or overlapping sites of penis and other male genital organs whose point of origin cannot be determined
  187.9 Male genital organ, site unspecified
    Male genital organ or tract NOS

188 Malignant neoplasm of bladder
Excludes carcinoma in situ (233.7)
  188.0 Trigone of urinary bladder
  188.1 Dome of urinary bladder
  188.2 Lateral wall of urinary bladder
  188.3 Anterior wall of urinary bladder
  188.4 Posterior wall of urinary bladder
  188.5 Bladder neck
    Internal urethral orifice
  188.6 Ureteric orifice
  188.7 Urachus
  188.8 Other specified sites of bladder
    Malignant neoplasm of contiguous or overlapping sites of bladder whose point of origin cannot be determined
  188.9 Bladder, part unspecified
    Bladder wall NOS

189 Malignant neoplasm of kidney and other and unspecified urinary organs
189.0 Kidney, except pelvis
Kidney NOS
Kidney parenchyma
189.1 Renal pelvis
Renal calyces
Ureteropelvic junction
189.2 Ureter
Excludes ureteric orifice of bladder (188.6)
189.3 Urethra
Excludes urethral orifice of bladder (188.5)
189.4 Paraurethral glands
189.8 Other specified sites of urinary organs
Malignant neoplasm of contiguous or overlapping sites of kidney and other urinary organs whose point of origin cannot be determined
189.9 Urinary organ, site unspecified
Urinary system NOS

MALIGNANT NEOPLASM OF OTHER AND UNSPECIFIED SITES (190 to 199)
Excludes carcinoma in situ (234.0 to 234.9)

190 Malignant neoplasm of eye
Excludes:
carcinoma in situ (234.0)
cartilage (171.0)
eyelid (skin) (172.1, 173.1)
optic nerve (192.0)
orbital bone (170.0)
190.0 Eyeball, except conjunctiva, cornea, retina, and choroid
Ciliary body
Crystalline lens
Iris
Sclera
Uveal tract
190.1 Orbit
Connective tissue of orbit
Extraocular muscle
Retrobulbar
Excludes bone of orbit (170.0)
190.2 Lacrimal gland
190.3 Conjunctiva
190.4 Cornea
190.5 Retina
190.6 Choroid
190.7 Lacrimal duct
Lacrimal sac
Nasolacrimal duct

190.8 Other specified sites of eye
Malignant neoplasm of contiguous or overlapping sites of eye whose point of origin cannot be determined
190.9 Eye, part unspecified

191 Malignant neoplasm of brain
Excludes:
cranial nerves (192.0)
retrobulbar area (190.1)
191.0 Cerebrum, except lobes and ventricles
Basal ganglia
Cerebral cortex
Corpus striatum
Globus pallidus
Hypothalamus
Thalamus
191.1 Frontal lobe
191.2 Temporal lobe
Hippocampus
Uncus
191.3 Parietal lobe
191.4 Occipital lobe
191.5 Ventricles
Choroid plexus
Floor of ventricle
191.6 Cerebellum NOS
Cerebellopontine angle
191.7 Brain stem
Cerebral peduncle
Medulla oblongata
Midbrain
Pons
191.8 Other parts of brain
Corpus callosum
Tapetum
Malignant neoplasm of contiguous or overlapping sites of brain whose point of origin cannot be determined
191.9 Brain, unspecified
Cranial fossa NOS

192 Malignant neoplasm of other and unspecified parts of nervous system
Excludes peripheral, sympathetic, and parasympathetic nerves and ganglia (171.0 to 171.9)
192.0 Cranial nerves
Olfactory bulb
192.1 Cerebral meninges
Dura mater
Falx (cerebelli, cerebri)

Meninges NOS
Tentorium
192.3 Spinal meninges
192.8 Other specified sites of nervous system
Malignant neoplasms of contiguous or overlapping sites of other parts of nervous system whose point of origin cannot be determined
192.9 Nervous system, part unspecified
Nervous system (central) NOS
Excludes meninges NOS (192.1)

193 Malignant neoplasm of thyroid gland
Sipple's syndrome
Thyroglossal duct
Use additional code, if desired, to identify any functional activity.

194 Malignant neoplasm of other endocrine glands and related structures
Use additional code, if desired, to identify any functional activity.
Excludes:
islets of Langerhans (157.4)
ovary (183.0)
testis (186.0 to 186.9)
thymus (164.0)
194.0 Adrenal gland
Adrenal cortex
Adrenal medulla
Suprarenal gland
194.1 Parathyroid gland
194.3 Pituitary gland and craniopharyngeal duct
Craniobuccal pouch
Hypophysis
Rathke's pouch
Sella turcica
194.4 Pineal gland
194.5 Carotid body
194.6 Aortic body and other paraganglia
Coccygeal body
Glomus jugulare
Para-aortic body
194.8 Other
Pluriglandular involvement NOS
Note: If the sites of multiple involvements are known, they should be coded separately.
194.9 Endocrine gland, site unspecified

195 Malignant neoplasm of other and ill-defined sites
Includes malignant neoplasms of contiguous sites, not elsewhere classified, whose point of origin cannot be determined
Excludes malignant neoplasm:
lymphatic and hematopoietic tissue (200.0 to 208.9)
secondary sites (196.0 to 198.8)
unspecified site (199.0 to 199.1)
195.0 Head, face, and neck
Cheek NOS
Jaw NOS
Nose NOS
Supraclavicular region NOS
195.1 Thorax
Axilla
Chest (wall) NOS
Intrathoracic NOS
195.2 Abdomen
Intra-abdominal NOS
195.3 Pelvis
Groin
Inguinal region NOS
Presacral region
Sacrococcygeal region
Sites overlapping systems within pelvis, such as:
rectovaginal (septum)
rectovesical (septum)
195.4 Upper limb
195.5 Lower limb
195.8 Other specified sites
Back NOS
Flank NOS
Trunk NOS

196 Secondary and unspecified malignant neoplasm of lymph nodes
Excludes:
any malignant neoplasm of lymph nodes, specified as primary (200.0 to 202.9)
Hodgkin's disease (201.0 to 201.9)
lymphosarcoma (200.1)
reticulosarcoma (200.0)
other forms of lymphoma (202.0 to 202.9)
196.0 Lymph nodes of head, face, and neck
Cervical
Cervicofacial
Scalene
Supraclavicular
196.1 Intrathoracic lymph nodes
Bronchopulmonary

Intercostal
Mediastinal
Tracheobronchial
196.2 Intra-abdominal lymph nodes
Intestinal
Mesenteric
Retroperitoneal
196.3 Lymph nodes of axilla and upper
limb
Brachial
Epitrochlear
Infraclavicular
Pectoral
196.5 Lymph nodes of inguinal region and
lower limb
Femoral
Groin
Popliteal
Tibial
196.6 Intrapelvic lymph nodes
Hypogastric
Iliac
Obturator
Parametrial
196.8 Lymph nodes of multiple sites
196.9 Site unspecified
Lymph nodes NOS

197 Secondary malignant neoplasm of respiratory and digestive systems
Excludes lymph node metastasis (196.0 to
196.9)
197.0 Lung
Bronchus
197.1 Mediastinum
197.2 Pleura
197.3 Other respiratory organs
Trachea
197.4 Small intestine, including duodenum
197.5 Large intestine and rectum
197.6 Retroperitoneum and peritoneum
197.7 Liver, specified as secondary
197.8 Other digestive organs and spleen

198 Secondary malignant neoplasm of other specified sites
Excludes lymph node metastasis (196.0 to
196.9)
198.0 Kidney
198.1 Other urinary organs
198.2 Skin
Skin of breast
198.3 Brain and spinal cord
198.4 Other parts of nervous system
Meninges (cerebral, spinal)

198.5 Bone and bone marrow
198.6 Ovary
198.7 Adrenal gland
Suprarenal gland
198.8 Other specified sites
198.81 Breast
Excludes skin of breast (198.2)
198.82 Genital organs
198.89 Other
Excludes retroperitoneal lymph nodes
(196.2)

199 Malignant neoplasm without specification of site
199.0 Disseminated, unspecified site
(primary, secondary)
Carcinomatosis
Generalized:
cancer
malignancy
Multiple cancer
199.1 Other, unspecified site (primary,
secondary)
Cancer
Carcinoma
Malignancy

MALIGNANT NEOPLASM OF LYMPHATIC AND HEMATOPOIETIC TISSUE (200 to 208)
Excludes:
secondary neoplasm of:
bone marrow (198.5)
spleen (197.8)
secondary and unspecified neoplasm of
lymph nodes (196.0 to 196.9)

The following fifth-digit subclassification is
for use with categories 200 to 202:
0 = unspecified site
1 = lymph nodes of head, face, and neck
2 = intrathoracic lymph nodes
3 = intra-abdominal lymph nodes
4 = lymph nodes of axilla and upper limb
5 = lymph nodes of inguinal region and
lower limb
6 = intrapelvic lymph nodes
7 = spleen
8 = lymph nodes of multiple sites.

200 Lymphosarcoma and reticulosarcoma
200.0 Reticulosarcoma
Lymphoma (malignant):
histiocytic (diffuse):
nodular
pleomorphic cell type
reticulum cell type
Reticulum cell sarcoma:
NOS
pleomorphic cell type
200.1 Lymphosarcoma
Lymphoblastoma (diffuse)
Lymphoma (malignant):
lymphoblastic (diffuse)
lymphocytic (cell type, diffuse)
lymphosarcoma type
Lymphosarcoma:
NOS
diffuse NOS
lymphoblastic (diffuse)
lymphocytic (diffuse)
prolymphocytic
Excludes:
lymphosarcoma:
follicular or nodular (202.0)
mixed cell type (200.8)
lymphosarcoma cell leukemia (207.8)
200.2 Burkitt's tumor or lymphoma
Malignant lymphoma, Burkitt's type
200.8 Other named variants
Lymphoma (malignant):
lymphoplasmacytoid type
mixed lymphocytic-histiocytic (diffuse)
Lymphosarcoma, mixed cell type (diffuse)
Reticulolymphosarcoma (diffuse)

201 Hodgkin's disease
201.0 Hodgkin's paragranuloma
201.1 Hodgkin's granuloma
210.2 Hodgkin's sarcoma
201.4 Lymphocytic-histiocytic predominance
201.5 Nodular sclerosis
Hodgkin's disease, nodular sclerosis:
NOS cellular phase
201.6 Mixed cellularity
201.7 Lymphocytic depletion
Hodgkin's disease, lymphocytic depletion:
NOS
diffuse fibrosis
reticular type

201.9 Hodgkin's disease, unspecified
Hodgkin's:
disease NOS
lymphoma NOS
Malignant:
lymphogranuloma
lymphogranulomatosis

202 Other malignant neoplasms of lymphoid and histiocytic tissue
202.0 Nodular lymphoma
Brill-Symmers disease
Lymphoma:
follicular (giant)
lymphocytic, nodular
Lymphosarcoma:
follicular (giant)
nodular
Reticulosarcoma, follicular or nodular
202.1 Mycosis fungoides
202.2 Sézary's disease
202.3 Malignant histiocytosis
Histiocytic medullary reticulosis
Malignant:
reticuloendotheliosis
reticulosis
202.4 Leukemic reticuloendotheliosis
Hairy-cell leukemia
202.5 Letterer-Siwe disease
Acute:
differentiated progressive histiocytosis
histiocytosis X (progressive)
infantile reticuloendotheliosis
reticulosis of infancy
Excludes:
Hand-Schüller-Christian disease (277.8)
histiocytosis (acute, chronic) (277.8)
histiocytosis X (chronic) (277.8)
202.6 Malignant mast cell tumors
Malignant:
mastocytoma
mastocytosis
Mast cell sarcoma
Systemic tissue mast cell disease
Excludes mast cell leukemia (207.8)
202.8 Other lymphomas
Lymphomas (malignant):
NOS
diffuse
Excludes benign lymphoma (229.0)
202.9 Other and unspecified malignant neoplasms of lymphoid and histiocytic tissue

Malignant neoplasm of bone marrow
NOS

203 Multiple myeloma and immunoproliferative neoplasms

The following fifth-digit subclassification is
for use with category 203:
0 = without mention of remission
1 = in remission.

203.0 Multiple myeloma
Kahler's disease
Myelomatosis
Excludes solitary myeloma (238.6)
203.1 Plasma cell leukemia
Plasmacytic leukemia
203.8 Other immunoproliferative neoplasms

204 Lymphoid leukemia
Includes leukemia:
lymphatic
lymphoblastic
lymphocytic
lymphogenous

The following fifth-digit subclassification is
for use with category 204:
0 = without mention of remission
1 = in remission.

204.0 Acute
Excludes acute exacerbation of chronic
lymphoid leukemia (204.1)
204.1 Chronic
204.2 Subacute
204.8 Other lymphoid leukemia
Aleukemic leukemia:
lymphatic
lymphocytic
lymphoid
204.9 Unspecified lymphoid leukemia

205 Myeloid leukemia
Includes:
leukemia:
granulocytic
myeloblastic
myelocytic
myelogenous
myelomonocytic
myelosclerotic
myelosis

The following fifth-digit subclassification is
for use with category 205:
0 = without mention of remission
1 = in remission.

205.0 Acute
Excludes acute exacerbation of chronic
myeloid leukemia (205.1)
205.1 Chronic
Eosinophilic leukemia
Neutrophilic leukemia
205.2 Subacute
205.3 Myeloid sarcoma
Chloroma
Granulocytic sarcoma
205.8 Other myeloid leukemia
Aleukemic leukemia:
granulocytic
myelogenous
myeloid
Aleukemic myelosis
205.9 Unspecified myeloid leukemia

206 Monocytic leukemia
Includes leukemia:
histiocytic
monoblastic
monocytoid

The following fifth-digit subclassification is
for use with category 206:
0 = without mention of remission
1 = in remission.

206.0 Acute
Excludes acute exacerbation of chronic
monocytic leukemia (206.1)
206.1 Chronic
206.2 Subacute
206.8 Other monocytic leukemia
Aleukemic:
monocytic leukemia
monocytoid leukemia
206.9 Unspecified monocytic leukemia

207 Other specified leukemia
Excludes:
leukemic reticuloendotheliosis (202.4)
plasma cell leukemia (203.1)

The following fifth-digit subclassification is
for use with category 207:
0 = without mention of remission
1 = in remission.

207.0 Acute erythremia and erythro-
leukemia
Acute erythremia myelosis
Di Guglielmo's disease
Erythremia myelosis
207.1 Chronic erythremia
Heilmeyer-Schöner disease
207.2 Megakaryocytic leukemia
Megakaryocytic myelosis
Thrombocytic leukemia
207.8 Other specified leukemia
Lymphosarcoma cell leukemia

208 Leukemia of unspecified cell type

The following fifth-digit subclassification is
for use with category 208:
0 = without mention of remission
1 = in remission.

208.0 Acute
Acute leukemia NOS
Blast cell leukemia
Stem cell leukemia
Excludes acute exacerbation of chronic
unspecified leukemia (208.1)
208.1 Chronic
Chronic leukemia NOS
208.2 Subacute
Subacute leukemia NOS
208.8 Other leukemia of unspecified cell
type
208.9 Unspecified leukemia
Leukemia NOS

BENIGN NEOPLASMS (210 to 229)

**210 Benign neoplasm of lip, oral cavity, and
pharynx**
Excludes cyst (of):
jaw (526.0 to 526.2, 526.89)
oral soft tissue (528.4)
radicular (522.8)
210.0 Lip
Frenulum labii
Lip (inner aspect, mucosa, vermilion border)
Excludes:
labial commissure (210.4)
skin of lip (216.0)
210.1 Tongue
Lingual tonsil

210.2 Major salivary glands
Gland:
parotid
sublingual
submandibular
Excludes benign neoplasms of minor
salivary glands:
NOS (210.4)
buccal mucosa (210.4)
lips (210.0)
palate (hard, soft) (210.4)
tongue (210.0)
tonsil, palatine (210.5)
210.3 Floor of mouth
210.4 Other and unspecified parts of
mouth
Gingiva
Gum (upper, lower)
Labial commissure
Oral cavity NOS
Oral mucosa
Palate (hard, soft)
Uvula
Excludes:
benign odontogenic neoplasms of
bone (213.0 to 213.1)
developmental odontogenic cysts
(526.0)
mucosa of lips (210.0)
nasopharyngeal (posterior, superior)
surface of soft palate (210.7)
210.5 Tonsil
Tonsil (faucial, palatine)
Excludes:
lingual tonsil (210.0)
pharyngeal tonsil (210.7)
tonsillar:
fossa (210.6)
pillars (210.6)
210.6 Other parts of oropharynx
Branchial cleft or vestiges
Epiglottis, anterior aspect
Fauces NOS
Mesopharynx NOS
Tonsillar:
fossa
pillars
Vallecula
Excludes epiglottis:
NOS (212.1)
suprahyoid portion (212.1)
210.7 Nasopharynx
Adenoid tissue
Lymphadenoid tissue

Pharyngeal tonsil
Posterior nasal septum
210.8 Hypopharynx
Arytenoid fold
Laryngopharynx
Postcricoid region
Pyriform fossa
210.9 Pharynx, unspecified
Throat NOS

211 Benign neoplasm of other parts of digestive system

211.0 Esophagus
211.1 Stomach
Body of stomach
Cardia of stomach
Fundus of stomach
Cardiac orifice
Pylorus
211.2 Duodenum, jejunum, and ileum
Small intestine NOS
Excludes:
ampulla of Vater (211.5)
ileocecal valve (211.3)
211.3 Colon
Appendix
Cecum
Ileocecal valve
Large intestine NOS
Excludes rectosigmoid junction (211.4)
211.4 Rectum and anal canal
Anal canal or sphincter
Anus NOS
Rectosigmoid junction
Excludes:
anus:
margin (215.6)
skin (216.5)
perianal skin (216.5)
211.5 Liver and biliary passages
Ampulla of Vater
Common bile duct
Cystic duct
Gallbladder
Hepatic duct
Sphincter of Oddi
211.6 Pancreas, except islets of Langer-hans
211.7 Islets of Langerhans
Islet cell tumor
Use additional code, if desired, to iden-tify any functional activity.
211.8 Retroperitoneum and peritoneum
Mesentery
Mesocolon

Omentum
Retroperitoneal tissue
211.9 Other and unspecified site
Alimentary tract NOS
Digestive system NOS
GI tract NOS
Intestinal tract NOS
Intestine NOS
Spleen NEC

212 Benign neoplasm of respiratory and intrathoracic organs

212.0 Nasal cavities, middle ear, and accessory sinuses
Cartilage of nose
Eustachian tube
Nares
Septum of nose
Sinus:
ethmoidal
frontal
maxillary
sphenoidal
Excludes:
auditory canal, external (216.2)
bone of:
ear (213.0)
nose (turbines) (213.0)
cartilage of ear (215.0)
ear (external, skin) (216.2)
nose NOS (229.8)
skin (216.3)
olfactory bulb (225.1)
polyp of:
accessory sinus (471.8)
ear (385.30-383.35)
nasal cavity (471.0)
posterior margin of septum and choanae (210.7)
212.1 Larynx
Cartilage:
arytenoid
cricoid
cuneiform
thyroid
Epiglottis (suprahyoid portion) NOS
Glottis
Vocal cords (false, true)
Excludes:
epiglottis, anterior aspect (210.6)
polyp of vocal cord or larynx (478.4)
212.2 Trachea
212.3 Bronchus and lung
Carina
Hilus of lung

212.4 Pleura
212.5 Mediastinum
212.6 Thymus
212.7 Heart
Excludes great vessels (215.4)
212.8 Other specified sites
212.9 Site unspecified
Respiratory organ NOS
Upper respiratory tract NOS
Excludes:
intrathoracic NOS (229.8)
thoracic NOS (229.8)

213 Benign neoplasms of bone and articular cartilage
Includes:
cartilage (articular, joint)
periosteum
Excludes:
cartilage of:
ear (215.0)
eyelid (215.0)
larynx (212.1)
nose (212.0)
exostosis NOS (726.91)
synovia (215.0 to 215.9)
213.0 Bones of skull and face
Excludes lower jaw bone (213.1)
213.1 Lower jaw bone
213.2 Vertebral column, excluding sacrum and coccyx
213.3 Ribs, sternum, and clavicle
213.4 Scapula and long bones of upper limb
213.5 Short bones of upper limb
213.6 Pelvic bones, sacrum, and coccyx
213.7 Long bones of lower limb
213.8 Short bones of lower limb
213.9 Bone and articular cartilage, site unspecified

214 Lipoma
Includes:
angiolipoma
fibrolipoma
hibernoma
lipoma (fetal, infiltrating, intramuscular)
myelolipoma
myxolipoma
214.0 Skin and subcutaneous tissue of face
214.1 Other skin and subcutaneous tissue
214.2 Intrathoracic organs
214.3 Intra-abdominal organs

214.4 Spermatic cord
214.8 Other specified sites
214.9 Lipoma, unspecified site

215 Other benign neoplasm of connective and other soft tissue
Includes:
blood vessel
bursa
fascia
ligament
muscle
peripheral, sympathetic, and parasympathetic nerves and ganglia
synovia
tendon (sheath)
Excludes:
cartilage:
articular (213.0 to 213.9)
larynx (212.1)
nose (212.0)
connective tissue of:
breast (217)
internal organ, except lipoma and hemangioma—code to benign neoplasm of the site
lipoma (214.0 to 214.9)
215.0 Head, face, and neck
215.2 Upper limb, including shoulder
215.3 Lower limb, including hip
215.4 Thorax
Excludes:
heart (212.7)
mediastinum (212.5)
thymus (212.6)
215.5 Abdomen
Abdominal wall
Hypochondrium
215.6 Pelvis
Buttock
Groin
Inguinal region
Perineum
Excludes uterine:
leiomyoma (218.0 to 218.9)
ligament, any (221.0)
215.7 Trunk, unspecified
Back NOS
Flank NOS
215.8 Other specified sites
215.9 Site unspecified

216 Benign neoplasm of skin
Includes:
blue nevus
dermatofibroma
hydrocystoma
pigmented nevus
syringoadenoma
syringoma
Excludes skin of genital organs (221.0 to 222.9)
216.0 Skin of lip
Excludes vermilion border of lip (210.0)
216.1 Eyelid, including canthus
Excludes cartilage of eyelid (215.0)
216.2 Ear and external auditory canal
Auricle (ear)
Auricular canal, external
External meatus
Pinna
Excludes cartilage of ear (215.0)
216.3 Skin of other and unspecified parts of face
Cheek, external
Eyebrow
Nose, external
Temple
216.4 Scalp and skin of neck
216.5 Skin of trunk, except scrotum
Axillary fold
Perianal skin
Skin of:
abdominal wall
anus
back
breast
buttock
chest wall
groin
perineum
Umbilicus
Excludes:
anal canal (211.4)
anus NOS (211.4)
skin of scrotum (222.4)
216.6 Skin of upper limb, including shoulder
216.7 Skin of lower limb, including hip
216.8 Other specified sites of skin
216.9 Skin, site unspecified

217 Benign neoplasm of breast
Breast (male, female):
connective tissue
glandular tissue
soft parts
Excludes:
adenofibrosis (610.2)
benign cyst of breast (610.0)
fibrocystic disease (610.1)
skin of breast (216.5)

218 Uterine leiomyoma
Includes:
fibroid (bleeding, uterine)
uterine:
fibromyoma
myoma
218.0 Submucous leiomyoma of uterus
218.1 Intramural leiomyomas of uterus
Interstitial leiomyoma of uterus
218.2 Subserous leiomyoma of uterus
Subperitoneal leiomyoma of uterus
218.9 Leiomyoma of uterus, unspecified

219 Other benign neoplasm of uterus
219.0 Cervix uteri
219.1 Corpus uteri
Endometrium
Fundus
Myometrium

220 Benign neoplasm of ovary
Use additional code, if desired, to identify any functional activity (256.0 to 256.1).
Excludes cyst:
corpus albicans (620.2)
corpus luteum (620.1)
endometrial (617.1)
follicular (atretic) (620.0)
graafian follicle (620.0)
ovarian NOS (620.2)
retention (620.2)

221 Benign neoplasm of other female genital organs
Includes adenomatous polyp, benign teratoma
Excludes cyst:
epophöron (752.11)
fimbrial (752.11)
Gartner's duct (752.11)
parovarian (752.11)
221.0 Fallopian tube and uterine ligaments
Oviduct
Parametrium

Uterine ligament (broad, rough, utero-
  sacral)
Uterine tube
221.1 Vagina
221.2 Vulva
  Clitoris
  External female genitalia NOS
  Greater vestibular (Bartholin's) gland
  Labia (majora, minora)
  Pudendum
  Excludes Bartholin's (duct, gland) cyst
    (616.2)
221.8 Other specified sites of female geni-
  tal organs
221.9 Female genital organ, site unspeci-
  fied
  Female genitourinary tract NOS

222 Benign neoplasm of male genital organs
  222.0 Testis
Use additional code, if desired, to identify
  any functional activity.
  222.1 Penis
    Corpus cavernosum
    Glans penis
    Prepuce
  222.2 Prostate
Excludes:
  adenomatous hyperplasia of prostate
    (600)
  prostatic:
    adenoma (600)
    enlargement (600)
    hypertrophy (600)
  222.3 Epididymis
  222.4 Scrotum
    Skin of scrotum
  222.8 Other specified sites of male genital
    organs
    Seminal vesicle
    Spermatic cord
  222.9 Male genital organ, site unspecified
    Male genitourinary tract NOS

**223 Benign neoplasm of kidney and other
  urinary organs**
  223.0 Kidney, except pelvis
    Kidney NOS
    Excludes renal:
      calyces (223.1)
      pelvis (223.1)
  223.1 Renal pelvis
  223.2 Ureter
    Excludes urethral orifice of bladder
      (223.3)

223.8 Other specified sites of urinary
  organs
  223.81 Urethra
    Excludes urethral orifice of bladder
      (223.3)
  223.89 Other
223.9 Urinary organ, site unspecified
  Urinary system NOS

224 Benign neoplasm of eye
Excludes:
  cartilage of eyelid (215.0)
  eyelid (skin) (216.1)
  optic nerve (225.1)
  orbital bone (213.0)
  224.0 Eyeball, except conjunctivae,
    cornea, retina, and choroid
    Ciliary body
    Iris
    Sclera
    Uveal tract
  224.1 Orbit
    Excludes bone of orbit (213.0)
  224.1 Lacrimal gland
  224.3 Conjunctiva
  224.4 Cornea
  224.5 Retina
    Excludes hemangioma of retina (228.03)
  224.6 Choroid
  224.7 Lacrimal duct
    Lacrimal sac
    Nasolacrimal duct
  224.8 Other specified parts of eye
  224.9 Eye, part unspecified

**225 Benign neoplasm of brain and other
  parts of nervous system**
Excludes:
  hemangioma (228.02)
  neurofibromatosis (237.7)
  peripheral, sympathetic, and parasympa-
    thetic nerves and ganglia (215.0 to
    215.9)
  retrobulbar (224.1)
  225.0 Brain
  225.1 Cranial nerves
  225.2 Cerebral meninges
    Meninges NOS
    Meningioma (cerebral)
  225.3 Spinal cord
    Cauda equina
  225.4 Spinal meninges
    Spinal meningioma
  225.8 Other specified sites of nervous sys-
    tem

225.9 Nervous system, part unspecified
Nervous system (central), NOS
Excludes meninges NOS (225.2)

226 Benign neoplasm of thyroid glands
Use additional code, if desired, to identify
any functional activity.

227 Benign neoplasm of other endocrine glands and related structures
Use additional code, if desired, to identify
any functional activity.
Excludes:
ovary (220)
pancreas (211.6)
testis (222.0)
227.0 Adrenal gland
Suprarenal gland
227.1 Parathyroid gland
227.3 Pituitary gland and craniopharyngeal duct (pouch)
Craniobuccal pouch
Hypophysis
Rathke's pouch
Sella turcica
227.4 Pineal gland
Pineal body
227.5 Carotid body
227.6 Aortic body and other paraganglia
Coccygeal body
Glomus jugulare
Para-aortic body
227.8 Other
227.9 Endocrine gland, site unspecified

228 Hemangioma and lymphangioma, any site
Includes:
angioma (benign, cavernous, congenital)
NOS
cavernous nevus
glomus tumor
hemangioma (benign, congenital)
Excludes:
benign neoplasm of spleen, except hemangioma and lymphangioma (211.9)
glomus jugulare (227.6)
nevus:
NOS (216.0 to 216.9)
blue or pigmented (216.0 to 216.9)
vascular (757.32)
228.0 Hemangioma, any site
228.00 Of unspecified site
228.01 Of skin and subcutaneous tissue
228.02 Of intracranial structures

228.04 Of intra-abdominal structures
Peritoneum
Retroperitoneal tissue
228.09 Of other sites
Systemic angiomatosis
228.1 Lymphangioma, any site
Congenital lymphangioma
Lymphatic nevus

229 Benign neoplasm of other and unspeci-fied sites
229.0 Lymph nodes
Excludes lymphangioma (228.1)
229.8 Other specified sites
Intrathoracic NOS
Thoracic NOS
229.9 Site unspecified

CARCINOMA IN SITU (230 to 234)
Includes:
Bowen's disease
erythroplasia
Queyrat's erythroplasia
Excludes leukoplakia

230 Carcinoma in situ of digestive organs
230.0 Lip, oral cavity, and pharynx
Gingiva
Hypopharynx
Mouth (any part)
Nasopharynx
Oropharynx
Salivary gland or duct
Tongue
Excludes:
aryepiglottic fold or interarytenoid
fold, laryngeal aspect (231.0)
epiglottis:
NOS (231.0)
suprahyoid portion (231.0)
skin of lip (232.0)
230.1 Esophagus
230.2 Stomach
Body of stomach
Cardia of stomach
Fundus of stomach
Cardiac orifice
Pylorus
230.3 Colon
Appendix
Cecum
Ileocecal valve
Large intestine NOS
Excludes rectosigmoid junction (230.4)

230.4 Rectum
Rectosigmoid junction
230.5 Anal canal
Anal sphincter
230.6 Anus, unspecified
Excludes:
anus
margin (232.5)
skin (232.5)
perianal skin (232.5)
230.7 Other and unspecified parts of intestine
Duodenum
Ileum
Jejunum
Small intestine NOS
Excludes ampulla of Vater (230.8)
230.8 Liver and biliary system
Ampulla of Vater
Common bile duct
Cystic duct
Gallbladder
Hepatic duct
Sphincter of Oddi
230.9 Other and unspecified digestive
organs
Digestive organ NOS
GI tract NOS
Pancreas
Spleen

231 Carcinoma in situ of respiratory system
231.0 Larynx
Cartilage:
arytenoid
cricoid
cuneiform
thyroid
Epiglottis:
NOS
posterior surface
suprahyoid portion
Vocal cords (false, true)
Excludes aryepiglottic fold or interarytenoid fold:
NOS (230.0)
hypopharyngeal aspect (230.0)
marginal zone (230.0)
231.1 Trachea
231.2 Bronchus and lung
Carina
Hilus of lung
231.8 Other specified parts of respiratory
system

Accessory sinus
Middle ear
Nasal cavities
Pleura
Excludes:
ear (external, skin, 232.2)
nose NOS (234.8)
skin (232.3)
231.9 Respiratory system, part unspecified
Respiratory organ NOS

232 Carcinoma in situ of skin
Includes pigment cells
232.0 Skin of lip
232.1 Eyelid, including canthus
232.2 Ear and external auditory canal
232.3 Skin of other and unspecified parts
of face
232.4 Scalp and skin of neck
232.5 Skin of trunk, except scrotum:
Anus, margin
Axillary fold
Perianal skin
Skin of:
abdominal wall
anus
back
breast
buttock
chest wall
groin
perineum
Umbilicus
Excludes:
anal canal (230.5)
anus NOS (230.6)
skin of genital organs (233.3, 233.5 to
233.6)
232.6 Skin of upper limb, including shoulder
232.7 Skin of lower limb, including hip
232.8 Other specified sites of skin
232.9 Skin, site unspecified

233 Carcinoma in situ of breast and genitourinary system
233.0 Breast
Excludes:
Paget's disease (174.0 to 174.9)
skin of breast (232.5)
233.1 Cervix uteri
233.2 Other and unspecified parts of
uterus

233.3 Other and unspecified female genital organs
233.4 Prostate
233.5 Penis
233.6 Other and unspecified male genital organs
233.7 Bladder
233.9 Other and unspecified urinary organs

234 Carcinoma in situ of other and unspecified sites
234.0 Eye
Excludes:
    cartilage of eyelid (234.8)
    eyelid (skin) (232.1)
    optic nerve (234.8)
    orbital bone (234.8)
234.8 Other specified sites
Endocrine gland (any)
234.9 Site unspecified
Carcinoma in situ NOS

NEOPLASMS OF UNCERTAIN BEHAVIOR (235 to 238)
Note: Categories 235 to 238 classify by site certain histomorphologically well-defined neoplasms, the subsequent behavior of which cannot be predicted from their present appearance.

235 Neoplasm of uncertain behavior of digestive and respiratory systems
235.0 Major salivary glands
Gland:
    parotid
    sublingual
    submandibular
Excludes minor salivary glands (235.1)
235.1 Lip, oral cavity, and pharynx
Gingiva
Hypopharynx
Minor salivary glands
Mouth
Nasopharynx
Tongue
Excludes:
    aryepiglottic fold or interarytenoid fold, laryngeal aspect (235.6)
    epiglottis:
        NOS (235.6)
        suprahyoid portion (235.6)
    skin of lip (238.2)

235.2 Stomach, intestines, and rectum
235.3 Liver and biliary passages
Ampulla of Vater
Bile ducts (any)
Gallbladder
Liver
235.4 Retroperitoneum and peritoneum
235.5 Other and unspecified digestive organs
Anal:
    canal
    sphincter
Anus NOS
Esophagus
Pancreas
Spleen
Excludes
    anus:
        margin (238.2)
        skin (238.2)
    perianal skin (238.2)
235.6 Larynx
Excludes aryepiglottic fold or interarytenoid fold:
    NOS (235.1)
    hypopharyngeal aspect (235.1)
    marginal zone (235.1)
235.7 Trachea, bronchus, and lung
235.8 Pleura, thymus, and mediastinum
235.9 Other and unspecified respiratory organs
Accessory sinuses
Middle ear
Nasal cavities
Respiratory organ NOS
Excludes:
    ear (external, skin) (238.2)
    nose (238.8)
    skin (238.2)

236 Neoplasm of uncertain behavior of genitourinary organs
236.0 Uterus
236.1 Placenta
Chorioadenoma (destruens)
Invasive mole
Malignant hydatid(iform) mole
236.2 Ovary
Use additional code, if desired, to identify any functional activity.
236.3 Other and unspecified female genital organs
236.4 Testis
Use additional code, if desired, to identify any functional activity.

236.5 Prostate
236.6 Other and unspecified male genital organs
236.7 Bladder
236.9 Other and unspecified urinary organs
  236.90 Urinary organ, unspecified
  236.91 Kidney and ureter
  236.99 Other

237 Neoplasm of uncertain behavior of endocrine glands and nervous system
237.0 Pituitary gland and craniopharyngeal duct
Use additional code, if desired, to identify any functional activity.
237.1 Pineal gland
237.2 Adrenal gland
Suprarenal gland
Use additional code, if desired, to identify any functional activity.
237.3 Paraganglia
Aortic body
Carotid body
Coccygeal body
Glomus jugulare
237.4 Other and unspecified endocrine glands
Parathyroid gland
Thyroid gland
237.5 Brain and spinal cord
237.6 Meninges
Meninges:
  NOS cerebral
  spinal
237.7 Neurofibromatosis
von Recklinghausen's disease
  237.70 Neurofibromatosis, unspecified
  237.71 Neurofibromatosis, Type 1 (von Recklinghausen's disease)
  237.72 Neurofibromatosis, Type 2 (acoustic neurofibromatosis)
237.9 Other and unspecified parts of nervous system
Cranial nerves
Excludes peripheral, sympathetic, and parasympathetic nerves and ganglia (238.1)

238 Neoplasm of uncertain behavior of other and unspecified sites and tissues
238.0 Bone and articular cartilage
Excludes:
cartilage:
  ear (238.1)

eyelid (238.1)
larynx (235.6)
nose (235.9)
synovia (238.1)
238.1 Connective and other soft tissue
Peripheral, sympathetic, and parasympathetic nerves and ganglia
Excludes:
cartilage of:
  articular (238.0)
  larynx (235.6)
  nose (235.9)
connective tissue of breast (238.3)
238.2 Skin
Excludes:
anus NOS (235.5)
skin of genital organs (236.3, 236.6)
vermilion border of lip (235.1)
238.3 Breast
Excludes skin of breast (238.2)
238.4 Polycythemia vera
238.5 Histiocytic and mast cells
Mast cell tumor NOS
Mastocytoma NOS
238.6 Plasma cells
Plasmacytoma NOS
Solitary myeloma
238.7 Other lymphatic and hematopoietic tissues
Disease:
  lymphoproliferative (chronic) NOS
  myeloproliferative (chronic) NOS
Idiopathic thrombocythemia
Megakaryocytic myelosclerosis
Myelosclerosis with myeloid metaplasia
Panmyelosis (acute)
Excludes:
  myelofibrosis (289.8)
  myelosclerosis NOS (289.8)
  myelosis:
    NOS (205.9)
    megakaryocytic (207.2)
238.8 Other specified sites
Eye
Heart
Excludes:
cartilage (238.1)
eyelid (skin) (238.2)
238.9 Site unspecified

**NEOPLASMS OF UNSPECIFIED NATURE
(239)**

239 Neoplasms of unspecified nature
Note: Category 239 classifies by site neoplasms of unspecified morphology and
behavior. The term "mass," unless otherwise stated, is not to be regarded as a
neoplastic growth.
Includes:
  "growth" NOS
  neoplasm NOS
  new growth NOS
  tumor NOS
  239.0 Digestive system
    Excludes:
      anus:
        margin (239.2)
        perianal skin (239.2)
      skin (239.2)
  239.1 Respiratory system
  239.2 Bone, soft tissue, and skin
    Excludes:
      anal canal (239.0)
      anus NOS (239.0)
      bone marrow (202.9)

cartilage:
  larynx (239.1)
  nose (239.1)
connective tissue of breast (239.3)
skin of genital organs (239.5)
vermilion border of lip (239.0
  239.3 Breast
    Excludes skin of breast (239.2)
  239.4 Bladder
  239.5 Other genitourinary organs
  239.6 Brain
    Excludes:
      cerebral meninges (239.7)
      cranial nerves (239.7)
  239.7 Endocrine glands and other parts of
    nervous system
    Excludes peripheral, sympathetic, and
      parasympathetic nerves and ganglia
      (239.2)
  239.8 Other specified sites
    Excludes:
      eyelid, skin (239.2)
      cartilage (239.2)
      great vessels (239.2)
      optic nerve (239.7)
  239.9 Site unspecified

Index

A

A-metha-Pred, 226-227
Abdominal and pelvic neoplasms, 59-94
  bladder cancer, 84-89
  colorectal cancer, 73-78
  esophageal cancer, 65-67
  gallbladder and bile duct cancers, 89-92
  gastric cancer, 59-65
  kidney cancer, 78-80
  liver cancer, 81-84
  pancreatic cancer, 67-73
ABVD chemotherapy protocol, 161, 239t
AC chemotherapy protocol, 239t
ACE (CAE) chemotherapy protocol, 239t
Acoustic neurinoma. *See* Schwannoma.
Acquired immunodeficiency syndrome (AIDS), Kaposi's sarcoma in, 153-156
Actimmune, 220-221
Actinic keratosis, 145t
  treating with topical fluorouracil, 147
Actinomycin D. *See* Dactinomycin.
Acute lymphoblastic leukemia. *See* Leukemia, acute.
Acute monoblastic leukemia. *See* Leukemia, acute.
Acute myeloblastic leukemia. *See* Leukemia, acute.
Adriamycin, 213-214
Adrucil, 216-217
Ak-Dex, 212-213
Aldesleukin, 200-201
Alkeran, 224
Alpha-fetoprotein, 4
Altretamine, 201
Amsacrine, 171
Analgesia, patient-controlled system, 14. *See also* Pain control in cancer patients.
Anal neoplasms, *ICD-9-CM* classification of, 266
Android F, 217-218
Ann Arbor staging system for Hodgkin's disease, 162i
AP chemotherapy protocol, 239t
ara-C. *See* Cytarabine.
Articular cartilage neoplasms, *ICD-9-CM* classification of, 269, 281
ASHAP chemotherapy protocol, 239t
Asparaginase, 171, 201-202
Astrocytoma, clinical features of, 18t

B

BACON chemotherapy protocol, 240
BACOP chemotherapy protocol, 240
Basal cell epithelioma, 141-143
  causes, 141
  diagnosis, 142
  signs and symptoms, 142
  special considerations, 143
  treatment, 142-143
BCNU. *See* Carmustine.
BCP chemotherapy protocol, 240
Bence Jones protein, 139
Benign tumors
  essential differences between malignant tumors and, 5t
  ICD-9-CM classification of, 279-284
BEP chemotherapy protocol, 240
BHD chemotherapy protocol, 240
BiCNU, 204-205
Bile duct cancer, 89-92
  causes, 90
  diagnosis, 91
  ICD-9-CM classification of extrahepatic, 266-267
    intrahepatic, 266
  signs and symptoms, 91
  special considerations, 92
  treatment, 91-92
Biological response modifiers, 10-11
Biopsy as diagnostic tool, 4
Biotherapy, 10-11
Bladder cancer, 84-89
  causes, 84-85
  comparing staging systems for, 86t
    Jewett-Strong-Marshall system, 86t
    TNM system, 86t
  diagnosis, 86
  ICD-9-CM classification of, 273
  signs and symptoms, 85
  special considerations, 88-89
  treatment, 85-87
Blenoxane, 202-203
Bleomycin sulfate, 100, 103, 122, 126, 161, 166, 168, 202-203
Blood and lymph neoplasms, 159-182
  acute leukemia, 168-174
  chronic granulocytic leukemia, 174-177
  chronic lymphocytic leukemia, 177-180
  Hodgkin's disease, 159-163
  malignant lymphomas, 163-166
  mycosis fungoides, 166-168
Blue nevi, 149
Bone tumors, benign, *ICD-9-CM* classification of, 281

Bone, skin, and soft-tissue neoplasms, 133-158
Bone tumors, primary malignant, 133-137
  causes, 135
  chemotherapy protocols for bony sarcoma
    AC, 239t
    CYVADIC, 247t
    HDMTX, 251t
    MAID, 253t
  comparison of types of, 134t
  diagnosis, 135
  ICD-9-CM classification of, 269
  signs and symptoms, 135
  special considerations, 136-137
  treatment, 135
Bowen's disease, 145t
Brain tumors, benign, *ICD-9-CM* classification of, 283-284
Brain tumors, malignant, 17-23
  causes, 17, 20
  chemotherapy protocols, pediatric
    MOP, 255t
    PCV, 256t
  comparison of, 18-20t
    astrocytoma, 18t
    ependymoma, 19t
    glioblastoma multiforme, 18t
    medulloblastoma, 19t
    meningioma, 19t
    oligodendroglioma, 18-19t
    schwannoma, 20t
  diagnosis, 20
  ICD-9-CM classification of, 274
  signs and symptoms, 20
  special considerations, 22-23
    care after craniotomy, 22-23
    care during hospitalization, 22
    other measures, 23
  treatment, 21
Breast cancer, 50-56
  causes, 50
  chemotherapy protocols for
    CAF (FAC), 241t
    CFM, 242t
    CFPT, 243t
    CMFVP, 244t
    FAC (CAF), 249t
    IMF, 252t
    VATH, 261t
  diagnosis, 52-53
  histologic classification of, 51
  ICD-9-CM classification of, 271-272
  pathophysiology, 50-51
  staging, 52
  signs and symptoms, 51
  special considerations, 54-56
    arm and hand care, 55
    postoperative care, 55-56
    preoperative care, 54-55
  treatment, 53-54

i refers to an illustration; t refers to a table

Breast, benign neoplasms of, *ICD-9-CM* classification of, 282
Bromocriptine, 26
Bronchial neoplasms, *ICD-9-CM* classification of, 268
Busulfan, 176, 203-204

C
CAF (FAC) chemotherapy protocol, 241t
CAMP chemotherapy protocol, 241t
Cancer
  causes of, 1-3
  diagnostic methods, 4
  differences between benign and malignant tumors, 5t
  hospice approach, 13-14
  immune tumor response, 3-4
  maintaining nutrition and fluid balance, 11-12
    providing tube feedings, 12
    total parenteral nutrition, 12-13
  major therapies, 6-11
    biotherapy, 10-11
    chemotherapy, 8-10
    hormonal therapy, 11
    radiation, 6-8
    surgery, 6
  pain control, 13
  psychological aspects, 15
  six most common sites of, 44i
  staging and grading, 4-5
CAP chemotherapy protocol, 241t
Carboplatin, 66, 204
Carcinoembryonic antigen, 4
Carcinogenesis, 1-3
  immune tumor response and, 3-4
Carcinoma in situ
  of breast and genitourinary system, 285-286
  of digestive organs, 284-285
  ICD-9-CM classification of, 284-286
  of respiratory system, 285
  of skin, 285
Carmustine (BCNU), 21, 23, 63, 140, 204
CAV (VAC) chemotherapy protocol, 241t
CAVe chemotherapy protocol, 242t
CC chemotherapy protocol, 242t
CCNU. *See* Lomustine.
CD (DC) chemotherapy protocol, 242t
CDC chemotherapy protocol, 242t
CeeNU, 223
Cerebellopontine angle tumor. *See* Schwannoma.
Cerubidine, 211-212
Cervical cancer, 104-109
  causes, 105
  diagnosis, 105-106
    staging, 106
  ICD-9-CM classification of, 272
  signs and symptoms, 105
  special considerations, 107-109
  treatment, 106-107

CF chemotherapy protocol, 242t
CFL chemotherapy protocol, 242t
CFM chemotherapy protocol, 242t
CFPT chemotherapy protocol, 243t
CHAP chemotherapy protocol, 243t
Chemotherapy. *See also under treatment for specific neoplasms.*
  acronyms and protocols (Appendix B), 239-262
  for cancer, 8-10
  chemotherapeutic drugs (Appendix A), 200-238
  special care needed during, 9-10
ChIVPP chemotherapy protocol, 243t
Chlorambucil, 80, 122, 179, 205-206
Chondrosarcoma, clinical features and treatment, 134t
CHOP chemotherapy protocol, 165, 243t
CHOP-Bleo chemotherapy protocol, 243t
Chordoma, clinical features and treatment, 134t
Chronic granulocytic leukemia. *See* Leukemia, chronic granulocytic.
Chronic lymphocytic leukemia. *See* Leukemia, chronic lymphocytic.
Chronic myelocytic leukemia. *See* Leukemia, chronic myelocytic.
Chronic myelogenous leukemia. *See* Leukemia, chronic granulocytic.
CISCA chemotherapy protocol, 244t
Cisplatin, 47, 48, 63, 66, 80, 87, 97, 100, 103, 111, 206-207
Cis-platinum. *See* Cisplatin.
Citrovorum factor. *See* Leucovorin calcium.
Cladribine, 207
Clark's staging system for malignant melanoma, 151i
Classification of neoplastic disorders, *ICD-9-CM* (Appendix C), 263-288. *See also* Staging of cancer.
CMF chemotherapy protocol, 244t
CMFVP chemotherapy protocol
  Cooper's, 244t
  SWOG, 244t
COAP chemotherapy protocol, 244t
COB chemotherapy protocol, 245t
Colonic neoplasms, *ICD-9-CM* classification of, 266. *See also* Colorectal cancer.
Colorectal cancer, 73-78
  causes, 73
  chemotherapy protocols for
    F-CL, 250t
    FAM, 249t
    FLe, 251t
    FMV, 251t
    MOF, 254t
  diagnosis, 74-75
    staging, 75
  ICD-9-CM classification of, 266
  signs and symptoms, 73-74
  special considerations, 76-77
  treatment, 76

COMLA chemotherapy protocol, 245t
Compound nevi, 149
Connective tissue neoplasms, *ICD-9-CM* classification of, 270, 281
COP chemotherapy protocol, 245t
COP-BLAM chemotherapy protocol, 245t
COPE chemotherapy protocol, 245t
COPP chemotherapy protocol, 246t
Cosmegen, 210-211
CP chemotherapy protocol, 246t
Craniotomy, care after
  in malignant brain tumors, 22-23
  in pituitary tumors, 27
Cryohypophysectomy, 27
Cutaneous reticulosis, malignant. *See* Mycosis fungoides.
CV chemotherapy protocol, 246t
CVEB chemotherapy protocol, 246t
CVI (VIC) chemotherapy protocol, 246t
CVP chemotherapy protocol, 247t
CVPP chemotherapy protocol, 247t
CYADIC chemotherapy protocol, 247t
CYVADIC chemotherapy protocol, 247t
Cyclophosphamide, 48, 54, 80, 87, 97, 122, 128, 140, 165, 167, 171, 207-208
Cyproheptadine, 26-27
Cytarabine, 171, 172, 208-209
Cytosar-U, 208-209
Cytosine arabinoside. *See* Cytarabine.
Cytoxan, 207-208

D
Dacarbazine, 135, 161, 209-210
Dactinomycin, 111, 122, 210-211
Dalalone, 212-213
Dalalone D.P., 212-213
Daunorubicin hydrochloride, 171, 172, 211-212
DC chemotherapy protocol, 248t
DCF. *See* Pentostatin.
DCPM chemotherapy protocol, 248t
DCT chemotherapy protocol, 248t
Decadrol, 212-213
Decadron, 212-213
Decadron phosphate, 212-213
Decaject-L.A., 212-213
Decameth L.A., 212-213
DepMedalone, 226-227
Depoject, 226-227
Depo-Medrol, 226-227
Depopred, 226-227
Depo-Predate, 226-227
Dermal nevi, 149
Dexacen-LA, 212-213
Dexacen LA-8, 212-213
Dexamethasone (systemic), 21, 212-213
Dexamethasone acetate, 212-213

i refers to an illustration; t refers to a table

Dexamethasone sodium phosphate, 212-213
Dexasone, 212-213
Dexasone-LA, 212-213
Dexon, 212-213
Dexone, 212-213
Dexone-LA, 212-213
DHAP chemotherapy protocol, 248t
Diagnostic methods for cancer, 4.
   See also under specific neoplasms.
Digestive organ neoplasms. See also Abdominal and pelvic neoplasms.
   ICD-9-CM classification of benign, 280
   malignant, 265-267
DNR. See Daunorubicin hydrochloride.
Doxorubicin hydrochloride, 48, 54, 63, 66, 71, 82, 87, 92, 95, 111, 122, 135, 140, 155, 161, 165, 167, 213-214
Drugs. See Chemotherapy.
DTIC-ACTD chemotherapy protocol, 248t
DTIC-Dome, 209-210
Dukes classification system for staging colorectal cancer, 75
Duodenal neoplasms, ICD-9-CM classification of, 266
Duralone, 226-227
Durameth, 226-227
DVP chemotherapy protocol, 248t
Dysplastic nevi, 149

E
Ear, middle, neoplasms of, ICD-9-CM classification of, 267-268
Efudex, 216-217
Elspar, 201-202
Emotional responses to cancer, 15
Endocrine gland neoplasms, ICD-9-CM classification of, 275, 284
Endometrial cancer. See Uterine cancer.
EP chemotherapy protocol, 248t
Ependymoma, clinical features of, 19t
Ergamisol, 222-223
Erythroplasia of Queyrat, 145t
ESHAP chemotherapy protocol, 249t
Esophageal cancer, 65-67
   causes, 65
   diagnosis, 65
   staging, 66
   signs and symptoms, 65
   special considerations, 66-67
   treatment, 66
Etoposide, 48, 97, 100, 111, 155, 167, 171, 214-215
Eulexin, 218
EVA chemotherapy protocol, 248t
Ewing's sarcoma
   clinical features and treatment, 134t
   T-2 chemotherapy protocol for, 259t

Exenteration, pelvic, management of in uterine cancer, 112
Extrahepatic bile duct cancer. See Bile duct cancer.
Eye neoplasms, ICD-9-CM classification of, 274, 283

F
FAC (CAF) chemotherapy protocol, 249t
F-CL chemotherapy protocol, 250t
Fallopian tube cancer, 127-129
   causes, 127
   diagnosis, 128
   signs and symptoms, 127
   special considerations, 128-129
   treatment, 128
FAM chemotherapy protocol, 249t
FAME chemotherapy protocol, 250t
FCE chemotherapy protocol, 250t
Female genital organs, neoplasms of. See Genital neoplasms.
Fibrosarcoma, clinical features and treatment, 134t
5-azacytidine, 171.
5 + 2 chemotherapy protocol, 250t
FL chemotherapy protocol, 250t
FLe chemotherapy protocol, 251t
Floxuridine, 82, 215
Fludara, 215-216
Fludarabine phosphate, 83, 215-216
Fluoroplex, 216-217
Fluorouracil, 47, 54, 63, 66, 71, 76, 80, 82, 87, 91, 216-217
   topical for actinic keratosis, 147
Fluoxymesterone, 217-218
Flutamide, 218
FMS chemotherapy protocol, 251t
FMV chemotherapy protocol, 251t
Folex, 225-226
Folinic acid. See Leucovorin calcium.
5-FU. See Fluorouracil.
FUDR, 215
FZ chemotherapy protocol, 251t

G
Gallbladder cancer, 89-92
   causes, 90
   diagnosis, 91
   ICD-9-CM classification of, 266-267
   signs and symptoms, 90-91
   special considerations, 92
   treatment, 91-92
Gastric cancer, 59-65
   causes, 59-61
   chemotherapy protocols
      FAM, 249t
      FAME, 250t
      FCE, 250t
   diagnosis, 61
      staging, 62
   signs and symptoms, 61
   sites of, 60i
   special considerations, 63-65
   treatment, 62-63

Gastrostomy tube feeding, 12
Genital neoplasms, 95-132
   cervical cancer, 104-109
   Fallopian tube cancer, 127-129
   ovarian cancer, 118-123
   penile cancer, 102-104
   prostate cancer, 95-99
   testicular cancer, 99-102
   uterine cancer, 109-115
   vaginal cancer, 115-118
   vulva, cancer of, 124-127
Genitourinary cancer. See also Bladder cancer and Genital neoplasms.
   chemotherapy protocols for treatment of
      BEP, 240t
      CAP, 241t
      CISCA, 244t
      CVEB, 246t
      FL, 250t
      FZ, 251t
      L-VAM, 252t
      m-PFL, 255t
      MVAC, 256t
      VAB, 260t
      VB, 261t
      VBP, 261t, 261t
      VIP, 262t
   ICD-9-CM classification of, 272-274
Giant cell tumor, malignant, clinical features and treatment, 134t
Glioblastoma multiforme, clinical features of, 18t
Goserelin acetate, 218-219
Grading, of cancer, 4-5
   essential differences between benign and malignant tumors, 5t
Granuloma fungoides. See Mycosis fungoides.
Grawitz's tumor. See Kidney cancer.
Gum neoplasms, ICD-9-CM classification of, 264
Gynecological cancers. See Genital neoplasms.

H
Halotestin, 217-218
HDAC chemotherapy protocol, 251t
HDMTX chemotherapy protocol, 251t
Head, neck, and spinal neoplasms, 18-42
   brain tumors, malignant, 17-23
   chemotherapy protocols
      CF, 242t
      CFL, 242t
      COB, 245t
      MAP, 253t
      MBC, 253t
      MF, 254t
      PFL, 257t
   laryngeal cancer, 28-32
   pituitary tumors, 24-28
   spinal neoplasms, 36-39
   thyroid cancer, 32-35

i refers to an illustration; t refers to a table

Heart neoplasms, *ICD-9-CM* classification of, 268
Hemangioma, *ICD-9-CM* classification of, 284
Hematopoietic tissue neoplasms, *ICD-9-CM* classification of, 276-279
Hepatic carcinoma. *See* Liver cancer.
Hexa-CAF chemotherapy protocol, 251t
Hexadrol, 212-213
Hexadrol phosphate, 212-213
Hexalen, 201
Hodgkin's disease, 159-163
  causes, 159
  chemotherapy protocols
    ABVD, 239t
    CAVe, 242t
    ChlVPP, 243t
    CVPP, 247t
    DHAP, 248t
    EVA, 249t
    MOPP, 255t
    MVPP, 256t
  diagnosis, 160-161
    Reed-Sternberg cells, 160
    staging, 162i
  ICD-9-CM classification of, 277
  signs and symptoms, 159-160
  special considerations, 163
  treatment, 161
Hormonal therapy, for cancer, 11
Hospice approach, 13-14
Hydrea, 219
Hydroxyurea, 176, 219
Hypernephroma. *See* Kidney cancer.
Hypopharyngeal neoplasms, *ICD-9-CM* classification of, 265
Hysterone, 217-218

I

ICD-9-CM classification of neoplastic disorders (Appendix C), 263-288
Ifex, 219-220
Ifosfamide, 71, 219-220
IMF chemotherapy protocol, 252t
Immune tumor response and carcinogenesis, 3-4
Immunotherapy. *See* Biotherapy.
Insulinomas, 69
Interferon alfa-2b, for AIDS-related Kaposi's sarcoma, 155
Interferon gamma-1b, 80, 220-221
Internal radiation treatment, safety precautions for use in uterine cancer, 114i
International Classification of Diseases, 9th revision, *Clinical Modification. See ICD-9-CM* classification.

International Federation for Gynecology and Obstetrics staging system
  for cervical cancer, 106
  for ovarian cancer, 121
  for uterine cancer, 111
  for vaginal cancer, 117
Islet cell tumors, 69

J

Jejunostomy feeding, 12
Jewett-Strong-Marshall system for staging bladder cancer, 86t
Junctional nevi, 149

K

Kaposi's sarcoma, 153-156
  causes, 153
  diagnosis, 154
    Laubenstein's stages, 154
  ICD-9-CM classification of, 272
  signs and symptoms, 153-154
  special considerations, 155-156
  treatment, 155
Kidney cancer, 78-80
  causes, 79
  diagnosis, 79
  ICD-9-CM classification of, 274
  signs and symptoms, 79
  special considerations, 80
  staging, 78
  treatment, 80
Kidneys, benign neoplasms of, *ICD-9-CM* classification of, 283
Kidrolase, 201-202

L

L-VAM chemotherapy protocol, 252t
Lanvis, 236
Laryngeal cancer, 28-32
  causes, 28
  diagnosis, 29
    staging, 30
  ICD-9-CM classification of, 268
  signs and symptoms, 28-29
  special considerations, 29, 31-32
    care after partial laryngectomy, 31
    care after total laryngectomy, 31-32
    care before laryngectomy, 29, 30
  treatment, 29
Laubenstein's stages in Kaposi's sarcoma, 154
Lentigo maligna, 149
Leucovorin calcium, 76, 100, 221
Leukemia, acute, 168-174
  causes, 169-170
    predisposing factors, 170
    what happens in leukemia, 171i
  diagnosis, 170-171

Leukemia, acute *(continued)*
  ICD-9-CM classification of, 278-279
  special considerations, 172-174
  treatment for acute lymphoblastic leukemia, 171
    induction chemotherapy protocols
      DVP, 248t
      VAP (VP + A) (pediatric), 260t
    maintenance chemotherapy protocols
      MM, 254t
  treatment for acute myeloblastic leukemia, 171
    induction chemotherapy protocols
      COAP, 244t
      DC (pediatric), 248t
      DCPM (pediatric), 248t
      MV, 256t
      7 + 3 (A + D), 258t
  treatment for acute monoblastic leukemia, 172
  treatment for acute nonlymphocytic leukemia, consolidation protocols
    CD (DC), 242t
    5 + 2, 250t
    HDAC, 251t
    MC, 253t
  treatment for acute nonlymphocytic leukemia, induction protocols
    DCT, 248t
    MC, 253t
  treatment for acute nonlymphocytic leukemia, maintenance protocols
    TC, 258t
Leukemia, chronic granulocytic, 174-177
  causes, 175
  diagnosis, 175-176
  signs and symptoms, 175
  special considerations, 176-177
  treatment, 176
Leukemia, chronic lymphocytic, 177-180
  causes, 178
  signs and symptoms, 178
  special considerations, 179-180
  treatment, 179
    CVP protocol for blast crisis, 247t
Leukeran, 205-206
Leukoplakia, 145t
Leuprolide acetate, 221-222
Leustatin, 207
Levamisole hydrochloride, 76, 222-223
Lip neoplasms, *ICD-9-CM* classification of
  benign, 279
  malignant, 263
Lipoma, *ICD-9-CM* classification of, 281

Liver cancer, 81-84
  causes, 81-82
  diagnosis, 82
  ICD-9-CM classification of, 266
  signs and symptoms, 82
  special considerations, 83-84
  treatment, 82-83
Lomustine, 21, 23, 80, 82, 91, 223
Lukes-Collins classification system
    for malignant lymphomas, 164t
Lung cancer, 43-49
  causes, 43-44
  chemotherapy protocols
    BACON, 240t
    CAV (VAC), 241t
    EP, 248t
    MICE (ICE), 254t
    PFL, 257t
  chemotherapy protocols for small-
      cell
    ACE (CAE), 239t
    COPE, 245t
    CV, 246t
    VAC, 260t
    VC, 261t
  chemotherapy protocols for non–
      small cell
    CAMP, 241t
    CAP, 241t
    CV, 246t
    CVI (VIC), 246t
    FAM, 249t
    MACC, 252t
    MVP, 256t
  diagnosis, 45-47
    staging, 46
  ICD-9-CM classification of, 268
  signs and symptoms, 44-45
  special considerations, 48-49
    care after thoracic surgery,
        48-49
    care before thoracic surgery,
        48
    care during chemotherapy and
        radiation, 49
  treatment, 47-48
Lupron, 221-222
Lymphangioma, *ICD-9-CM* classifi-
    cation of, 284
Lymphatic system. See Blood and
    lymph neoplasms.
Lymphatic tissue neoplasms,
    ICD-9-CM classification of,
    276-279
Lymphedema, avoiding with postop-
    erative arm and hand care in
    breast cancer patients, 55
Lymph node neoplasms, *ICD-9-CM*
    classification of, 275-276
Lymphomas, malignant, 163-166
  causes, 165
  chemotherapy protocols
    ASHAP, 239t
    BACOP, 240t
    CHOP, 243t
    CHOP-Bleo, 243t
    COMLA, 245t

Lymphomas, malignant *(continued)*
    COP-BLAM, 245t
    COPO, 245t
    COPP, 246t
    CVP, 247t
    ESHAP, 249t
    m-BACOD, 253t
    MACOP-B, 252t
    MINE, 254t
    OPEN, 256t
    ProMACE, 257t
    ProMACE/cytaBOM, 258t
  classification of, 164t
  diagnosis, 165
  ICD-9-CM classification of, 277
  signs and symptoms, 165
  special considerations, 166
  treatment, 165-166
Lymphosarcomas. See Lymphomas,
    malignant.
Lysodren, 228-229

M
MACC chemotherapy protocol, 252t
MACOP-B chemotherapy protocol,
    252t
MAID chemotherapy protocol, 253t
Male genital organs, *ICD-9-CM*
    classification of benign neo-
    plasms of, 283. See also Geni-
    tal neoplasms.
Malignant melanoma. See Mela-
    noma, malignant.
Malignant plasmacytosis. See Multi-
    ple myeloma.
Malignant tumors, essential differ-
    ences between benign tumors
    and, 5t
MAP chemotherapy protocol, 253t
Matulane, 233
m-BACOD chemotherapy protocol,
    253t
MBC chemotherapy protocol, 253t
MC chemotherapy protocol, 253t
Mechlorethamine hydrochloride,
    161, 167, 223-224
Mediastinal neoplasms, *ICD-9-CM*
    classification of, 268
Medralone, 226-227
Medrol, 226-227
Medrone, 226-227
Medulloblastoma, clinical features
    of, 19t
Melanoma, malignant, 147-153
  causes, 148
  chemotherapy protocols
    BHD, 240t
    DTIC-ACTD, 248t
    VBC, 261t
    VDP, 262t
  diagnosis, 150-152
    staging, 151
  ICD-9-CM classification of,
    270-271

Melanoma, malignant *(continued)*
  signs and symptoms, 148-150
    recognizing potentially malig-
        nant nevi, 149
  special considerations, 152-153
  treatment, 152
Melphalan, 122, 224
Meningioma, clinical features of, 19t
Meprolone, 226-227
Mercaptopurine, 224-225
Mesna, 225
Mesnex, 225
Methotrexate, 21, 54, 63, 66, 76,
    82, 100, 103, 122, 166,
    225-226
Methyl CCNU. See Semustine.
Methylprednisolone, 226-227
Methylprednisolone acetate,
    226-227
Methylprednisolone sodium succi-
    nate, 226-227
Meticorten, 232-233
Mexate, 225-226
MF chemotherapy protocol, 254t
MICE (ICE) chemotherapy protocol,
    254t
MINE chemotherapy protocol, 254t
Mithracin, 231-232
Mithramycin, 231-232
Mitomycin, 47, 63, 83, 228
Mitotane, 228-229
Mitoxantrone hydrochloride, 171,
    229
MM chemotherapy protocol, 254t
MOF chemotherapy protocol, 254t
Moles. See Nevi *and* Melanoma, ma-
    lignant.
MOP chemotherapy protocol, 255t
MOPP chemotherapy protocol, 161,
    255t
Mouth neoplasms, *ICD-9-CM* classi-
    fication of, 264
MP chemotherapy protocol, 255t
m-PFL chemotherapy protocol, 255t
M-Prednisol, 226-227
M-2 chemotherapy protocol, 255t
Multiple myeloma, 138-141
  causes, 138
  chemotherapy protocols
    BCP, 240t
    MP, 255t
    M-2, 255t
    VAD, 260t
    VBAP, 261t
    VCAP, 261t
  diagnosis, 139-140
    Bence Jones protein, 139
  ICD-9-CM classification of, 278
  signs and symptoms, 138-139
  special considerations, 140-141
  treatment, 140
Mustargen, 223-224
Mutamycin, 228
MVAC chemotherapy protocol, 256t
MV chemotherapy protocol, 256t
MVP chemotherapy protocol, 256t
MVPP chemotherapy protocol, 256t

i refers to an illustration; t refers to a table

Mycosis fungoides, 166-168
  causes, 166
  diagnosis, 167
  signs and symptoms, 166-167
  special considerations, 168
  treatment, 167
Myelomatosis. *See* Multiple myeloma.
Myleran, 203-204

N

Narcotic analgesics in advanced
  cancer, 13
Nasal cavity neoplasms, *ICD-9-CM*
  classification of, 267
Nasogastric tube feeding, 12
Nasopharyngeal neoplasms, *ICD-9-
  CM* classification of, 265
National Cancer Institute classification system for malignant lymphomas, 164t
NCI. *See* National Cancer Institute.
Neck, neoplasms of. *See* Head,
  neck, and spinal neoplasms.
Neoplasms of uncertain behavior,
  ICD-9-CM classification of,
  286-287
Neoplasms of unspecified nature,
  ICD-9-CM classification of,
  288
Neosar, 207-208
Nephrocarcinoma. *See* Kidney cancer.
Nervous system neoplasms,
  ICD-9-CM classification of,
  274-275
Neurilemoma. *See* Schwannoma.
Nevi, recognizing potentially malignant, 149. *See also* Melanoma,
  malignant.
Nitrogen mustard. *See* Mechlorethamine hydrochloride.
Nitrosoureas for malignant brain tumors, 21
Nolvadex, 234-235
Non-Hodgkin's lymphomas. *See*
  Lymphomas, malignant.
Novantrone, 229
Nutrition in cancer patients
  maintaining nutrition and fluid
    balance, 11-12
  providing tube feedings, 12
  total parenteral nutrition, 12-13

O

Oligodendroglioma, clinical features
  of, 18-19t
Oncovin, 238
OPEN chemotherapy protocol, 256t
Oral cavity neoplasms, *ICD-9-CM*
  classification of
  benign, 279
  malignant, 263-265
Orasone, 232-233

Oropharyngeal neoplasms, *ICD-9-
  CM* classification of, 264-265
Osteogenic sarcoma, clinical features and treatment, 134t
Ovarian cancer, 118-123
  causes, 119
  chemotherapy protocols for epithelial
    AP, 239t
    CAP (PAC), 241t
    CC, 242t
    CDC, 242t
    CHAP, 243t
    CP, 246t
    Hexa-CAF, 251t
  chemotherapy protocols for germ
    cell
    VAC, 260t
  diagnosis, 120
    staging, 121
  ICD-9-CM classification of, 273
  signs and symptoms, 119-120
  special considerations, 122-123
  treatment, 120, 122
Ovarian neoplasms, benign, *ICD-9-
  CM* classification of, 282

PQ

PAC chemotherapy protocol, 241t
Paclitaxel, 122, 229-230
Pain control in cancer patients, 13
  narcotic analgesics in advanced
    cancer, 13
  patient-controlled analgesia system, 14
  transcutaneous electrical nerve
    stimulation, 38
Panasol, 232-233
Pancreatic cancer, 67-73
  causes, 67-68
  chemotherapy protocols
    FAM, 249t
    FMS, 251t
  diagnosis, 69-70
    staging, 70
  ICD-9-CM classification of, 267
  islet cell tumors, 69
  signs and symptoms, 68-69
  special considerations, 71-73
  treatment, 70-71
  types of, 68t
    body and tail of pancreas, 68t
    head of pancreas, 68t
Paraplatin, 204
Parosteal osteogenic sarcoma, clinical features and treatment,
  134t
Patient-controlled analgesia system,
  14
PCV chemotherapy protocol, 256t
Pelvic exenteration, management of
  in uterine cancer, 112
Pelvic neoplasms. *See* Abdominal
  and pelvic neoplasms.

Penile cancer, 102-104
  causes, 102
  diagnosis, 103
  ICD-9-CM classification of, 273
  signs and symptoms, 103
  special considerations, 103-104
  treatment, 103
Pentostatin, 230-231
Peritoneal neoplasms, *ICD-9-CM*
  classification of, 267
PFL chemotherapy protocol, 257t
Pharyngeal neoplasms, *ICD-9-CM*
  classification of
  benign, 279
  malignant, 264-265
L-Phenylalanine mustard. *See* Melphalan.
Pipobroman, 231
Pituitary tumors, 24-28
  causes, 24
  diagnosis, 25
  signs and symptoms, 24-25
  special considerations, 27-28
    postcraniotomy care, 27
  treatment, 25-27
    transsphenoidal pituitary surgery, 26i
Placental neoplasms, *ICD-9-CM*
  classification of, 272
Plasma cell myeloma. *See* Multiple
  myeloma.
Plasmacytoma, malignant. *See* Multiple myeloma.
Platinol, 206-207
Pleural neoplasms, *ICD-9-CM* classification of, 268
Plicamycin, 231-232
Prednicen-M, 232-233
Prednisone, 54, 140, 161, 165,
  166, 171, 175, 232-233
Premalignant skin lesions, causes,
  clinical signs, and treatment,
  145t
  actinic keratosis, 145t
  Bowen's disease, 145t
  erythroplasia of Queyrat, 145t
  leukoplakia, 145t
Procarbazine hydrochloride, 21, 23,
  161, 233
Proleukin, 200-201
ProMACE chemotherapy protocol,
  257t
ProMACE-cytaBOM chemotherapy
  protocol, 258t
Prostate cancer, 95-99
  causes, 95
  diagnosis, 96
  ICD-9-CM classification of, 273
  signs and symptoms, 96
  special considerations, 97-99
  staging, 97
  treatment, 96-97
Psychological aspects of cancer
  care, 15

Pulse VAC chemotherapy protocol, 258t
Purinethol, 224-225

R
Radiation therapy. *See also under treatment for specific neoplasms.*
  adverse effects of, 8t
  for cancer, 6-8
  internal radiation safety precautions in uterine cancer, 114i
  preparing the patient for external, 6
Rappaport classification system for malignant lymphomas, 164t
Rectal cancer. *See* Colorectal cancer.
Rectosigmoid junction neoplasms, *ICD-9-CM* classification of, 266
Rectal neoplasms, *ICD-9-CM* classification of, 266. *See also* Colorectal cancer.
Reed-Sternberg cells in Hodgkin's disease, 160i
Renal cell carcinoma. *See* Kidney cancer.
Rep-Pred, 226-227
Reproductive system neoplasms. *See* Genital neoplasms.
Respiratory and intrathoracic organ neoplasms, *ICD-9-CM* classification of. *See also* Thoracic neoplasms.
  benign, 280-281
  malignant, 267-269
Reticulosarcoma, *ICD-9-CM* classification of, 277
Retroperitoneum, neoplasms of, *ICD-9-CM* classification of, 267

S
Salivary gland neoplasms, *ICD-9-CM* classification of, 264
Sarcomas, comparing primary malignant bone tumors, 134t
Schwannoma, clinical features of, 20t
Secondary malignancies, *ICD-9-CM* classification of, 275-276
Semustine, 233-234
7 + 3 (A + D) chemotherapy protocol, 258t
6-MP. *See* Mercaptopurine.
6-TG. *See* Thioguanine.
Sk-Dexamethasone, 212-213
Skin, benign neoplasms of, *ICD-9-CM* classification of, 282

Skin cancer, 141-156
  basal cell epithelioma, 141-143
  ICD-9-CM classification of, 270-271
  Kaposi's sarcoma, 153-156
  malignant melanoma, 147-153
  premalignant skin lesions, 145t
  squamous cell carcinoma, 143-147
Sk-Prednisone, 232-233
Small intestine, neoplasms of, *ICD-9-CM* classification of, 266
Soft-tissue neoplasms. *See also* Bone, skin, and soft-tissue neoplasms.
  chemotherapy protocols
    CYADIC for sarcomas, 247t
    CYVADIC for sarcomas, 247t
    (pulse) VAC protocol for sarcoma, 258t
  ICD-9-CM classification of, 270, 281
Solu-Medrol, 226-227
Solurex, 212-213
Solurex-LA, 212-213
Spinal neoplasms, 36-39
  causes, 36
  diagnosis, 37
  signs and symptoms, 36-37
  special considerations, 38-39
  treatment, 37-38
Spongioblastoma multiforme. *See* Glioblastoma multiforme.
Squamous cell carcinoma, 143-147
  causes, 144
  premalignant skin lesions, 145t
  diagnosis, 144
  staging, 146
  signs and symptoms, 144
  special considerations, 146-147
  treatment, 144-146
    of actinic keratosis with topical fluorouracil, 147
Staging of cancer, 4-5
  using Ann Arbor system for Hodgkin's disease, 162i
  using Clark's system for malignant melanoma, 151i
  using Dukes system for colorectal cancer, 75
  using International Federation of Gynecology and Obstetrics system
    cervical cancer, 106
    ovarian cancer, 121
    uterine cancer, 111
    vaginal cancer, 117
  using Jewett-Strong-Marshall system for bladder cancer, 86t
  using Laubenstein's system for Kaposi's sarcoma, 154
  using NCI, Rappaport, and Lukes-Collins systems for malignant lymphomas, 164t

Staging of cancer *(continued)*
  using TNM system
    bladder cancer, 86t
    breast cancer, 52
    esophageal cancer, 66
    gastric cancer, 62
    kidney cancer, 78
    laryngeal cancer, 30
    lung cancer, 46
    malignant melanoma, 151
    pancreatic cancer, 70
    prostate cancer, 97t
    squamous cell carcinoma, 146
    testicular cancer, 101
    thyroid cancer, 34
  of the vulva, 125
Stomach cancer, *ICD-9-CM* classification of, 265-266. *See also* Gastric cancer.
Streptozocin, 71, 76, 82, 234
Surgery for cancer, 6. *See also under treatment for specific neoplasms.*

T
Tamoxifen citrate, 54, 80, 234-235
Taxol (paclitaxel), 48, 54, 229-230
TC chemotherapy protocol, 258t
Teniposide, 80, 235
Teslac, 236
TESPA, 236-237
Testicular cancer, 99-102
  causes, 99
  diagnosis, 99-100
  ICD-9-CM classification of, 273
  signs and symptoms, 99
  special considerations, 100-102
  staging, 101
  treatment, 100
Testolactone, 236
Therapies for cancer
  biotherapy, 10-11
  chemotherapy, 8-10
  hormonal therapy, 11
  radiation, 6-8
    adverse effects of, 8t
    preparing the patient for external, 6
  surgery, 6
Thioguanine, 172, 236
Thiotepa, 122, 236-237
Thoracic neoplasms, 43-58
  breast cancer, 50-56
  lung cancer, 43-49
Thymic neoplasms, *ICD-9-CM* classification of, 268
Thyroid cancer, 32-35
  causes, 33
  diagnosis, 33-34
  staging, 34
  ICD-9-CM classification of, 275
  signs and symptoms, 33
  special considerations, 35
  treatment, 34-35
Thyroid neoplasms, benign, *ICD-9-CM* classification of, 284

i refers to an illustration; t refers to a table

TNM staging system, definition, 4-5.
See also Staging of cancer.
Tongue, neoplasms of, *ICD-9-CM*
classification of malignant,
263-264
Total parenteral nutrition, 12-13
TPN. *See* Total parenteral nutrition.
Tracheal neoplasms, *ICD-9-CM* clas-
sification of, 268
Transcutaneous electrical nerve
stimulation, 38.
Transsphenoidal pituitary surgery,
26i
TSPA, 236-237
T-2 chemotherapy protocol, 259t
Tube feeding, 12
2-Chlorodeoxyadenosine. *See* Cladri-
bine.
2'-Deoxycoformycin. *See* Pentosta-
tin.

U
Uterine adnexa neoplasms, *ICD-9-
CM* classification of, 273
Uterine cancer, 109-115
causes, 109
diagnosis, 110
staging, 111
ICD-9-CM classification of, 272
signs and symptoms, 110
special considerations, 111-115
internal radiation safety precautions, 114i
treatment, 110-111
managing pelvic exenteration,
112
Uterine neoplasms, benign, *ICD-9-
CM* classification of, 282

V
VA chemotherapy protocol, 259t
VAB chemotherapy protocol, 260t
VAC chemotherapy protocol, 260t
VAD chemotherapy protocol, 260t
Vaginal cancer, 115-118
causes, 115-116
diagnosis, 116
staging, 117
signs and symptoms, 116
treatment, 117-118
VAP (VP + A) chemotherapy proto-
col, 260t
VATH chemotherapy protocol, 261t
VB chemotherapy protocol, 261t
VBAP chemotherapy protocol, 261t
VBC chemotherapy protocol, 261t
VBP chemotherapy protocol, 261t
VC chemotherapy protocol, 261t
VCAP chemotherapy protocol, 261t
VDP chemotherapy protocol, 262t
Velban, 237-238
VePesid, 214-215
Vercyte, 231

Vinblastine sulfate, 80, 100, 122,
155, 161, 237-238
Vincristine sulfate, 47, 48, 54, 80,
100, 122, 135, 155, 161,
165, 166, 238-239
Vindesine, 47, 97, 100
VIP chemotherapy protocol, 262t
VLB. *See* Vinblastine sulfate.
VM-26. *See* Teniposide.
VP-16. *See* Etoposide.
Vulva, cancer of, 124-127
causes, 124
diagnosis, 124-125
staging, 125
signs and symptoms, 124
special considerations, 126-127
treatment, 125-126
Vumon, 235

WXY
Wellcovorin, 221
Wilms' tumor, chemotherapy proto-
cols for. *See also* Kidney can-
cer.
VA, 259t
VAC, 260t.

Z
Zanosar, 234
Zoladex, 218-219

i refers to an illustration; t refers to a table